LASER SYSTEMS IN FLOW MEASUREMENT

LASER SYSTEMS IN FLOW MEASUREMENT

Tariq S. Durrani
University of Strathclyde
Glasgow, Scotland

and

Clive A. Greated
University of Edinburgh
Edinburgh, Scotland

PLENUM PRESS • NEW YORK AND LONDON

Library of Congress Cataloging in Publication Data

Durrani, Tariq S   1943-
  Laser systems in flow measurement.

  Bibliography: p.
  Includes index.
  1. Laser Doppler velocimeter. I. Greated, Clive A., 1940-   joint author. II.
Title.
TA357.D86   620.1'064'028   76-26093
ISBN 0-306-30857-6

© 1977 Plenum Press, New York
A Division of Plenum Publishing Corporation
227 West 17th Street, New York, N.Y. 10011

Printed in the United States of America

Preface

It is now well established that laser flow-measuring systems have important advantages over more conventional techniques both for industrial and laboratory applications. These fundamental advantages are indicated by the enormous research effort which has gone into their development over the last decade and by the number of commercial systems which have become available. Although the field is still developing, the most important theoretical results required for relating the system outputs to the fluid flow parameters have now been formulated and a book on the subject therefore seems timely.

In the text we have tried to collect together the most important results both from our own papers and from publications by other authors and to present these in a concise and easily readable form. Emphasis has been placed on the fundamental theory and limitations associated with the various techniques rather than on detailed description of specific systems. We have also included a number of new results on areas such as photon counting in turbulent and periodic flows, frequency domain and time domain analysis of laser Doppler velocimeter signals, effect of background noise on system performance, and on cross-correlation techniques for diffusing flows.

Since the subject matter of this book is interdisciplinary in nature, we anticipate that its readers will be from wide-ranging backgrounds, for instance, electronic and mechanical engineers, physicists, mathematicians, fluid dynamicists, and others. To make the text self-contained and easily understandable to these readers, it has been necessary to include a substantial introductory section. We have assumed that readers with, say, a mathematical background will skip over Section 1.2, while Sections 1.3

and 1.4 would not be required by fluid dynamicists or optics experts. Although we have attempted to give a comprehensive list of the most pertinent references, the literature on laser anemometry is so vast that a completely exhaustive collection of references would have detracted from the main theme. However, a bibliography listing over 600 papers has been published as a technical memorandum by DISA Elektronik, Herlev, Copenhagen, Denmark.

We are indebted to a large number of people who have assisted us in this venture, particularly Mrs. A. Lampard for typing the main portion of the text, Mr. D. Stewart-Robinson for drafting the illustrations, and to Plenum Press for skillful editing and production of the book. Messrs. J. J. Allan, G. Dowrick, Q. I. Daudpota and D. Molyneux were of great assistance in the preparation of diagrams and proofreading. Finally, we would like to thank our wives for their encouragement and understanding during this project.

T. S. Durrani
C. A. Greated

Contents

Notation

Chapter 1

a_m Modulation amplitude for a periodic flow

a Rectangular aperture width

$\mathbf{C_{xx}}$ Covariance matrix

c Depth of rectangular apertures in mask

$\mathrm{cov}\,[\ ]$ Covariance

$\{dN(t)\}$ Increment process

d_p Particle diameter

$E[\ ]$ Expectation operation

$E[x|y]$ Conditional expectation of x given y

E_{ij} Three-dimensional energy spectrum

$\mathscr{E}(x, y)$ Complex light amplitude at coordinates x and y

$F_\xi(x)$ Probability distribution of event $\{\xi \leq x\}$

$f(r)$ Eulerian longitudinal correlation coefficient (spatial)

$g(r), g_2(r), g_3(r)$ Eulerian transverse correlation coefficients (spatial)

$I(x, y)$ Optical intensity

i_0 Mean current from photodetector

j $\sqrt{-1}$

k, k_1, k_2, k_3 Wave numbers

L Focal length of lens

$M_x(\eta)$ Characteristic function of argument η for a random variable x

$\{N(0, t)\}$ (Poisson) counting process

$P_\xi(x)$ Probability of event $\{\xi = x\}$ or probability distribution of a random variable

$p(\ )$ — Probability density function

$p(\mathbf{r};t)$ — Probability density function for a displacement $\mathbf{r}$ in time t

$p(\ |\ )$ — Conditional probability density function

$R_i(\mathbf{r},t)$ — Space–time correlation function for ith component of velocity

R_{ij} — Covariance tensor

$R_x(\ )$ — Autocorrelation of random variable x

$R_{xy}(\ )$ — Cross correlation between two random variables x and y

$\mathbf{r}$ — Separation vector between two points in the flow

T — Sample time

U — Flow velocity in a specified direction

U_i, U_i' — Velocity in ith coordinate direction, when tensor notation is employed

u_i, u_i' — Velocity fluctuation in the ith coordinate direction, when tensor notation is employed

V — Particle velocity in a specified direction

$\text{var}\,[\ ]$ — Variance

$\{x(t)\}$ — Stochastic process

x_1, x_2, x_3 — Coordinate directions when tensor notation is employed

$x_p(t)$ — Coordinate position of a particle, in mean flow direction

α — Overall quantum efficiency of photodetector fitted with a discriminator

α' — Quantum efficiency of photodetector

δ_{ij} — Kronecker delta: $\delta_{ij} = 1$ for $i = j$, $\delta_{ij} = 0$ otherwise

$\delta(x)$ — Dirac delta function

$\Phi_x(\omega)$ — Spectral density function of process x at frequency ω (rad/sec)

η — Photodetector sensitivity

Λ — Lagrangian integral time scale for the downstream component of velocity

Λ_f — Eulerian longitudinal integral scale of turbulence

λ — Optical wavelength

λ_f — Eulerian longitudinal microscale

$\lambda_0, \lambda(t)$ — Rate parameters of Poisson counting process

ρ — Normalized covariance or correlation coefficient

$\rho_i(\tau)$ — Lagrangian autocorrelation coefficient for the ith component of velocity

$\rho_E(\tau)$ — Eulerian autocorrelation coefficient of the downstream component of velocity

ρ_0 Fluid density

ρ_p Particle density

$\rho_L(\tau)$ Lagrangian autocorrelation coefficient for the downstream component of velocity

σ_u rms value of the velocity fluctuation in a chosen direction

rect (x) equals 1 for $|x| \leq \frac{1}{2}$, equals 0 otherwise

Chapter 2

a Rectangular-aperture width

b Distance between apertures

c Rectangular-aperture depth

C_{sc} Scattering cross section of particle

d Distance between beams

d_i Distance between observation volume and collecting lens

d_0 Distance between collecting lens and detector surface

$\mathscr{E}_I, \mathscr{E}_R, \mathscr{E}_s, \mathscr{E}(\mathbf{r})$ Incident, reference, and scattered optical fields and optical field at location $\mathbf{r}$

F_0 Focal point

f Focal length of collecting lens

f_0 Doppler frequency in Hz

f_s Frequency shift in Hz

I Intensity of optical radiation

$i_F, i_{DH}, i(t)$ Fringe, Doppler heterodyne, and time-varying photocurrent

K_p Variable dependent on particle size

L Focal length of beam-focusing lens

M Magnification factor

N_F Number of fringes in observation volume

r_a Radius of circular aperture

r_0, r_u Radius of laser beam at waist and of unapertured laser beam

r_p Particle radius

sinc x $\dfrac{\sin x}{x}$

$\mathbf{U}$ Velocity vector

U Uniform flow velocity

$u_1(t), u(t)$ Velocity fluctuation in direction of mean flow (the subscript 1 is omitted when only one component is considered)

$u_2(t)$ Velocity fluctuation in direction perpendicular to the mean flow

$V_p(t)$ Velocity of pth scatterer at time t

$W(t)$ Weighting function

$x_p(t)$ Instantaneous position of pth scatterer at time t

β Coefficient associated with weighting function; dimensions: $(\text{length})^{-1}$

γ, ρ, μ Parameters associated with weighting function for various optical configurations

η Sensitivity of photodetector

Δt Passage time of scatterers across observation volume

$\Delta x, \Delta y, \Delta z$ Dimensions of observation volume

ω_0 Doppler frequency (rad/sec)

σ (Scattering) amplitude function of particle

θ Half-angle between incident beams

Chapter 3

$a(t), b(t)$ Orthogonal components of filtered Doppler signal

b_0 Average Doppler signal power

C_0, C_1 Mean and mean square value of K_p [Equations (2.6.51) and (2.6.52)]

D Velocity-to-(radial) frequency conversion factor

$F[x]$ Fourier transform of x

f_b Output low-pass filter bandwidth

f_0 Mean Doppler frequency in Hz

g_0 Mean number of particles crossing observation volume per unit time for unit flow velocity

g Mean concentration of scatterers in flow (numbers/unit volume)

$H(t)$ Envelope of filtered Doppler signal

$i(t)$ Photocurrent

K_p Variable dependent on particle size

N_p Expected number of particles per second $(= g_0 U)$

$n(t)$ Noise

$R_L(\tau)$ Lagrangian autocorrelation of flow velocity fluctuations

$R_u(z; \tau)$ Space–time correlation of flow velocity

$R_w(\beta z)$ Spatial correlation of weighting function

$R_w(\tau)$ (Time) autocorrelation of weighting function $[R_w(\tau) = R_w(\beta U \tau)/U]$

$R_x(\tau)$ Autocorrelation of $x(t)$ for lag value τ

$R_{\dot\phi}(\tau)$ Autocorrelation of ambiguity noise for lag τ

$\mathcal{T}$ Turbulence micro time scale

U Uniform flow velocity

$U(t), U_0$ Turbulent velocity and its mean value

$U_a(t)$ Velocity observed by LDV

$U(\xi, t)$ Instantaneous fluid velocity at location ξ and time t

$u_1(t), u_2(t)$ Velocity fluctuations in directions along and transverse to the flow, perpendicular to the optical axis

$V_p(t)$ Instantaneous velocity of pth particle

$W(\beta z)$ Spatially defined weighting function

$W(t)$ Weighting function (in general a function of flow velocity)

$x(t)$ Photodetector signal

$x_i(t)$ Doppler signal due to ith particle

β Coefficient in weighting function with dimensions $(\text{length})^{-1}$

Δf Doppler signal bandwidth in Hz

$\Delta\omega$ Spectral width of power spectrum (if not indicated otherwise) of Doppler signal with constant flow velocity

$\Phi_x(f)$ Power spectrum of $x(t)$

$\Phi_u(\omega, k)$ Frequency wave number spectrum of flow

$\dot\phi(t)$ Ambiguity noise

κ Weighting constant

$\Lambda(x)$ $\begin{cases} 1 - |x|, & |x| \le 1 \\ 0, & \text{otherwise} \end{cases}$

μ $\omega_0/2(b/a)$

$\Omega(\tau)$ Autocorrelation of instantaneous particle displacement

ω_m Frequency deviation in rad/sec

$\omega_i(t)$ Instantaneous frequency of Doppler signal in rad/sec

$\rho_u(\tau)$ Normalized correlation function of velocity fluctuations

$\rho_w(\tau)$ Normalized autocorrelation of weighting function

σ_u rms velocity fluctuation

θ Half-angle between converging beams

$\xi_p(t), \zeta_p(t + \tau)$ Position of pth particle at times t and $t + \tau$

Chapter 4

A, A_i Weighting constants

a_m Amplitude of sinusoidal modulation

D Velocity-to-frequency conversion constant

$dN(\ )$ Stochastic differential (or increment process)

$I(t)$ Light intensity

M Number of correlation products accumulated

m Time integral of intensity ($m_0 = E[m]$)

N_p Expected number of particles per second

$N(kT, \overline{k+1}T)$ Number of counts in the interval $(kT, \overline{k+1}T)$

$q(t)$ Instantaneous phase

$\mathbf{R}$ Correlation matrix

$R_\psi(\tau), R_I(\tau)$ Nonnormalized autocorrelations of the intensity

$\tilde{R}_a(sT), R_a(sT)$ Nonnormalized and normalized count correlation $[r_a(sT) = M\tilde{R}_a(sT)]$

$R_w(\tau)$ Autocorrelation function of $W(t)$

T Sample time

U_0 Mean value of turbulent velocity

$U(t)$ Instantaneous flow velocity $[U(t) = U_0 + u(t)]$

$v(t)$ Instantaneous deviation of Doppler frequency from the mean $[v(t) = Du(t)]$

α Overall quantum efficiency of the photodetector

$\Phi(\omega)$ Power or energy spectrum

Λ Lagrangian integral time scale of turbulence

μ Optical parameter in mask system $[\mu = \omega_0 a/(2b)]$

ω_0 Doppler frequency in rad/sec

ω_m Frequency of sinusoidal modulation

ω_s Frequency shift

ρ Passage time across the beam

$\rho_E(\tau), \rho_v(\tau)$ Normalized autocorrelation functions of $u(t)$ and $v(t)$

σ_u rms turbulent velocity fluctuation $\{\sigma_u^2 = E[u^2(t)]\}$

$\psi(t), \psi_i(t)$ Light intensity

Chapter 5

B Bandwidth of signals from detectors 1 and 2

B_0, B_1 Constants characterizing particle size distribution in the flow: $B_0 = E[\beta_i], B_1 = E[\beta_i^2]$

d Distance traveled by particle in time d_0/U_0

d_0 Distance between beams

I_0 Intensity at center of focal spot

$I_1(\mu), I_2(\mu)$ Intensities integrated over the surfaces of detectors 1 and 2

$M(kT, \overline{k+1}T),$ Number of counts in time interval kT to $\overline{k+1}T$ in channels
$N(kT, \overline{k+1}T)$ 1 and 2, respectively

N_p Mean number of particles passing each beam per second

$R_1(\xi), R_2(\xi)$ Autocorrelation function for the integrated intensities over detectors 1 and 2, respectively

$R_{12}(\xi)$ Cross-correlation function for the intensities integrated over the surfaces of detectors

$\hat{R}_{12}(\xi)$ Estimated value of $R_{12}(\xi)$

$\hat{R}_c(sT)$ Nonnormalized counting cross-correlation function

r_0 Waist radius of diffraction-limited spot

r_u Waist radius of unapertured laser beam

r_y Semiaxis of beam intensity profile in y direction

T_m Measuring time or sample time

t_k Random arrival times of particles in the beams

α Overall quantum efficiency of detectors

β_i Random variable characterizing size distribution of particles in the flow

ε Mean square error in $\hat{R}_{12}(\xi)$

η Sensitivity of detectors

Λ Lagrangian integral time scale of the turbulence

$\rho_L(\tau)$ Lagrangian autocorrelation coefficient for the downstream component of the velocity fluctuation

σ_u rms velocity fluctuation

τ_k Random arrival times of particles in the beams

ξ Passage time between two beams distance d_0 apart $(\xi_0 = d_0/U_0)$

ξ_p Time lag corresponding to the peak of the cross-correlation function

Chapter 6

The symbols used here are the same as those for Chapters 4 and 5.

Chapter 1

INTRODUCTION

1.1 Historical Developments

Due to the complexity of fluid motion phenomena and the difficulties involved in applying equations of motion to even the simplest of realistic situations, fluid dynamicists rely heavily on experimental techniques of flow measurement for application both in the laboratory and in field studies. Precise knowledge of how the instrumental records are related to the various fluid dynamic parameters is of course essential if experimental results are to be meaningful, and in general it is a complex task to determine the manner in which a particular system responds under specified flow conditions. This is particularly the case with turbulent flows, and the majority of natural phenomena fall into this category. Thus the development of new measuring techniques has also led to an important field for theoretical research.

Limitations of Conventional Anemometers

Flow velocity is the most important parameter in nearly all fluid dynamic problems, and this book will be entirely devoted to velocity measurement. Because of its simplicity and reliability, the Pitot tube is probably still the most widely used fluid-velocity-measuring instrument. However, in the study of rapidly fluctuating flows it is of little use since its frequency response and spatial resolution are far too poor to resolve the small-scale eddy structure that is of major importance in the study of turbulence. To achieve this an instrument is required that has a very short response time, typically of the order 1 msec, and that averages the velocity field over only a very small volume, typically of the order of 1 mm^3. The hot-wire anemometer was developed to achieve this order of resolution and has for many years been the standard apparatus for the study of turbulence, only now being rivaled by more sophisticated optical techniques. This statement should be qualified by noting that flow visualization can often be used to resolve fine eddy structure, but, for quantitative analysis, extensive data reduction by computer is usually involved. Early hot-wire probes suffered the disadvantage that they could not be used in liquids or in fact in any flow environments more hostile than the standard laboratory wind tunnel. This problem has now been partly overcome by the introduction of coated probes (or hot-film probes), although these are generally more bulky and have a poorer frequency response than the more delicate uncoated wires. Because of the difficulties associated with using hot-wire anemometers for measuring in liquids, miniature propeller meters are frequently used, especially in the hydraulics laboratory, where the scales of the apparatus tend to be large. With these meters the velocity is obtained by recording the rate of revolution of the propeller blades, normally using an electronic counting mechanism; with suitable processing equipment the output record essentially can be in the form of instantaneous velocity. However, even though the propellers can be made extremely small, down to 4 or 6 mm in diameter, the spatial resolution is not generally good enough for resolving the microstructure of turbulence fluctuations. Also, the frequency response tends to be very poor, due partly to inertial effects and partly to the fact that a count is only recorded every instant a blade passes the electrode on the propeller mounting. Thus a time-averaged velocity is obtained, the integration time being the time taken for two successive blades to pass the electrode. The upper limit of frequency response is typically of the order 10 Hz, which does not in any way match the hot-wire anemometer.

Despite the effectiveness of the hot-wire anemometer in resolving turbulence structure, there are a number of problems associated with the instrument, some of which are rather fundamental in nature. These have limited its application to certain types of flow situations and also inevitably have led researchers to seek new and more sophisticated measuring techniques. The foremost problem is that of probe interference, i.e., insertion of the instrument perturbs the flow, and false readings result. This is common to all conventional velocity meters and can lead to significant errors especially in small-scale experiments or where arrays of probes are to be employed. An equally fundamental problem is concerned with calibration. Since all wire probes are slightly different, they must be calibrated against some standardized instrument to determine the output voltage characteristics as functions of flow velocity. Pitot tubes are generally used as calibration references. Thus, the hot-wire anemometer gives a comparison rather than an absolute measurement. This is a disadvantage of rather academic importance in the measurement of low-speed air flows, where the Pitot tube is known to give highly reliable readings. However, in, for example, the measurement of non-Newtonian liquid flows, calibration can prove a major problem since Pitot tube measurements cannot be relied upon.

The output from a hot-wire anemometer is not a linear function of velocity; in fact the output voltage varies approximately as the fourth root of velocity. This complicates the analysis of records considerably and usually means that for accurate measurements of turbulence, some form of linearizer must follow the anemometer which takes account of the calibration curve for the particular wire being used. For more approximate results it is often assumed that over small velocity ranges the calibration curve is linear. One of the other difficulties of interpreting results in a turbulent flow is that in a three-dimensional flow field the wire does not respond to the instantaneous velocity component in any one given direction. All velocity fluctuations in a plane perpendicular to the wire affect the rate of heat loss and, hence, the voltage output. Again, approximate results can be used to overcome this difficulty when turbulence levels are low (Hinze, 1959).

Hot-wire anemometers can be applied most easily to steady flows or to flows that have a steady mean velocity superimposed by small turbulent fluctuations whose rms value does not exceed about 10% of the mean. For the reasons just outlined, interpolation of results at higher turbulence levels is extremely difficult. An instrument designed for measuring in high-turbulence situations is the pulsed hot wire (Bradshaw, 1971). In essence, this is a probe on which three thin wires are mounted short distances apart, the two outside, receiving, wires being parallel to each other and at right angles to the central, transmitting, wire. The transmitting wire is heated periodically with a pulsatile current, and the resulting streaks of heated fluid are convected downstream by the flow. The receiving wires operate in the same manner as the normal hot-wire anemometer and are sensitive to small temperature changes. Thus the passage time of each hot streak between transmitting and receiving wire is recorded electronically and converted to velocity by multiplying the reciprocal of the passage time by the distance between the wires. The sign of the velocity is determined by noting which of the two outside wires receives the pulse. Note that the pulsed-wire technique gives a direct measurement of velocity, the calibration being independent of the detailed properties of the fluid, and thus it overcomes one of the fundamental problems of hot-wire anemometry. In fact, experience has shown that it can be used successfully to measure velocities in very high turbulence and reversing flows such as might occur behind a step or a blunt body. However, there are also serious limitations to its application. First, its spatial resolution tends to be rather poorer than the single hot wire, and of course it does not overcome the problem of probe interference with the flow patterns. Second and more important, its frequency response is poor since the time interval between pulses cannot in practice be less than the smallest passage time between wires if confusion due to inductive pickup is to be avoided. This in general rules out the possibility of recording continuous velocity traces for use in spectral and correlation analysis.

Development of Optical Techniques

Flow visualization by photographing, or simply observing visually, the paths of marker particles or dye introduced into the flow is one of the earliest and still one of the most powerful flow measurement techniques. The great problem of flow visualization lies in the quantitative analysis of data, since this involves tracking the motions of thousands of particles through the flow, which is difficult even with the aid of a modern computer. Some of the most useful results have been obtained by recording cine films of hydrogen bubbles in water, the advantage of this technique being that strings of bubbles can be released at precisely known positions and time intervals and consequently that computer analysis of the films can be simplified. Even so, one cannot avoid the problem of having to analyze a three-dimensional flow field from a series of two-dimensional photographs. Various attempts have been made at analyzing stereoscopic photographs to reconstruct three-dimensional flow patterns (Christie *et al.*, 1972), but this still further increases the quantity of data to be handled. Note that there are various ways in which flow visualization photographs can be analyzed, e.g., one can record the motions of successive particles passing through fixed points in space from which Eulerian velocity records can be reconstructed, or one can track the Lagrangian motions of individual particles as they pass across the flow field. Generally speaking, the Eulerian information is the more useful. Frequently particle velocities are determined by using carefully timed exposures and noting the lengths of streaks traced out by the individual particles.

The most obvious attraction of optical flow measuring techniques such as flow visualization is that they avoid the necessity of introducing probes into the measuring region and hence do not perturb the flow. However, the photographic methods just described tend to be most useful for determining the large-scale structure of turbulence. In order to observe the microstructure of turbulent fluctuations one needs to track the motions of microscopically small marker particles that will faithfully follow the high-frequency fluctuations. Fage and Townend (1932) developed an ultramicroscope (dark-field microscope) system for visual observation of these small-scale motions. This in fact employs some of the techniques used in modern laser anemometers. The principle of the ultramicroscope depends on the fact that microscopic particles, naturally present in most fluids, become visible when illuminated by an intense beam and viewed against a dark background even though they are invisible against a bright background. By employing a rotating objective they were able to observe the microscopic motions from a frame of reference moving with the mean fluid velocity. The modern laser anemometers, which are the subject of this book, derive their signals by remotely detecting the light scattered from these microscopic particles.

Schlieren optical systems have been standard equipment in aerodynamics laboratories for many years. Like the shadowgraph and Mach Zehnder interferometer methods, they rely on refractive index gradients within the flow region to deflect the beam and cause varying intensities over the plane of the photographic plate, rather than on the presence of marker particles to scatter the incident light. A characteristic of all of these three commonly used techniques of flow visualization is that they give an integrated picture through the flow region, as opposed to point information. This makes quantitative analysis of results extremely difficult. Point information on refractive index and hence density gradients can be obtained if two separate narrow beams (usually laser beams) are employed. Both beams pass through the flow region and then pass over knife edges onto photodetectors. Refractive index gradients then cause deflection of the beams and hence varying photodetector signals, each signal being caused by the integrated effect along the beam's length. If, for example, the beams are perpendicular to each other and intersect at a point in the flow, information on refractive index fluctuations at this point can be extracted by cross-correlating the two detector signals. By moving the beams at various separations quantitative data on the spatial structure of turbulence can also be determined. This technique is known as crossed-beam correlation and is described in detail by Fisher and Krause (1967). Note, however, that it can only be used in an indirect manner to give velocity information.

Laser Systems

The introduction of the laser has made possible the development of the modern optical point velocity measuring systems which have now become one of the most powerful tools in experimental fluid dynamics. The first laser Doppler demonstration was described by Yeh and Cummins (1964), and since then there have been numerous developments of both the optics and processing electronics. A major part of the book will be concerned with the analysis of this technique, which we will see has the high spatial and temporal resolution associated with hot-wire anemometry and in addition some fundamental advantages. First, there is no flow interference since the probing is purely optical. Second, since the instrument records velocity in a direct manner (like the pulsed-wire anemometer) no calibration is required. Third, the instrument measures the component of velocity in a specified direction, the output being a linear function of this velocity component. Quite clearly these are three fundamental advantages. Hence the great interest and rapid development of laser Doppler systems. There are also other advantages over hot-wire methods of flow measurement. For example, the method can be used in very high turbulence flows and over velocity ranges from a few millimeters per minute to supersonic quantities. Also, it can be easily adapted to enable three velocity components to be measured simultaneously.

Following the success of the laser Doppler anemometer an interest has arisen in the development of other laser velocity measuring methods that rely on the scattering of light by microscopic particles in the flow. The most important example is the two-beam cross-correlation method. This is very similar in concept to the pulsed-wire anemometer since it measures the time of flight between two beams focused into the flow. Cross-correlation techniques will be discussed in Chapter 5.

An important development in laser anemometry has been the introduction of photon counting techniques. These have been used in various branches of physics for some years but have only very recently been applied to flow measurement. In a photon counting experiment one seeks to detect digitally the arrival times of individual photons in a beam; the advantage of this procedure is the greatly improved sensitivity over the more commonly known analog methods. With a photon counting detector it is possible to work with extremely low intensities of scattered radiation, which opens a completely new range of problems to which laser anemometry can be applied, e.g., in biological fluid dynamics, where the use of high laser powers is often intolerable.

We have said that the laser anemometers to be described in this book rely for their operation on the detection of scattered light from some tracer elements in the flow, generally microscopic dust or seeding particles. This important point deserves some further explanation. Light is scattered whenever it passes through an inhomogeneous medium, and since the fluid itself consists of discrete molecules, there will always be some degree of scattering. The two most generally useful theories of scattering (Van de Hulst, 1957) are due to Rayleigh and Mie. However, Rayleigh's theory only applies to scattering diameters smaller than about one tenth of the incident radiation wavelength, e.g., to diameters less than $0.06\,\mu$m for HeNe radiation. In practical application there will always be particles in the flow, either seeded or naturally occurring, of the order 1 or $2\,\mu$m in size. Scattering from these particles will completely dominate molecular scattering and Rayleigh scattering from smaller particles. Thus, it is generally assumed that the Mie theory should be used for scattering calculations in laser anemometry. Since marker particles are normally separated many diameters apart in the fluid, they can be treated independently to a good approximation; i.e., the independent single scattering condition can be assumed to hold. Ashley and Cobb (1958) and Jonsson (1974) have tabulated and sketched the angular distribution of scattered radiation from polystyrene spheres in water according to the Mie theory. The main features of these results are as follows. In the forward direction, scattering is over a wide angle when the particles are small, but for larger particles the scattered intensity falls off very rapidly with angular deviation from the optical axis. For particles whose diameter is of the same order as the wavelength of incident light the total scattering in the forward direction (integrated intensity) is about three orders of magnitude greater than the total backscattered radiation.

1.2. Mathematical Preliminaries

This section covers the basic mathematical relationships to be employed throughout the text. A working acquaintance of the reader with statistics and probability theory is assumed. Nevertheless, some definitions and concepts are included here for completeness and self-sufficiency. For a detailed and rigorous treatment, the reader is referred to standard works (Parzen, 1962; Cramer, 1963; Papoulis, 1965).

A physical process that has some random element involved in its structure and that develops in time controlled by probabilistic rather than deterministic laws is called a *stochastic process*. Thus the phenomenon of Brownian motion, the fluctuating current in an electronic circuit due to thermal or shot-noise effects, and growth of populations represent some well-known stochastic processes. An important stochastic process with which we will be closely concerned is the velocity field in a turbulent fluid. This process involves random parameters of both space and time.

A stochastic process is defined as a collection $\{x(t), t \in T\}$ of random variables (to be defined below). The set T is the index set of the process. When the index set consists of discrete elements, $T = \{0, \pm 1, \pm 2, \ldots\}$, the stochastic process is called a stochastic sequence or discrete-parameter process, and when $T = \{t; -\infty < t < \infty\}$ the process is a continuous-parameter process. A physical record of the random variables $\{x(t)\}$ is referred to as a realization of the random process.

Random Variables and Their Probability Distributions

To study stochastic processes, we should define precisely random variables and the probability laws that govern them.

Consider a definite random experiment $\mathscr{E}$ which is repeatable under identical (controlled) conditions a large number of times. Let Ω be the space of all possible outcomes of the experiment. Let ω be a subset in the space Ω, called an event, which is said to occur if and only if the observed outcome of the experiment belongs to the set ω. The class of subsets ω form a Borel algebra $\mathscr{F}$. A random variable is defined as a real-valued function of the elementary outcomes (or whatever we may assign as the outcomes of the experiment):

$$\xi = \xi(\omega), \qquad \omega \in \Omega \tag{1.2.1}$$

Thus if at a particular trial of the experiment, $\mathscr{E}$ a single outcome x is observed, then the event ω is said to occur if it contains the element x. Further, we state that the random variable ξ has a probability

$$P_\xi(x) = P(\xi = x)$$

of assuming the realized value x, i.e., the probability of an outcome of a trial of the experiment being equal to x is $P_\xi(x)$. Thus, probability is defined as a number that is associated with a possible outcome of the random experiment $\mathscr{E}$. $P_\xi(x)$ is equal to or greater than 0, but cannot exceed 1. $P_\xi(x) = 0$ implies that ξ takes the value x in a negligible fraction of the total number of trials in the ensemble of possible runs, while $P_\xi(x) = 1$ is interpreted as the certainty that ξ takes the value x on all (but a negligible portion of the total possible number of) trials in the ensemble.

/ More rigorously, a set function $\mathscr{P}$ is defined on the algebra $\mathscr{F}$, and the triplet $(\Omega, \mathscr{F}, \mathscr{P})$ is called a probability space. Ω is a nonempty set with elements that are usually interpreted as outcomes of a random experiment, while $\mathscr{F}$ is a Borel algebra of subsets of Ω. It consists of elements called events. $\mathscr{P}$ is a (probability) measure on $\mathscr{F}$. /

[Measure (or Lebesgue measure) is a technical term for a concept which has all the characteristics of probability. We do not propose to enter here into the analytic refinements necessary to define measure, and suggest Doob (1953) as a classic reference on the rigorous theory of applied probability and stochastic processes.]

Random variables may be described as either discretely or continuously distributed variables. A discrete variable ξ takes only a finite (or denumerable) number of different values of x with corresponding probabilities $P_\xi(x) = P(\xi = x)$. Here $\{\xi = x\}$ represents the event that ξ takes the value x. The probability of the event $\{x_1 \leq \xi \leq x_2\}$ that ξ takes one of the values of x lying in $x_1 \leq x \leq x_2$ on any given trial of the experiment $\mathscr{E}$ is

$$P_\xi\{x_1 \leq x \leq x_2\} = \sum_{x_1}^{x_2} P_\xi(x)$$

where the summation covers all the finite or denumerable values of x which the variable ξ may take. $P_\xi(x)$ as a function of all possible values x of the random variable ξ is called the *probability distribution* of this variable. / .

/ A function $F_\xi(x)$ that is defined as the probability that ξ takes any one of the allowed values of x, or less, on any given trial of the experiment $\mathscr{E}$ is called its *distribution function*; thus we have

$$F_\xi(x) = P\{\xi \leq x\}, \qquad -\infty < x < \infty. \; /$$

The distribution function possesses the following general properties: /

(1) $F_\xi(x) \geq 0, \qquad -\infty < x < \infty$

(2) $0 \leq F_\xi(x) \leq 1, \qquad F_\xi(\infty) = 1, \qquad F_\xi(-\infty) = 0$ /

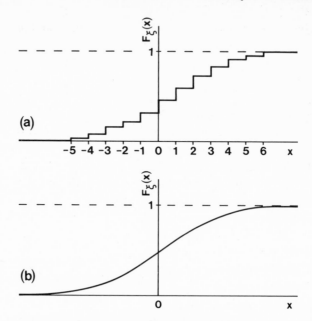

Figure 1.2.1. Typical distribution functions for (a) a discrete
random variable; (b) a continuous random variable.

(3) It is a nondecreasing function. For any x_1 and x_2, with $x_2 > x_1$,
we have

$$P_\xi\{x_1 \leq \xi \leq x_2\} = F_\xi(x_2) - F_\xi(x_1)$$

The distribution function $F_\xi(x)$ of a discrete random variable ξ is
piecewise constant (Figure 1.2.1a).

If the distribution function $F_\xi(x)$ of the random variable ξ is continuous,
then the variable ξ takes any single value x only with probability 0. If the
distribution function is not only continuous but also differentiable, then

$$p_\xi(x) = \frac{d}{dx} F_\xi(x) = \lim_{\Delta x \to 0} \frac{P\{x \leq \xi \leq x + \Delta x\}}{\Delta x} \qquad (1.2.2)$$

is called the *probability density function* and ξ is called a continuously
distributed random variable. The probability density function is a nonnegative function such that for any x_1 and x_2 with $x_2 > x_1$, we have

$$P\{x_1 \leq \xi \leq x_2\} = \int_{x_1}^{x_2} p_\xi(x) \, dx$$

and obviously

$$P\{-\infty \le \xi \le \infty\} = \int_{-\infty}^{\infty} p_\xi(x)\, dx = 1$$

Similarly, if ξ is a discrete random variable that can take on finite values $\{x_k; k = 1, 2, \ldots, N, \text{ say}\}$, we have

$$\sum_{k=1}^{N} P_\xi(x_k) = 1$$

Figure 1.2.1b gives a distribution function for a continuous random variable. It is a monotonic and continuous distribution such that $F_\xi(-\infty) = 0$ and $F_\xi(\infty) = 1$.

The above definitions can be extended to cover families of random variables or a random vector $\boldsymbol{\xi} = (\xi_1, \xi_2, \ldots, \xi_n)$. Thus for discrete random variables $\xi_1, \ldots, \xi_n$, a finite probability may be defined for the event $\{\xi_1 = x_1, \xi_2 = x_2, \ldots, \xi_n = x_n\}$, in that the variables $\xi_1, \ldots, \xi_n$ take the values $x_1, \ldots, x_n$ on any given trial of an experiment. Hence, we have

$$P(x_1, \ldots, x_n) = P\{\xi_1 = x_1, \xi_2 = x_2, \ldots, \xi_n = x_n\}$$

The probabilities $P(x_1, \ldots, x_n)$ where the variables $x_1, \ldots, x_n$ take all possible values of the random variables $\xi_1, \ldots, \xi_n$ form the *joint probability distribution* of these variables. The probability of the event $\{x'_1 \le \xi_1 \le x''_1, x'_2 \le \xi_2 \le x''_2, \ldots, x'_n \le \xi_n \le x''_n\}$ that the random variables $\xi_1, \ldots, \xi_n$ lie within the intervals $\{x'_1 \le \xi_1 \le x''_1, \ldots, x'_n \le \xi_n \le x''_n\}$ is given by

$$P\{x'_1 \le \xi_1 \le x''_1, \ldots, x'_n \le \xi_n \le x''_n\} = \sum_{x'_1}^{x''_1} \cdots \sum_{x'_n}^{x''_n} P(x_1, \ldots, x_n)$$

If the random variables $\xi_1, \ldots, \xi_n$ are continuous, for which a *joint distribution* can be defined as

$$F_{\xi_1, \ldots, \xi_n}(x_1, \ldots, x_n) = P\{\xi_1 \le x_1, \ldots, \xi_n \le x_n\}$$

where $\xi_1, \ldots, \xi_n$ can take on any allowed values in the range $-\infty < \xi_1 < x_1, \ldots, -\infty < \xi_n < x_n$, then a nonnegative function called the *joint probability density function* of the random variables $\xi_1, \ldots, \xi_n$ may be defined as

$$p(x_1, \ldots, x_n) = \frac{d^n}{dx_1 \cdots dx_n} F_{\xi_1, \ldots, \xi_n}(x_1, \ldots, x_n) \qquad (1.2.3)$$

The probability of the event $\{x'_1 \leq \xi_1 \leq x''_1, \ldots, x'_n \leq \xi_n \leq x''_n\}$ for continuous random variables $\{\xi_1, \ldots, \xi_n\}$ is given by

$$P\{x'_1 \leq \xi_1 \leq x''_1, \ldots, x'_n \leq \xi_n \leq x''_n\} = \int_{x'_1}^{x''_1} \cdots \int_{x'_n}^{x''_n} p(x_1, \ldots, x_n)\, dx_1 \cdots dx_n$$

The random variables $\xi_1, \ldots, \xi_n$ are called independent random variables if all possible events of the form $\{x'_1 \leq \xi_1 \leq x''_1, \ldots, x'_n \leq \xi_n \leq x''_n\}$ are mutually independent. Discrete random variables are independent if and only if their joint distribution is separable, i.e.,

$$P(x_1, \ldots, x_n) = P_{\xi_1}(x_1) \cdots P_{\xi_n}(x_n)$$

where $P_{\xi_k}(x_k)$ is the distribution of any single variable $\xi_k,\ k = 1, \ldots, n$. Similarly, continuous random variables are independent if and only if the density of their joint distribution is such that

$$p(x_1, \ldots, x_n) = p_{\xi_1}(x_1) \cdots p_{\xi_n}(x_n)$$

where $p_{\xi_k}(x_k)$ is the probability density function of a single random variable $\xi_k,\ k = 1, \ldots, n$.

Expectation, Variance, and Correlation

The expected value or mean value of a random variable (rv) is defined as

$$E[x] = \begin{cases} \displaystyle\int_{-\infty}^{\infty} x\, dF(x) \\[2ex] \displaystyle\sum_{k=-\infty}^{\infty} x_k P(x_k) & \text{for discrete rv} \\[2ex] \displaystyle\int_{-\infty}^{\infty} x p(x)\, dx & \text{for continuous rv} \end{cases} \qquad (1.2.4)$$

depending upon whether it is specified by its distribution function, its probability distribution, or its probability density function. The first integral is referred to as a Lebesgue–Steiltjes integral as $F(x)$ is of bounded variation in $(-\infty < x < \infty)$. [An excellent treatment of such integrals is given by Cramer (1963)]. Conceptually, we have:

(a) For a discrete random variable,

$$F(x) = \sum_k P(x_k) U(x - x_k)$$

where $U(x)$ is a unit step function: $U(x) = 1$ for $x \geq 0$, $U(x) = 0$ for $x < 0$.

(b) For a continuous random variable

$$F(x) = \int_{-\infty}^{x} p(x)\, dx$$

is an absolutely continuous function.

More specifically, we have

$$dF(x) = \begin{cases} \sum_{k} P(x_k)\delta(x - x_k)\, dx & \text{for discrete rv} \\[2mm] p(x)\, dx & \text{for continuous rv} \end{cases}$$

such that in either case

$$F(x) = \int_{-\infty}^{x} dF(x) \tag{1.2.5}$$

Here the random variable x is synonymous with ξ_1 in that $P(x_k) = P_\xi(x_k)$, with the discrete variable taking values $\{x_k; k = 0, \pm 1, \ldots\}$, and similarly $p(x) = p_\xi(x)$, $F(x) = F_\xi(x)$.

The operator E shall be used throughout the text to denote mathematical expectation. For a random variable z that is a function of the random variables $x_1, \ldots, x_n$, i.e., $z = \phi(x_1, \ldots, x_n)$, we have

$$E[z] = \begin{cases} \displaystyle\int_{-\infty}^{\infty} \cdots \int_{-\infty}^{\infty} \phi(x_1, \ldots, x_n)\, dF(x_1, \ldots, x_n) \\[3mm] \displaystyle\sum_{-\infty}^{\infty} \cdots \sum_{-\infty}^{\infty} \phi(x_1, \ldots, x_n) P(x_1, \ldots, x_n) & \text{discrete rv} \\[3mm] \displaystyle\int_{-\infty}^{\infty} \cdots \int_{-\infty}^{\infty} \phi(x_1, \ldots, x_n) p(x_1, \ldots, x_n)\, dx_1 \cdots dx_n & \text{continuous rv} \end{cases}$$

The properties of expectation are

(1) $E[a] = a$ for any constant
(2) $E[cx] = cE[x]$ for any constant c
(3) $E[x_1 + x_2] = E[x_1] + E[x_2]$ for any two rv's x_1, x_2
(4) $E[x_1 x_2] = E[x_1]E[x_2]$ if the rv's x_1 and x_2 are independent

The variance of a random variable is defined as

$$\text{var}\,[x] = E[(x - \mu_x)^2] \tag{1.2.6}$$

where $\mu_x = E[x]$. The variance has the following properties:

(1) var $[a] = 0$ for constant a
(2) var $[cx] = c^2$ var $[x]$ for any constant c
(3) var $[x_1 + x_2] =$ var $[x_1] +$ var $[x_2]$ for any two independent rv's

Sometimes the symbols μ_x and σ_x^2 are used to denote the mean value and variance of the random variable x.

Higher-order moments of a random variable are defined as

$$\mu_n(x) = \begin{cases} \displaystyle\int_{-\infty}^{\infty} x^n \, dF(x) & \\[2ex] \displaystyle\sum_k x_k^n P(x_k) & \text{for discrete rv} \\[2ex] \displaystyle\int_{-\infty}^{\infty} x^n p(x) \, dx & \text{for continuous rv} \end{cases} \tag{1.2.7}$$

Usually these moments can be conveniently obtained from the *characteristic function* or moment-generating function of a random variable. The characteristic function is defined for any real variable η as

$$M_x(\eta) = \begin{cases} \displaystyle\int_{-\infty}^{\infty} e^{-j\eta x} \, dF(x) & \\[2ex] \displaystyle\sum_k e^{-j\eta x_k} P(x_k) & \text{discrete rv} \\[2ex] \displaystyle\int_{-\infty}^{\infty} e^{-j\eta x} p(x) \, dx & \text{continuous rv} \end{cases} \tag{1.2.8}$$

In all cases

$$\mu_n(x) = \frac{\partial^n}{(-j\partial\eta)^n} M_x(\eta)\big|_{\eta=0}$$

with the properties $M_x(0) = 1$ and $|M_x(\eta)| \leq 1$ for all η and

$$M_{x_1 x_2}(\eta_1, \eta_2) = M_{x_1}(\eta_1) M_{x_2}(\eta_2)$$

for independent random variables x_1 and x_2. Since the characteristic function is the Fourier transform of the probability density function and the discrete Fourier transform of the probability distribution for discrete-integer-valued random variables $\{x_k = 0, 1, 2, \ldots\}$, we have the following inversion formulas:

$$p(x) = \frac{1}{2\pi} \int_{-\infty}^{\infty} e^{j\eta x} M_x(\eta)\, d\eta, \quad -\infty < x < \infty$$

$$P(x = k) = \frac{1}{2\pi} \int_{-\pi}^{\pi} e^{j\eta k} M_x(\eta)\, d\eta \tag{1.2.9}$$

For random variables which take on only positive real (or integer) values, moment-generating functions may be defined as

$$\phi_x(z) = \begin{cases} \displaystyle\sum_{k=0}^{\infty} P(x = k)z^{-k} & \text{discrete rv } (|z| < 1) \\[2ex] \displaystyle\int_0^{\infty} e^{-zx} p(x)\, dx & \text{continuous rv } (0 < z < \infty) \end{cases} \tag{1.2.10}$$

with

$$\mu_n(x) = \begin{cases} \left. \left(-z\dfrac{\partial}{\partial z}\right)^n \phi_x(z) \right|_{z=1} & \text{discrete case} \\[2ex] \left. (-1)^n \dfrac{\partial^n}{\partial z^n} \phi_x(z) \right|_{z=0} & \text{continuous case} \end{cases} \tag{1.2.11}$$

Since the moment-generating functions are the z transform and Laplace transforms of probability distributions, these may be conveniently inverted by standard techniques to obtain $P(x)$ and $p(x)$, respectively.

Table I contains the definitions described above. Their extension to the case of several-variable (multivariate) distributions is straightforward. We list some of these for the distributions of continuous random variables in Table II.

Correlation between any two random variables x_1 and x_2 is defined as

$$R(x_1, x_2) = E[x_1 x_2] \tag{1.2.12}$$

and the *covariance* between the variables as

$$\text{cov}\,[x_1 x_2] = E[(x_1 - \mu_1)(x_2 - \mu_2)] \tag{1.2.13}$$

$$= R(x_1, x_2) - \mu_1 \mu_2$$

with the normalized covariance, also called the *correlation coefficient*, defined as

$$\rho = \frac{\text{cov}\,[x_1 x_2]}{\sigma_1 \sigma_2} \tag{1.2.14}$$

Table I. *Fundamental Characteristics of Distribution Functions*

Characteristics	Random variables	
	Continuous	Discrete
Mean value or expectation	$\mu_x = E[x] = \int_{-\infty}^{\infty} x p(x)\, dx$	$\mu_x = \sum_k x_k P(x_k)$
Variance	$\sigma_x^2 = \int_{-\infty}^{\infty} (x - \mu_x)^2 p(x)\, dx$	$\sigma_x^2 = \sum_k (x_k - \mu_x)^2 P(x_k)$
nth moment about the origin	$\mu_n = \int_{-\infty}^{\infty} x^n p(x)\, dx$	$\mu_n = \sum_k x_k^n P(x_k)$
Characteristic function	$M_x(\eta) = \int_{-\infty}^{\infty} e^{-j\eta x} p(x)\, dx$	$M_x(\eta) = \sum_k e^{-j\eta x_k} P(x_k)$
Inversion formula	$p(x) = \dfrac{1}{2\pi} \int_{-\infty}^{\infty} e^{j\eta x} M_x(\eta)\, dx$	$P(x_k) = \int_{-\pi}^{\pi} e^{j\eta x_k} M_x(\eta)\, d\eta/2\pi$ (for x_k an integer)
Expectation of a function $f(x)$	$E[f(x)] = \int_{-\infty}^{\infty} f(x) p(x)\, dx$	$E[f(x)] = \sum_k f(x_k) P(x_k)$

where

$$\mu_1 = E[x_1], \qquad \mu_2 = E[x_2], \qquad \text{var}\,[x_1] = \sigma_1^2, \qquad \text{var}\,[x_2] = \sigma_2^2$$

For independent random variables x_1 and x_2, equations (1.2.13) and (1.2.14) are zero, and the variables are called uncorrelated. The correlation or the correlation coefficient characterizes the degree of linear dependence of x_1 and x_2. In general, ρ lies within the range $\{-1 \leq \rho \leq 1\}$.

Conditional Distributions and Densities

The *conditional distribution* $F_\xi(x_1|\mathcal{U})$ of the random variable x given an event $\mathcal{U}$ in the event set $\mathcal{F}$, is defined as the conditional probability of the event $\{x \leq x_1\}$, i.e.,

$$F_\xi(x_1|\mathcal{U}) = P\{x \leq x_1|\mathcal{U}\} = \frac{P\{x \leq x_1, \mathcal{U}\}}{P\{\mathcal{U}\}} \qquad (1.2.15)$$

where x is any real-valued function of the outcome ξ of the experiment $\mathcal{E}$,

Table II. Fundamental Characteristics of Continuous Multivariate Distributions

Given: $\mathbf{X} = (x_1, x_2, \ldots, x_n)^T$, a random vector of dimension n

Properties	Definition
Mean value	$\mu(\mathbf{X}) = \displaystyle\int_{-\infty}^{\infty} \int_{-\infty}^{\infty} \cdots \int_{-\infty}^{\infty}$
	$\times (x_1, x_2, x_3, \cdots, x_n)^T p(x_1, x_2, \cdots, x_n)\, dx_1\, dx_2 \cdots dx_n$
	or $\quad \mu(\mathbf{X}) = \displaystyle\int_{-\infty}^{\infty} \underset{n\,\text{fold}}{\cdots} \int_{-\infty}^{\infty} \mathbf{X}p(\mathbf{X}) \prod_{k=1}^{n} dx_k$
Second moment	$\mathbf{C_{XX}} = E[\mathbf{XX}^T] = \displaystyle\int_{-\infty}^{\infty} \cdots \int_{-\infty}^{\infty} (\mathbf{XX}^T)p(\mathbf{X}) \prod_{k=1}^{n} dx_k$
Covariance	$\text{cov}(\mathbf{X}) = \displaystyle\int_{-\infty}^{\infty} \underset{n\,\text{fold}}{\cdots} \int_{-\infty}^{\infty} (\mathbf{X} - \mu(\mathbf{X}))(\mathbf{X} - \mu(\mathbf{X}))^T p(\mathbf{X}) \prod_{k=1}^{n} dx_k$
	$= E[(\mathbf{X} - \mu(\mathbf{X}))(\mathbf{X} - \mu(\mathbf{X}))^T]$
Characteristic function	$M(\mathbf{\eta}) = E[\exp(-j\mathbf{\eta}^T\mathbf{X})]$
	$= \displaystyle\int_{-\infty}^{\infty} \underset{n\,\text{fold}}{\cdots} \int_{-\infty}^{\infty} \exp(-j\mathbf{\eta}^T\mathbf{X})p(\mathbf{X}) \prod_{k=1}^{n} dx_k$
Inversion formula	$p(\mathbf{X}) = \dfrac{1}{(2\pi)^n} \displaystyle\int_{-\infty}^{\infty} \underset{n\,\text{fold}}{\cdots} \int_{-\infty}^{\infty} \exp(j\mathbf{X}^T\mathbf{\eta})M(\mathbf{\eta}) \prod_{k=1}^{n} d\eta_k$

and $\{x \leq x_1, \mathcal{U}\}$ is the event consisting of all outcomes such that $x(\xi) \leq x_1$ and $\xi \in \mathcal{U}$.

The conditional distribution has the following properties:

$$F_\xi(\infty|\mathcal{U}) = 1, \qquad F_\xi(-\infty|\mathcal{U}) = 0$$

$$F_\xi(x_2|\mathcal{U}) - F_\xi(x_1|\mathcal{U}) = P\{x_1 < x < x_2|\mathcal{U}\}$$

$$= \frac{P\{x_1 < x < x_2, \mathcal{U}\}}{P\{\mathcal{U}\}}$$

which are the same as for ordinary distributions.

For a continuous random variable a probability density function can be defined as

$$p(x|\mathcal{U}) = \frac{dF(x|\mathcal{U})}{dx} \qquad (1.2.16)$$

such that

$$\int_{-\infty}^{\infty} p(x|\mathcal{U})\, dx = 1$$

Some Probability Distributions

Tables III and IV list some well-known probability distributions and density functions, along with various parameters used to define them. Of particular interest to us is the Poisson probability distribution of the form

$$P(s) = \frac{\lambda^s}{s!} e^{-\lambda}, \qquad s = 0, 1, 2, \ldots \qquad (1.2.17)$$

It is determined by a unique positive parameter λ called the rate parameter or the intensity parameter of the distribution.

The most common distribution associated with real random variables is the *Gaussian* (or *normal*) *distribution*. It is of paramount importance in the study of probability theory because many random variables that arise in practical applications can be considered to be approximately normally distributed. It has the further advantage that it is exceedingly convenient and analytically simple to handle.

The Gaussian distribution is determined by two parameters μ and σ, and its probability density function is expressed as

$$p(x) = \frac{1}{(2\pi\sigma^2)^{1/2}} \exp\left[-\frac{(x-\mu)^2}{2\sigma^2} \right] \qquad -\infty < x < \infty \qquad (1.2.18)$$

A normally distributed random variable x has a mean value $E[x] = \mu$ and a variance σ^2. The notation $N\{\mu, \sigma^2\}$ is often used to denote a *normal probability density function* with mean μ and variance σ^2.

Stochastic Processes

Referring to a given experiment $\mathscr{E}$ specified by (i) its outcome ξ, which is an element in the space Ω, (ii) its events ω, which form a subset in Ω and form the Borel algebra $\mathscr{F}$, and (iii) a probability measure $\mathscr{P}$ for the events that gives a probability space $(\Omega, \mathscr{F}, \mathscr{P})$, we may assign to each outcome ξ of the experiment a real or complex time function $x(t, \xi)$, just as earlier we had assigned a random variable $x(\xi)$ to every outcome ξ. Then $\{x(t, \xi), t \in T\}$ represents a family or ensemble of time-dependent functions, one for each outcome ξ. A stochastic process is thus a function of two variables ξ and t.

While the outcomes ξ belong to Ω, t belongs to the index set T of real numbers.

For each particular outcome ξ_k, $x(t, \xi_k)$ is a function of time and is called a sample function or member function of the ensemble, or a realization or representation of the process. For any particular value of $t = t_k$, $x(t_k, \xi)$ depends upon the outcomes ξ and is therefore a random variable, while $x(t_k, \xi_k)$ is a particular number.

We shall use the notation $\{x(t)\}$ to define a stochastic process; the dependence on ξ will be taken as implicit.

As stated earlier, the index set T defines the type of stochastic process. For t discrete we have a stochastic sequence, and if t is continuous then $\{x(t)\}$ is called a continuous-parameter stochastic process. In the rest of this section we shall only be concerned with the latter, and the term "stochastic process" will refer to a continuous-parameter stochastic process.

For any real-valued stochastic process $\{x(t)\}$, at any specific time t, $x(t)$ is a random variable with a distribution function $F(x; t)$ which, in general, will depend upon t. By definition,

$$F(x; t) = P\{x(t) \le x\}$$

i.e., $F(x; t)$ is equal to the probability of the event $\{x(t) \le x\}$ for all outcomes ξ in which the (random) functions $x(t)$ of the stochastic process do not exceed the real number x at the specified time t.

The function $F(x; t)$ is called the first-order distribution of the process $\{x(t)\}$. If the continuous derivative $\partial F/\partial x$ exists for all points in the interval $-\infty \le x \le \infty$, then the probability density function for the process is given by

$$p(x; t) = \frac{\partial F(x; t)}{\partial x} \tag{1.2.19}$$

which is similar to equation (1.2.2).

Extending this definition to consider two time instants t_1 and t_2, we have the random variables $x(t_1)$ and $x(t_2)$. We can then define the probability of the event $\{x(t_1) \le x_1, x(t_2) \le x_2\}$ as the *joint distribution function*

$$F(x_1, x_2; t_1, t_2) = P\{x(t_1) \le x_1, x(t_2) \le x_2\} \tag{1.2.20}$$

$F(x_1, x_2; t_1, t_2)$ is called the *second-order distribution* of the process. The *joint probability density function* associated with this distribution is

$$p(x_1, x_2; t_1, t_2) = \frac{\partial^2 F(x_1, x_2; t_1, t_2)}{\partial x_1 \, \partial x_2} \tag{1.2.21}$$

Note the similarity to equation (1.2.3).

Table III. Some Well-Known Discrete Probability Distributions

Name	Expression	Range or condition	Mean	Variance	Characteristic function
Single point or degenerate $[x_k = \text{constant } (\mu)]$	$\delta(x_k - \mu)$	$-\infty < \mu < \infty$	μ	0	$e^{-j\eta\mu}$
Binary valued $(\pm\alpha)$	$\frac{1}{2}[\delta(x_k + \alpha) + \delta(x_k - \alpha)]$	$0 \leq \alpha < \infty$	0	α^2	$\cos\eta\alpha$
Binomial (probability of occurrence $= v$ for $x_k = s,\ s = 0, 1, 2, \ldots, N)$	$\binom{N}{s} v^s(1-v)^{N-s}$	$0 < v < 1$	Nv	$Nv(1-v)$	$(1 - v + v\,e^{-j\eta})^N$
Poisson, $x_k = s,\ s = 0, 1, 2, \ldots, \infty$; mean rate $= \lambda$	$\dfrac{\lambda^s}{s!}e^{-\lambda}$	$0 < \lambda < \infty$	λ	λ	$e^{-\lambda(1 - e^{-j\eta})}$

Table IV. *Some Well-Known Probability Density Functions for Continuous Random Variables*

Name	Expression	Range or condition	Mean	Variance	Characteristic function
Uniform or rectangular	$\dfrac{1}{2a}$	$-a \leq x \leq a$	0	$\dfrac{a^2}{3}$	$\dfrac{\sin a\eta}{a\eta}$
Exponential	$\dfrac{1}{\lambda} \exp\left(-\dfrac{x-\mu}{\lambda} \right)$	$\mu < x < \infty$ $0 < \lambda < \infty$	$\mu + \lambda$	λ^2	$\dfrac{e^{-j\eta\mu}}{1 + j\eta\lambda}$
Gaussian, $N\{\mu, \sigma^2\}$	$\dfrac{1}{(2\pi\sigma^2)^{1/2}} \exp\left[-\dfrac{1}{2}\left(\dfrac{x-\mu}{\sigma}\right)^2 \right]$	$-\infty < x < \infty$ $-\infty < \mu < \infty$ $0 < \sigma < \infty$	μ	σ^2	$\exp\left(-j\mu\eta - \tfrac{1}{2}\sigma^2\eta^2 \right)$
Chi-square with n degrees of freedom	$\dfrac{x^{n/2 - 1}\, e^{-x/2}}{2^{n/2}\, \Gamma(n/2)}$	$0 < x < \infty$ $1 < n < \infty$	n	$2n$	$\dfrac{1}{(1 + 2\eta)^{n/2}}$ (moment-generating function)
Bivariate Gaussian between two Gaussian random variables (x_1, x_2), each $N\{0, \sigma^2\}$, with correlation $= \rho$	$\dfrac{1}{2\pi\sigma^2(1 - \rho^2)^{1/2}} \exp\left[-\dfrac{x_1^2 - 2x_1 x_2 \rho + x_2^2}{2\sigma^2(1 - \sigma^2)} \right]$	$-\infty < x_1 < \infty$ $-\infty < x_2 < \infty$ $0 < \sigma < \infty$ $0 < \rho < 1$	0	$\sigma^2 \begin{pmatrix} 1 & \rho \\ \rho & 1 \end{pmatrix}$ (covariance matrix)	$M(\eta, \lambda)$ $= \exp[-\tfrac{1}{2}\sigma^2(\eta^2 + 2\eta\lambda\rho + \lambda^2)]$
Multivariate Gaussian for n-dimensional vector variable $N\{\mu, \mathbf{C_{xx}}\}$	$\dfrac{1}{(2\pi)^{n/2}|\mathbf{C_{xx}}|^{1/2}} \exp[-\tfrac{1}{2}(\mathbf{X} - \mu)^T \mathbf{C_{xx}}^{-1}(\mathbf{X} - \mu)]$		μ	$\mathbf{C_{xx}}$	$\exp(-j\eta^T\mu - \tfrac{1}{2}\eta^T\mathbf{C_{xx}}\eta)$

The following properties may be easily verified:

(1) $F(x_1, x_2; t_1, t_2) \geq 0$, for $-\infty < x_1 < \infty$, $-\infty < x_2 < \infty$,
    for all t_1, t_2

(2) $0 \leq F(x_1, x_2; t_1, t_2) \leq 1$, $F(\infty, \infty; t_1, t_2) = 1$,
    $F(-\infty, -\infty, t_1, t_2) = 0$

(3) $F(x_1, \infty; t_1, t_2) = F(x_1, t_1)$

(4) $p(x_1, t_1) = \int_{-\infty}^{\infty} p(x_1, x_2; t_1, t_2)\, dx_2$ for all t_2

A *conditional probability distribution* for the stochastic process $x(t)$ is defined as

$F(x_1, t_1 | x_2, t_2)$

$$= \frac{P\{x(t_1) \leq x_1, x(t_2) = x_2\}}{P\{x(t_2) = x_2\}}$$

$$= \lim_{\Delta x_2 \to 0} \frac{P\{x(t_1) \leq x_1, x(t_2) \leq x_2 + \Delta x_2\} - P\{x(t_1) \leq x_1, x(t_2) \leq x_2\}}{P\{x(t_2) \leq x_2 + \Delta x_2\} - P\{x(t_1) \leq x_2\}}$$

$$= \frac{(\partial/\partial x_2) F(x_1, x_2; t_1, t_2)}{(\partial/\partial x_2) F(x_2, t_2)} \tag{1.2.22}$$

which is the probability of the event $\{x(t_1) \leq x_1$ given $x(t_2) = x_2\}$, and it leads to the *conditional probability density function*

$$p(x_1, t_1 | x_2, t_2) = \frac{p(x_1, x_2; t_1, t_2)}{p(x_2; t_2)} \tag{1.2.23}$$

The above relationships can be extended to cover two stochastic processes $\{x(t)\}$ and $\{y(t)\}$. A *joint distribution function* can be defined as the probability of the event $\{x(t_1) \leq x_1; y(t_2) \leq y_1\}$:

$$F(x_1, y_1; t_1, t_2) = P\{x(t) \leq x_1, y(t_2) \leq y_1\}$$

and a *joint probability density function* defined as the continuous derivative

$$p(x_1, y_1; t_1, t_2) = \frac{\partial^2 F(x_1, y_1; t_1, t_2)}{\partial x_1 \partial y_1} \tag{1.2.24}$$

An *n*th-order distribution function of a stochastic process $\{x(t)\}$ is defined as

$$F(x_1, x_2, \ldots, x_n; t_1, t_2, \ldots, t_n) = P\{x(t_1) \leq x_1, x(t_2) \leq x_2, \ldots, x(t_n) \leq x_n\}$$

for any n and $t_1, \ldots, t_n$. Corresponding to this we have the *n*th-order probability density function $p(x_1, \ldots, x_n; t_1, \ldots, t_n)$ as the *n*th-order derivative of

F with respect to $x_1, \ldots, x_n$. The hierarchy of distributions

$$F(x_1; t_1), F(x_1, x_2; t_1, t_2), \ldots, F(x_1, \ldots, x_n; t_1, \ldots, t_n)$$

or equivalently

$$p(x_1, t_1), p(x_1, x_2; t_1, t_2), \ldots, p(x_1, \ldots, x_n; t_1, \ldots, t_n)$$

as $n \to \infty$ provide a complete statistical description of the stochastic process.

Moments of a Stochastic Process

The expected value or mean value of a stochastic process is the expected value of the random variable $x(t)$:

$$E[x(t)] = \begin{cases} \displaystyle\int_{-\infty}^{\infty} x \, dF(x; t) \\ \displaystyle\int_{-\infty}^{\infty} xp(x; t) \, dx \end{cases} \tag{1.2.25}$$

which in general is a function of time.

The variance of the process at any time instant t is defined as

$$\mathrm{var}\,[x(t)] = \begin{cases} \displaystyle\int_{-\infty}^{\infty} \{x - E[x(t)]\}^2 \, dF(x; t) \\ \displaystyle\int_{-\infty}^{\infty} x^2 p(x; t) \, dx - E^2[x(t)] \end{cases} \tag{1.2.26}$$

The *autocorrelation function* $R_x(t_1, t_2)$ of a stochastic process is the joint moment of the random variables $x(t_1)$ and $x(t_2)$, and is given by

$$R_x(t_1, t_2) = E[x(t_1)x(t_2)] = \begin{cases} \displaystyle\int_I x_1 x_2 \, dF(x_1, x_2; t_1, t_2) \\ \displaystyle\int_{-\infty}^{\infty} x_1 x_2 p(x_1, x_2; t_1, t_2) \, dx_1 \, dx_2 \end{cases} \tag{1.2.27}$$

where I is the rectangle of the (x_1, x_2) plane. $R_x(t_1, t_2)$ is a function of t_1 and t_2.

The autocovariance of the stochastic process is defined as

$$\mathrm{cov}\,[x(t_1)x(t_2)] = E[\{x(t_1) - E[x(t_1)]\}\{x(t_2) - E[x(t_2)]\}]$$

$$= R_x(t_1, t_2) - E[x(t_1)]E[x(t_2)] \tag{1.2.28}$$

The normalized autocovariance function of the process is expressed as

$$\rho_x(t_1, t_2) = \frac{\text{cov}\,[x(t_1)x(t_2)]}{\{\text{var}\,[x(t_1)]\,\text{var}\,[x(t_2)]\}^{1/2}} \qquad (1.2.29)$$

For an uncorrelated random process, $\text{cov}\,[x(t_1)x(t_2)] = 0$ for all t_1 and t_2 as $p(x_1, x_2; t_1, t_2) = p(x_1; t_1)p(x_2; t_2)$.

The cross correlation between two stochastic processes $\{x(t)\}$, $\{y(t)\}$ is the joint moment between the random variables $x(t_1)$ and $y(t_2)$:

$$R_{xy}(t_1, t_2) = E[x(t_1)y(t_2)] = \begin{cases} \displaystyle\int_I xy\,dF(x, y; t_1, t_2) \\[2ex] \displaystyle\int\!\!\!\int_{-\infty}^{\infty} xyp(x, y; t_1, t_2)\,dx\,dy \end{cases} \qquad (1.2.30)$$

from equation (1.2.24); I is the rectangle of the (x, y) plane. In general $R_{xy}(t_1, t_2)$ is a function of t_1 and t_2.

The cross covariance between the two stochastic processes is defined as

$$\text{cov}\,[x(t_1)y(t_2)] = R_{xy}(t_1, t_2) - E[x(t_1)]E[y(t_2)] \qquad (1.2.31)$$

Similarly the normalized cross covariance or cross-correlation coefficient is given by

$$\rho_{xy}(t_1, t_2) = \frac{\text{cov}\,[x(t_1)y(t_2)]}{\{\text{var}\,[x(t_1)]\,\text{var}\,[x(t_2)]\}^{1/2}} \qquad (1.2.32)$$

For zero mean stochastic processes, i.e., $E[x(t)] = 0$, $E[y(t)] = 0$ for all t, the autocorrelation function is equal to the autocovariance function, and cross correlation equals the cross-covariance function.

Stationarity

A stochastic process $\{x(t)\}$ is said to be stationary in the strict sense if its statistics (distributions or densities) do not depend upon the time reference. Thus for a strictly stationary process the statistics of $x(t)$ and $x(t + \tau)$ are identical, for any value of τ. Further, for any n, the nth-order probability density function of a stationary process is such that

$$p(x_1, \ldots, x_n; t_1, \ldots, t_n) = p(x_1, \ldots, x_n; t_1 + \tau, \ldots, t_n + \tau) \quad (1.2.33)$$

for any τ.

Similarly, two stochastic processes $\{x(t)\}$ and $\{y(t)\}$ are jointly stationary in the strict sense if the joint distributions (densities) of $x(t)$, $y(t)$ are the same as the joint distributions (densities) of $x(t + \tau)$, $y(t + \tau)$ for any τ.

From equation (1.2.33), $p(x; t) = p(x; t + \tau)$ for any τ, so that the probability density function of a stationary stochastic process is time-independent. Hence we have

$$p(x; t) = p(x)$$

which indicates that the mean value $E[x(t)]$ of equation (1.2.25) is a constant for a stationary process. Also, for strict stationarity, the joint probability density function is such that

$$p(x_1, x_2; t_1, t_2) = p(x_1, x_2; t_1 + \varepsilon, t_2 + \varepsilon) = p(x_1, x_2; \tau) \quad (1.2.34)$$

for $\tau = t_2 - t_1$ and any ε and depends only upon the time difference τ. Hence $p(x_1, x_2; \tau)$ may be taken as the joint probability density function of the random variables $x(t + \tau)$ and $x(t)$.

Employing equation (1.2.34) in equation (1.2.27), we see that the auto-correlation function $R_x(t_1, t_2)$ of a stationary stochastic process is only a function of the time interval or lag $(t_2 - t_1)$, and in general

$$R_x(\tau) = E[x(t + \tau)x(t)] = R_x(-\tau)$$

$$\rho_x(\tau) = \frac{\text{cov}\,[x(t)x(t + \tau)]}{\text{var}\,[x(t)]} \quad (1.2.35)$$

For two jointly stationary stochastic processes, we have a similar relationship for the cross-correlation function:

$$R_{xy}(\tau) = E[x(t + \tau)y(t)]$$

$$R_{yx}(\tau) = E[x(t)y(t + \tau)] \quad (1.2.36)$$

A stochastic process is said to be wide-sense stationary if it satisfies the following conditions

(a) $E[x^2(t)] < \infty$

(b) $E[x(t)] = \mu$ is a constant

(c) $E[(x(t) - \mu)(x(s) - \mu)]$ depends only upon $t - s$

Wide-sense stationary processes are termed as second-order stationary as they involve only second-order moments or distributions.

Any two stochastic processes are jointly stationary in the wide sense if each satisfies the above three conditions, and their cross-correlation function depends only on the lag value, i.e.,

$$E[x(t + \tau)y(t)] = R_{xy}(\tau)$$

Ergodicity and Time Averages

A stochastic process $\{x(t)\}$ is said to be ergodic if all its statistics can be determined from a single realization of the process. This is due to the *ergodic theorem* (Wong, 1971), details of which are beyond the scope of this text. The property of ergodicity is a useful link between the mathematical description of a stochastic process and its physical record.

Given a finite record $\{x(t), -T \leq t \leq T\}$ of a stationary stochastic process $\{x(t)\}$, if the process is ergodic, then for any function $g(x(t))$ the ensemble average (i.e., the expectation value) equals the time average,

$$E[g(x(t))] = \lim_{T \to \infty} \frac{1}{2T} \int_{-T}^{T} g(x(t))\, dt \qquad (1.2.37)$$

provided certain conditions (called metric transitivity) are satisfied. Very crudely, these require that the variance of the estimator, as given by equation (1.2.37) tends to zero as $T \to \infty$. Usually these conditions are satisfied in all practical circumstances. Thus the property of ergodicity allows most parameters of interest in a stochastic process to be determined from a long enough record of the process.

For a stochastic process $\{x(t)\}$, we consider three important statistics which may be determined from a record $\{x(t), -T \leq t \leq T\}$:

(a) The time-averaged mean value is

$$\mu_T = \frac{1}{2T} \int_{-T}^{T} x(t)\, dt \qquad (1.2.38)$$

Thus $E[\mu_T] = E[x(t)] = \mu$, a constant. The variance of μ_T may be determined as

$$\operatorname{var}[\mu_T] = \frac{1}{(2T)^2} \int_{-T}^{T} \int_{-T}^{T} E[x(t_1)x(t_2)]\, dt_1\, dt_2 - \mu^2$$

$$= \frac{1}{(2T)^2} \int_{-T}^{T} \int_{-T}^{T} R_x(t_1 - t_2)\, dt_1\, dt_2 - \mu^2, \qquad \text{due to stationarity of}$$
$$\{x(t)\}$$

$$= \frac{1}{2T} \int_{-2T}^{2T} \left(1 - \frac{|\tau|}{2T}\right) R_x(\tau)\, d\tau - \mu^2 \qquad (1.2.39)$$

According to the ergodic property of $\{x(t)\}$, $\mu_T \to E[x(t)]$ as $T \to \infty$ if and only if $\operatorname{var}[\mu_T] \to 0$ as $T \to \infty$. Then the condition for equivalence is

$$\lim_{T \to \infty} \frac{1}{2T} \int_{-2T}^{2T} R_x(\tau)\, d\tau = \mu^2 \qquad (1.2.40)$$

As such, the ergodicity of the mean value is usually not very difficult to test.

(b) The time-averaged autocorrelation function is given by

$$\hat{R}_x(\tau) = \frac{1}{2T - |\tau|} \int_{-T}^{T - |\tau|} x(t + \tau)x(t)\, dt, \qquad 0 \le \tau < 2T \qquad (1.2.41)$$

Obviously $E[\hat{R}_x(\tau)] = R_x(\tau)$. The estimator $\hat{R}_x(\tau)$ is ergodic, in that $\hat{R}_x(\tau) \rightarrow R_x(\tau)$ as $T \rightarrow \infty$, provided the following condition is satisfied:

$$\lim_{T \to \infty} \text{var}\,[\hat{R}_x(\tau) = 0$$

or

$$\lim_{T \to \infty} \frac{1}{(2T)^2} \int_{-T}^{T} \int_{-T}^{T} E[x(t_1 + \tau)x(t_1)x(t_2 + \tau)x(t_2)]\, dt_1\, dt_2 = R_x^2(\tau) \qquad (1.2.42)$$

To test the ergodicity of the autocorrelation function we require the fourth-order moments of the stochastic process. These in general are difficult to evaluate. If however the process $\{x(t)\}$ has a Gaussian probability density function, with a mean value $E[x(t)] = \mu$, then

$$E[x(t_1 + \tau)x(t_1)x(t_2 + \tau)x(t_2)] = R_x^2(\tau) + R_x^2(t_1 - t_2)$$
$$+ R_x(t_1 - t_2 + \tau)R_x(t_1 - t_2 - \tau) - 2\mu_x^4$$

(see Gaussian process, p. 28), and the above condition reduces to

$$\lim_{T \to \infty} \frac{1}{2T} \int_{-2T}^{2T} \left(1 - \frac{|t|}{2T}\right)[R_x^2(t) + R_x(t + \tau)R_x(t - \tau)]\, dt = 2\mu_x^4 \qquad (1.2.43)$$

(c) If finite realizations $\{x(t), y(t), -T \le t \le T\}$ of two jointly stationary stochastic processes $\{x(t), y(t)\}$ are available, then an estimate of the cross-correlation function is given by the time-averaged value

$$\hat{R}_{xy}(\tau) = \frac{1}{2T - |\tau|} \int_{-T}^{T - |\tau|} x(t + \tau)y(t)\, dt, \qquad 0 \le \tau \le 2T \qquad (1.2.44)$$

Thus $E[\hat{R}_{xy}(\tau)] = R_{xy}(\tau)$ and the estimate is ergodic if and only if

$$\text{var}\,[\hat{R}_{xy}(\tau)] \rightarrow 0 \quad \text{as} \quad T \rightarrow \infty$$

In other words

$$\lim_{T \to \infty} \frac{1}{2T} \int_{-T}^{T} \int_{-T}^{T} E[x(t_1 + \tau)y(t_1)x(t_2 + \tau)y(t_2)]\, dt_1\, dt_2 = R_{xy}^2(\tau)$$

For jointly stationary Gaussian-distributed processes for which $E[x(t)] = E[y(t)] = 0$, this condition reduces to

$$\lim_{T \to \infty} \frac{1}{2T} \int_{-2T}^{2T} \left(1 - \frac{|t|}{2T}\right)[R_x(t)R_y(t) + R_{xy}(t + \tau)R_{yx}(t - \tau)]\, dt = 0$$

Some simple bounds may be derived for the autocorrelation and cross-correlation functions. For any two real-valued stochastic processes the following squared quantity is always nonnegative, irrespective of t_1, t_2:

$$E\left[\left(\frac{x(t_1)}{\sqrt{E[x^2(t_1)]}} - \frac{y(t_2)}{\sqrt{E[y^2(t_2)]}}\right)^2\right] \geq 0$$

On expanding this we obtain

$$|R_{xy}(t_1, t_2)| \leq \sqrt{E[x^2(t_1)]}\sqrt{E[y^2(t_2)]}$$

Similarly we have

$$|R_x(t_1, t_2)| \leq \sqrt{E[x^2(t_1)]}\sqrt{E[x^2(t_2)]}$$

For a stationary stochastic process these inequalities become

$$|R_{xy}(\tau)| \leq (R_x(0)R_y(0))^{1/2}$$
$$|R_x(\tau)| \leq R_x(0) \tag{1.2.45}$$

These indicate that for zero mean stationary processes, the normalized covariances $|\rho_x(\tau)|$ and cross covariances $|\rho_{xy}(\tau)|$ lie in the interval $(0, 1)$.

Gaussian Process

Several randomly occurring phenomena associated with physical systems can be closely characterized as Gaussian random processes, e.g., the random noise current in an electronic circuit due to shot or thermal noise effects. Also, the randomly fluctuating velocity in most turbulent flows can be considered as a normally distributed stochastic process.

A process $\{x(t)\}$ is said to be *normal* if the random variables $x(t_1), \ldots, x(t_n)$ are jointly normally distributed for any n and $t_1, \ldots, t_n$, i.e., they possess the multivariate probability density function

$$p(x_1, \ldots, x_n; t_1, \ldots, t_n)$$

$$= \frac{1}{(2\pi)^{n/2}|\mathbf{C_{XX}}|^{1/2}} \exp\left\{-\tfrac{1}{2}(\mathbf{X} - \boldsymbol{\mu})^T \mathbf{C_{XX}^{-1}}(\mathbf{X} - \boldsymbol{\mu})\right\} \tag{1.2.46}$$

for $n \geq 1$, where

$$\mathbf{X}^T = (x_1, \ldots, x_n)$$

$$\boldsymbol{\mu} = E[\mathbf{X}]$$

$$\mathbf{C_{XX}} = \text{cov}[\mathbf{XX}^T] = E[\mathbf{XX}^T] - \boldsymbol{\mu}\boldsymbol{\mu}^T$$

and T denotes transposition; $\mathbf{C_{XX}}$ is the covariance matrix of the random variables in the vector $\mathbf{X}$, with any element $\mathbf{C_{XX}}(j, k) = \text{cov}\,[x(t_j)x(t_k)]$. If the process is wide-sense stationary, then $\mathbf{C_{XX}}(j, k) = R_x(|t_j - t_k|) - \mu^2$, where $E[x(t)] = \mu$ for all t. Since the probability density function of equation (1.2.46) for the normal process depends upon $(t_1, \ldots, t_n)$ only through the covariance function $\mathbf{C_{XX}}(j, k)$ for any $\{t_j, t_k\}$, it follows that if $\{x(t)\}$ is wide-sense stationary, it is also strictly stationary. The process is described completely by the hierarchy of normal density functions for $n = 1, 2, \ldots$ of equation (1.2.46), which in their turn are expressed in terms of the mean value μ, and the autocorrelation function $\{R_x(\tau)\}$ for all τ. Thus the statistics of a stationary Gaussian process are completely specified if its mean value and autocorrelation function are known.

The characteristic function associated with the Gaussian density function is

$$M_{\mathbf{X}}(\boldsymbol{\eta}) = E[\exp\,(-j\eta^T x)]$$

$$= \exp\,(-j\boldsymbol{\eta}^T\boldsymbol{\mu} - \tfrac{1}{2}\boldsymbol{\eta}^T\mathbf{C_{XX}}\boldsymbol{\eta}), \qquad n > 1 \qquad (1.2.47)$$

where $\boldsymbol{\eta}^T = (\eta_1, \ldots, \eta_n)$. A useful relationship can be derived from this for the joint moment of the process:

$$E[x(t_1)x(t_2)x(t_3)x(t_4)] = \frac{\partial^4}{\partial\eta_1\partial\eta_2\partial\eta_3\partial\eta_4}M_x(\eta_1, \eta_2, \eta_3, \eta_4)\Big|_{\eta_1,\ldots,\eta_4 = 0}$$

$$= R_x(t_1 - t_2)R_x(t_3 - t_4) + R_x(t_1 - t_3)R_x(t_2 - t_4)$$

$$+ R_x(t_1 - t_4)R_x(t_2 - t_3) - 2\mu^4 \qquad (1.2.48)$$

Poisson Process

Poisson distributions and Poisson processes will play a central role in the developments to follow below. We shall discuss some of the important features associated with such processes and shall touch upon other relevant properties as they appear.

Consider that within a time interval of duration t the occurrence of some events is registered by means of an integer-valued process $\{N(0, t)\}$, called *counting process*, which counts the number of events as they occur. Thus for $t > 0$, $N(0, t)$ represents the number of events within the interval $(0, t)$. The occurrence times of the events are considered to be random.

If the flow of events or, equivalently, the counting process has the following properties, then the counting process is called a *homogeneous Poisson process*:

(a)   The number of events occurring in nonoverlapping time intervals
      are mutually independent random variables. Thus for any $t_1 < t_2$
      $< t_3 < t_4$, the variables $N(t_1, t_2)$ and $N(t_3, t_4)$ representing the
      number of events in the intervals (t_1, t_2) and (t_3, t_4), respectively,
      are random and independent.

(b)   The counting process $\{N(0, t); t > 0\}$ has stationary increments;
      i.e., the random variables $N(t_1, t_1 + \tau)$ and $N(t_2, t_2 + \tau)$ are
      identically distributed.

(c)   The probability that more than one event occurs in a short time
      interval Δt is $O(\Delta t)$, where $O(\Delta t)$ tends to 0 faster than Δt.

(d)   If the events are counted in an interval beginning at time $t = 0$,
      then $N(0, 0) = 0$.

Poisson processes can also be defined for all real values of t

$$\{-\infty < t < \infty\}$$

under the assumption that the events registered by the counting process
started a long time ago.

Poisson processes are characterized by a rate (or intensity) parameter,
which is the mean number of events per unit time, i.e., the rate of counts. If
this rate parameter is a constant, we have a homogeneous Poisson process.
However, if it varies with time as the counting process proceeds, then the
counting process is called a *nonhomogeneous Poisson process*. A nonhomogeneous Poisson process with a nonrandom rate parameter possesses
properties (a), (c), and (d). However its increments are nonstationary; i.e.,
random variables $N(t_1, t_1 + \tau)$ and $N(t_2, t_2 + \tau)$ do not have the same
probability distribution. Finally, for a nonhomogeneous Poisson process
with a random rate parameter, only properties (c) and (d) are valid.

We shall now develop the statistics of a Poisson process. Let the
probability of a single event occurring within a short time interval $(t, t + \Delta t)$
be $\lambda(t)\Delta t + O(\Delta t)$, where $\lambda(t)$ is a real (positive) variable. If $\lambda(t) = \lambda_0$, a
constant, i.e., the probability of occurrence of an event depends only upon
the time interval Δt and not on the time instant t, then the underlying process
is a homogeneous Poisson process. If $\lambda(t)$ is time-varying, i.e., the probability of an event depends not only on the interval Δt, but also on the
time instant t, then we have a nonhomogeneous Poisson process. $\lambda(t)$ is
called the rate parameter (or intensity) of the Poisson process. In the following
discussion we shall assume that $\lambda(t)$ is not a random variable.

Let the probability of exactly k counts in the interval $(0, t)$ be given by $P(k, t)$, which is the same as $P(N(0, t) = k)$. Then the following equation governs the counting distribution:

$$P(k, t + \Delta t) = P(k, t)[1 - \lambda(t)\,\Delta t] + P(k - 1, t)\lambda(t)\,\Delta t \qquad (1.2.49)$$

For $\Delta t \to 0$, this may be recast into

$$\frac{dP(k, t)}{dt} = -\lambda(t)[P(k, t) - P(k - 1, t)]$$

with the initial condition $P(k, 0) = 0$. Using the generating function

$$M(z, t) = \sum_{k=0}^{\infty} P(k, t)z^{-k}$$

we have

$$\frac{dM(z, t)}{dt} = -\lambda(t)(1 - z^{-1})M(z, t)$$

This leads to

$$M(z, t) = \exp\left[-(1 - z^{-1})\int_0^t \lambda(\tau)\,d\tau\right] \qquad (1.2.50)$$

and, on inversion, to

$$P(k, t) = \frac{1}{k!}\left(\frac{\partial}{\partial z^{-1}}\right)^k M(z, t)\bigg|_{z=\infty} = \frac{1}{k!}\left[\int_0^t \lambda(\tau)\,d\tau\right]^k \exp\left[-\int_0^t \lambda(\tau)\,d\tau\right] \qquad (1.2.51)$$

For a homogeneous Poisson process this reduces to

$$P(N(0, t) = k) = \frac{1}{k!}(\lambda_0 t)^k\, e^{-\lambda_0 t}$$

It follows from equations (1.2.50) and (1.2.51) that

$$E[N(0, t)] = \int_0^t \lambda(\tau)\,d\tau$$

$$E[\{N(0, t)\}^2] = \left[\int_0^t \lambda(\tau)\,d\tau\right]^2 + \int_0^t \lambda(\tau)\,d\tau \qquad (1.2.52)$$

The mean value of the Poisson process always equals its variance. Thus for a homogeneous Poisson process (mean value = variance = $\lambda_0 t$), λ_0 is seen as giving the mean number of events per unit time or the mean rate of occurrence of events; hence the name "rate parameter."

By an analysis similar to the above it may be easily shown that for a nonhomogeneous Poisson process, the probability distribution of counts over any interval (t_1, t_2) is given by

$$P(N(t_1, t_2) = k) = \frac{1}{k!}\left[\int_{t_1}^{t_2} \lambda(\tau)\, d\tau\right]^k \exp\left[-\int_{t_1}^{t_2} \lambda(\tau)\, d\tau\right] \quad (1.2.53)$$

Autocorrelation of a Poisson Process

Considering nonoverlapping time intervals $t_1 < t_2 < t_3 < t_4$ by property (a) quoted earlier, we have

$$E[N(t_1, t_2)N(t_3, t_4)] = E[N(t_1, t_2)]E[N(t_3, t_4)] = \int_{t_1}^{t_2}\int_{t_3}^{t_4} \lambda(\tau_1)\lambda(\tau_2)\, d\tau_1\, d\tau_2$$

If the intervals under consideration (t_1, t_2) and (t_3, t_4) are overlapping, i.e., $t_1 < t_3 < t_2 < t_4$, then property (a) cannot be directly applied. However it is not too difficult to see that

$$N(t_1, t_2) = N(t_1, t_3) + N(t_3, t_2)$$
$$N(t_3, t_4) = N(t_3, t_2) + N(t_2, t_4)$$

where the intervals (t_1, t_3), (t_3, t_2), and (t_2, t_4) are now nonoverlapping, as such:

$$E[N(t_1, t_2)N(t_3, t_4)] = E[N(t_1, t_3)N(t_3, t_2)] + E[N(t_3, t_2)N(t_2, t_4)]$$
$$+ E[N(t_1, t_3)N(t_2, t_4)] + E[\{N(t_3, t_2)\}^2]$$

Three terms in the above equation consist of products of uncorrelated random variables. After some algebraic manipulation of equation (1.2.52) it may be shown that

$$E[N(t_1, t_2)N(t_3, t_4)] = \int_{t_1}^{t_2}\int_{t_3}^{t_4} \lambda(\tau_1)\lambda(\tau_2)\, d\tau_1\, d\tau_2 + \int_{t_3}^{t_2} \lambda(\tau)\, d\tau \quad (1.2.54)$$

If $t_1 = t_3 = 0, t_4 > t_2$, we have

$$R(t_4, t_2) = E[N(0, t_2)N(0, t_4)] = \left[\int_0^{t_2} \lambda(\tau)\, d\tau\right]\left[1 + \int_0^{t_4} \lambda(\tau)\, d\tau\right]$$

For a homogeneous Poisson process we have

$$R(t_a, t_b) = \lambda_0 t_b + \lambda_0^2 t_a t_b, \qquad t_a > t_b > 0$$

An interesting case arises if the rate parameter of the Poisson process is itself a random variable. Then the probability distributions of equations

(1.2.51) and (1.2.53) and the statistics in equations (1.2.52) and (1.2.54) are all conditional variables, conditioned on the functional

$$\left\{ \int_0^t \lambda(\tau)\, d\tau \right\}$$

For instance, for random $\{\lambda(t)\}$, equation (1.2.52) may be rewritten as

$$E[N(0, t)|m] = m$$

$$E[\{N(0, t)\}^2|m] = m^2 + m$$

where

$$m = \int_0^t \lambda(\tau)\, d\tau$$

To obtain unconditional expected values, we should take moments about the distribution of m. Thus, we have

$$E[g(m)] = \int_0^\infty g(m)p(m)\, dm$$

where $p(m)$ is the probability density function of m; $\{g(m)\}$ could be $E[P(N(0, t) = k)|m]$ or $E[N(0, t)|m]$ or var $[N(0, t)|m]$ or any other related function. To determine unconditional values of the counting autocorrelation, we require the joint probability density function of

$$\int_{t_1}^{t_2} \lambda(\tau)\, d\tau \quad \text{and} \quad \int_{t_3}^{t_4} \lambda(\tau)\, d\tau$$

For further details see Chapter 4.

Poisson Increments and Impulses

Let us denote the occurrence times of events by $t_1, t_2, \ldots$, such that the kth event occurs at time t_k; $\{t_1, t_2, \ldots\}$ are called waiting times of the Poisson process, and the time differences $t_2 - t_1 = \tau_1$, $t_3 - t_2 = \tau_2$, etc., are the interarrival times of the process. Figure 1.2.2a shows the counting process $\{N(0, t)\}$; note the process is stepwise continuous and incremented each time an event occurs. The sequence of δ functions of Figure 1.2.2b are the Poisson impulses of unit height, and they represent the occurrence times (or waiting times). We can express the counting process as

$$N(0, t) = \sum_k U(t - t_k) \tag{1.2.55}$$

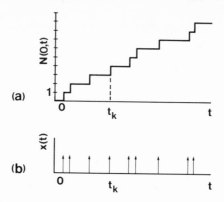

Figure 1.2.2. Poisson process.

where $U(\ )$ is a unit step function. The Poisson impulse process may be written as

$$x(t) = \sum_k \delta(t - t_k) \tag{1.2.56}$$

Defining an increment process $\{dN(t) = N(t, t + dt), \text{ for all } t\}$, it is obvious that

$$\frac{dN(t)}{dt} = x(t), \qquad dN(t) = \sum_k \delta(t - t_k)\,dt \tag{1.2.57}$$

By taking limits, we obtain from equations (1.2.52)–(1.2.54),

$$E[dN(t)] = \lambda(t)\,dt$$

which is the probability that an event will occur in the interval $(t, t + dt)$, and

$$E[dN(t_1)\,dN(t_2)] = \lambda(t_1)\lambda(t_2)\,dt_1\,dt_2 + \lambda(t_1)\,dt_1\,\delta(t_2 - t_1) \tag{1.2.58}$$

It follows that the statistics of the Poisson impulse process are given by

$$E[x(t)] = \lambda(t)$$
$$E[x(t_1)x(t_2)] = \lambda(t_1)\lambda(t_2) + \lambda(t_1)\delta(t_2 - t_1) \tag{1.2.59}$$

For a homogeneous Poisson process, we need to replace $\lambda(t)$ by λ_0.

Extension of the above analysis to counting processes defined over all real values of t, $\{-\infty < t < \infty\}$, is straightforward and leads to identical results.

From equation (1.2.58) since

$$\text{cov}\,[dN(t_1)\,dN(t_2)] = \lambda(t_1)\delta(t_1 - t_2)$$

$\{dN(t)\}$ represents an orthogonal increment process. Another well-known stochastic process $\{\xi(t)\}$ which has orthogonal increments, i.e., one for which $\xi(t_1) - \xi(t_2)$ and $\xi(s_1) - \xi(s_2)$ have zero covariance if the intervals (t_1, t_2) and (s_1, s_2) are nonoverlapping, is the Wiener process or the Brownian motion process. The increments of a Wiener process are normally distributed, with zero mean value and variance proportional to the interval length.

Shot Noise Processes and Campbell's Theorem

Processes which arise as linear operations on Poisson processes are called *filtered Poisson processes*. A classic example of this is the *shot-noise process* in which an electron on arrival at the electrode of a valve (or at the cathode surface of a photodetector) generates a signal, such that the signal is $g(\tau)$ at time τ after the arrival at the electrode. The electrons arrive at random on the electrode surface, and the total signal produced at any time is the sum (or superposition) of the signals generated by each electron and is given by

$$z(t) = \sum_{k=-\infty}^{\infty} g(t - t_k) \tag{1.2.60}$$

where $\{t_k\}$ are the arrival times of the electrons. $\{z(t)\}$ may be considered as the response of a linear system to a Poisson-distributed input sequence $\{x(t)\}$, cf. equation (1.2.56), $\{g(t)\}$ being the impulse response of the system.

We are particularly interested in processes like $\{z(t)\}$, and we shall show later that signals arising in laser Doppler velocimeters can be modeled in this form, although the underlying Poisson processes would be more complicated than those discussed here.

Equation (1.2.60) may be recast into a Steiltjes integral:

$$z(t) = \int_{-\infty}^{\infty} g(t - \tau) \sum_{k=-\infty}^{\infty} \delta(\tau - t_k) \, d\tau$$

$$= \int_{-\infty}^{\infty} g(t - \tau) \, dN(\tau) \tag{1.2.61}$$

If $\{dN(t)\}$ is an increment process arising from a homogeneous Poisson process with rate parameter λ_0, we have, by using equation (1.2.58),

$$E[z(t)] = \lambda_0 \int_{-\infty}^{\infty} g(\tau) \, d\tau \tag{1.2.62}$$

$$E[z(t_1)z(t_2)] = \left[\lambda_0 \int_{-\infty}^{\infty} g(\tau) \, d\tau \right]^2 + \lambda_0 \int_{-\infty}^{\infty} g(\tau)g(t_2 - t_1 + \tau) \, d\tau$$

$$\text{cov}\,[z(t_1)z(t_2)] = \lambda_0 R_g(t_2 - t_1) \tag{1.2.63}$$

where $R_g(t_2 - t_1)$ is the autocorrelation of the function $\{g(t)\}$, with

$$R_g(\tau) = \int_{-\infty}^{\infty} g(u)g(u + \tau)\, du \tag{1.2.64}$$

We see that for a homogeneous Poisson impulse process, $\{z(t)\}$ is a second-order stationary stochastic process.

Equations (1.2.62)–(1.2.64) are an analytic statement of Campbell's theorem (Rice, 1944), where the mean value and covariance of a shot-noise process is expressed in terms of the rate parameter λ_0 and the impulse response $\{g(t)\}$.

If the underlying process is a nonhomogeneous process with a non-random rate parameter $\lambda(t)$, then we have for $\{z(t)\}$

$$
\begin{aligned}
E[z(t)] &= \int_{-\infty}^{\infty} \lambda(\tau)g(t - \tau)\, d\tau \\[2mm]
\mathrm{cov}\,[z(t_1)z(t_2)] &= \int_{-\infty}^{\infty} \lambda(\tau)g(t_1 - \tau)g(t_2 - \tau)\, d\tau
\end{aligned}
\tag{1.2.65}
$$

Spectral Representation of a Stochastic Process

The power spectral density function forms an important concept in the study of stationary stochastic processes. Its practical utility lies in the apparent ease with which it can be estimated from a realization of the process and in its relationship with the other relevant statistics of the process, i.e., its autocorrelation function.

By definition, the spectral density function (or spectrum) $\Phi_x(\omega)$ is the Fourier transform of the autocorrelation $R_x(\tau)$ of a stationary stochastic process $\{x(t)\}$,

$$\Phi_x(\omega) = \int_{-\infty}^{\infty} e^{-j\omega\tau} R_x(\tau)\, d\tau, \qquad -\infty < \omega < \infty \tag{1.2.66}$$

which on inversion leads to

$$R_x(\tau) = \frac{1}{2\pi} \int_{-\infty}^{\infty} e^{j\omega\tau} \Phi_x(\omega)\, d\omega, \qquad -\infty < \tau < \infty \tag{1.2.67}$$

The area under the power spectral density function gives the mean square value or power of the process $\{x(t)\}$, hence its name. (Since we shall be largely concerned with electrical signals, the term "power" should create no ambiguity.)

Since $R_x(\tau) = R_x(-\tau)$, $\Phi_x(\omega)$ is a real-valued function. Also $\Phi_x(\omega) \geq 0$, since $\Phi_x(\omega)\,d\omega$ is the power content of the process in the frequency band $(\omega, \omega + d\omega)$ and the power content is always a positive quantity for any ω.

For any two stationary stochastic processes $\{x(t)\}$ and $\{y(t)\}$ a cross-power spectral density function is defined as

$$\Phi_{xy}(\omega) = \int_{-\infty}^{\infty} R_{xy}(\tau)\,e^{-j\omega\tau}\,d\tau, \qquad -\infty < \omega < \infty \qquad (1.2.68)$$

where $R_{xy}(\tau)$ is the cross correlation between the two processes. $\Phi_{xy}(\omega)$ and $R_{xy}(\tau)$ form a Fourier transform pair:

$$R_{xy}(\tau) = \frac{1}{2\pi}\int_{-\infty}^{\infty} e^{j\omega\tau}\Phi_{xy}(\omega)\,d\omega, \qquad -\infty < \tau < \infty \qquad (1.2.69)$$

Since $R_{xy}(\tau)$ is not necessarily an even function, the cross-spectral density function can be complex-valued, with the real and imaginary parts called the cospectrum and quadrature spectrum, respectively.

An estimate of the power spectral density function can be obtained from a record $\{x(t),\ -T < t < T\}$ of a process by the following:

$$\Phi_x(\omega) = \frac{1}{2T}\left|\int_{-T}^{T} x(t)\,e^{-j\omega t}\,dt\right|^2 \qquad (1.2.70)$$

Then

$$E[\Phi_x(\omega)] = \frac{1}{2T}\int_{-T}^{T}\int_{-T}^{T} R_x(t_1 - t_2)\,e^{-j\omega(t_1 - t_2)}\,dt_1\,dt_2$$

$$= \frac{1}{2T}\int_{-2T}^{2T} (2T - |\tau|)R_x(\tau)\,e^{-j\omega\tau}\,d\tau$$

For a large record we have

$$E[\Phi_x(\omega)] = \lim_{T\to\infty}\left[\int_{-2T}^{2T} R_x(\tau)\,e^{-j\omega\tau}\,d\tau - \frac{1}{2T}\int_{-2T}^{2T} \tau R_x(\tau)\,e^{-j\omega\tau}\,d\tau\right] \qquad (1.2.71)$$

Thus $E[\Phi_x(\omega)] \to \Phi_x(\omega)$ if and only if

$$\int_{-\infty}^{\infty} |\tau R_x(\tau)|\,d\tau < \infty$$

This condition is satisfied by all such processes which do not contain any deterministic components, i.e., processes which have a rational power spectral density function such that $|d\Phi_x(\omega)/d\omega| < \infty$ for all ω. For details of the variance of $\Phi_x(\omega)$, see Blackman and Tukey (1958).

It may be seen that a complete statistical description of a stationary Gaussian process is available if its spectral density function is known. Therefore, in practice, it is sufficient to measure the power spectrum of a process to specify it completely once it is ascertained that the underlying distribution is Gaussian.

Harmonic Analysis

If a time-varying signal $x(t)$ is periodic with period T_0, then a Fourier series such as

$$x(t) = \sum_{k=-\infty}^{\infty} a_k \, e^{j(2\pi kt/T_0)} \tag{1.2.72}$$

gives a decomposition of the signal into discrete frequency components, provided $x(t)$ satisfies the Dirichlet conditions of being single-valued and finite, with a finite number of discontinuities and maxima and minima within the period T_0.

If $x(t)$ is not periodic, but (roughly) decays to zero as $t \to \infty$, i.e., it satisfies the condition of absolute integrability

$$\int_{-\infty}^{\infty} x^2(t) \, dt < \infty$$

then it can be represented by

$$x(t) = \frac{1}{2\pi} \int_{-\infty}^{\infty} e^{j\omega t} A(\omega) \, d\omega, \qquad -\infty < t < \infty \tag{1.2.73}$$

where $A(\omega)$ is the Fourier integral of $x(t)$, and it forms a continuous function in the frequency domain.

A Fourier-type (harmonic) representation for stochastic processes is given by a generalized integral that contains equations (1.2.72) and (1.2.73) as special cases. Thus any time-varying signal (periodic, nonperiodic, or a zero mean, second-order stationary process) can be expressed as

$$x(t) = \frac{1}{2\pi} \int_{-\infty}^{\infty} e^{j\omega t} \, dG(\omega) \tag{1.2.74}$$

where $\{G(\omega)\}$ is uniquely determined by the general form of $x(t)$. If $x(t)$ is a periodic function, then $G(\omega)$ is stepwise continuous:

$$G(\omega) = \sum_{k} a_k U(\omega - 2\pi k/T_0)$$

or

$$dG(\omega) = \sum_k a_k \delta(\omega - 2\pi k/T_0)\, d\omega$$

If $x(t)$ is nonperiodic but is absolutely integrable, then

$$dG(\omega) = A(\omega)\, d\omega, \qquad \text{for all } \omega$$

If, however, $\{x(t)\}$ is a zero mean, stationary process, then $dG(\omega)$ is a random variable and $\{G(\omega)\}$ is an orthogonal increment process such that

$$E[dG(\omega)] = 0, \qquad\qquad \text{for all } \omega$$

$$E[dG(\omega_1)\, dG^*(\omega_2)] = \begin{cases} \Phi_x(\omega_1)\, d\omega_1, & \omega_1 = \omega_2 \\ 0, & \text{otherwise} \end{cases} \qquad (1.2.75)$$

where * denotes complex conjugate. From equations (1.2.74) and (1.2.75) we see that

$$R_x(\tau) = E[x(t)x(t + \tau)]$$

$$= \frac{1}{2\pi} \int_{-\infty}^{\infty} e^{j\omega\tau}\Phi_x(\omega)\, d\omega, \qquad -\infty < \omega < \infty \qquad (1.2.76)$$

This is the celebrated *Wiener–Khintchine theorem* that relates the auto-correlation function of a stationary stochastic process to its spectral density function.

A converse relationship exists for equation (1.2.74), which states that if a process has the spectral representation of equation (1.2.74), with $G(\omega)$ orthogonal, then it may be shown that $\{x(t)\}$ is a stationary process.

Corresponding to the three cases considered here, a spectral distribution function $\{F(\omega)\}$ can be defined that gives a complete description of $\{x(t)\}$ in the frequency domain:

$$R_x(\tau) = \frac{1}{2\pi} \int_{-\infty}^{\infty} e^{j\omega\tau}\, dF(\omega) \qquad (1.2.77)$$

where

(i) for a periodic signal, $R_x(\tau)$ is a circular correlation given by

$$R_x(\tau) = \frac{1}{T_0} \int_{-T_0/2}^{T_0/2} x(t)x(t + \tau)\, dt$$

$$dF(\omega) = \sum_k |a_k|^2 \delta(\omega - 2\pi k/T_0)\, d\omega \qquad (1.2.78)$$

$F(\omega)$ is therefore stepwise continuous.

(ii) For a nonperiodic signal we have

$$R_x(\tau) = \int_{-\infty}^{\infty} x(t)x(t + \tau)\, d\tau, \qquad -\infty < \tau < \infty$$

$$dF(\omega) = |A(\omega)|^2\, d\omega \tag{1.2.79}$$

Here $F(\omega)$ is a continuous function.

(iii) For a stochastic process

$$dF(\omega) = \Phi_x(\omega)\, d\omega$$

For a mixed process, the spectral distribution function would consist of any combination of the three functions described here.

The spectral distribution function $F(\omega)$ has the following properties:

(1) $F(\omega) \geq 0$ for all ω
(2) $F(-\infty) = 0$, $F(\infty) = \sigma_x^2$ [mean square value of $x(t)$]
(3) $F(\omega)$ is a monotonic function in ω
(4) For any $\omega_2 > \omega_1$, $F(\omega_2) - F(\omega_1) \geq 0$ is the power content of $\{x(t)\}$ in the frequency range (ω_2, ω_1)

White Noise

A Gaussian-distributed stationary stochastic process which has a uniform power spectral density function over a wide range of frequencies is called a *white noise process*. Mathematically, $\{x(t)\}$ is a white noise process if its spectral density function is

$$\Phi_x(\omega) = K_0 \qquad \text{for all } \omega \tag{1.2.80}$$

where, K_0 is a constant, and for its autocorrelation function we have $R_x(\tau) = K_0\delta(\tau)$. Physically, such a process is not possible since its power spectral density function is not integrable (which suggests infinite power). Several limiting approximations exist for a white noise process, a convenient one being a Gaussian process which has a correlation function

$$R_x(\tau) = \tfrac{1}{2}K_0\lambda\, e^{-\lambda|\tau|}$$

with λ so large that $R_x(\tau) \to K_0\delta(\tau)$ and $\Phi_x(\omega) \to K_0$.

Convolution, Frequency Response, and Moments

The convolution $z(t)$ between any two signals $\{x(t)\}, -\infty < t < \infty\}$ and $\{y(t), -\infty < t < \infty\}$ is defined as

$$z(t) = \begin{cases} \displaystyle\int_{-\infty}^{\infty} x(t-\tau)y(\tau)\, d\tau \\[2em] \displaystyle\int_{-\infty}^{\infty} x(\tau)y(t-\tau)\, d\tau \end{cases} \tag{1.2.81}$$

Symbolically, the convolution operation is expressed as $z(t) = x(t) * y(t)$. If the conditions of causality are not imposed, then the output $z(t)$ of any linear system with impulse response $h(t)$ for an input signal $x(t)$ is given by

$$z(t) = \int_{-\infty}^{\infty} h(t-\tau)x(\tau)\, d\tau \tag{1.2.82}$$

which on Fourier transformation leads to

$$Z(j\omega) = H(j\omega)X(j\omega)$$

where the definitions of $Z(j\omega)$, $H(j\omega)$, $X(j\omega)$ are obvious. $H(j\omega)$ is called the frequency response of the linear system. If $\{x(t)\}$ is a stationary stochastic process, then a similar relationship holds between the spectral density functions,

$$\Phi_z(\omega) = |H(j\omega)|^2 \Phi_x(\omega) \tag{1.2.83}$$

Also,

$$z(t) = \int_{-\infty}^{\infty} e^{j\omega t} H(j\omega)\, dG(\omega)$$

where $x(t)$ is as defined in equation (1.2.78).

In general, for any $x(t)$ and $y(t)$ which are absolutely integrable, we have from equation (1.2.81)

$$\int_{-\infty}^{\infty} z(t)\, dt = \int_{-\infty}^{\infty} x(t)\, dt \int_{-\infty}^{\infty} y(t)\, dt$$

$$Z(0) = X(0)Y(0)$$

where $Y(j\omega)$ is the Fourier transform of $y(t)$. Further, the following set of relationships may be easily verified:

$$\mu_z = \frac{\int_{-\infty}^{\infty} t z(t)\, dt}{\int_{-\infty}^{\infty} z(t)\, dt} = \text{normalized mean value}$$

$$\sigma_z^2 = \frac{\int_{-\infty}^{\infty} t^2 z(t)\, dt}{\int_{-\infty}^{\infty} z(t)\, dt} - \mu_z^2 = \text{normalized variance}$$

Then

$$\mu_z = \mu_x + \mu_y$$

and

$$\sigma_z^2 = \sigma_x^2 + \sigma_y^2 \qquad (1.2.84)$$

Furthermore, for any integrable set of functions, if

$$z(t) = x_1(t) * x_2(t) * \cdots * x_n(t)$$

then for any n

$$\mu_z = \sum_{k=1}^{n} \mu_{x_k}$$

$$\sigma_z^2 = \sum_{k=1}^{n} \sigma_{x_k}^2 \qquad (1.2.85)$$

and obviously

$$Z(j\omega) = \prod_{k=1}^{n} X_k(j\omega)$$

For nonnegative functions $\{x_k(t) \geq 0$, for all $k, t\}$ as $n \to \infty$, $z(t)$ tends to a normal curve with mean μ_z and variance σ_z^2:

$$z(t) \to \frac{Z(0)}{(2\pi\sigma_z^2)^{1/2}} \exp\left[-\frac{(t - \mu_z)^2}{2\sigma_z^2} \right] \qquad (1.2.86)$$

Equation (1.2.86) is a statement of the *central limit theorem.*

1.3 Statistical Parameters in Turbulence

In this section we will outline some of the most important flow parameters and turbulence characteristics that will be encountered by the experimentalist engaged in laser anemometry. For detailed treatises on statistical fluid dynamics the reader is referred to the texts by Hinze (1959),

Townsend (1956), Monin and Yaglòm (1971), and Tennekes and Lumley (1972). Since all of the flow-measuring techniques to be described later in the book rely on the assumption that small seeding particles present in the flow will faithfully follow the fluid motions, the question of particle trackability will also be considered. Another question of interest, which we will just briefly touch upon, is the effect of refractive index changes on the propagation of a laser beam through a turbulent fluid.

Equations of Motion

The starting point for most fluid dynamic calculations is the Navier–Stokes equation, which in Cartesian tensor notation (Leslie, 1973) is

$$\frac{\partial U_i}{\partial t} + \frac{\partial U_i}{\partial x_j} U_j = -\frac{1}{\rho_0} \frac{\partial P_0}{\partial x_i} + \frac{\mu_0}{\rho_0} \frac{\partial^2 U_i}{\partial x_j \partial x_j} + g_i \qquad (1.3.1)$$

where U_i ($i = 1, 2, 3$) are the velocity components in the three coordinate directions, ρ_0 is the fluid density, μ_0 the fluid viscosity, and P_0 the normal pressure. It has been assumed in writing the above equation that the only external forces acting on the fluid elements are due to the gravitational field g_i, although of course g_i can easily be replaced by a more general expression if there are other external applied forces. The Navier–Stokes equation is only valid for Newtonian fluids, e.g., water and air, and additional terms are required to account for the non-Newtonian characteristics of fluids such as polymer solutions and fiber suspensions (Brodkey, 1967; McComb, 1973).

Solutions to equation (1.3.1) can be obtained most easily when the fluid can be regarded as incompressible, in which case the continuity condition is

$$\frac{\partial U_i}{\partial x_i} = 0 \qquad (1.3.2)$$

On combining equations (1.3.1) and (1.3.2) we have

$$\frac{\partial U_i}{\partial t} + \frac{\partial}{\partial x_j}(U_i U_j) = -\frac{1}{\rho_0} \frac{\partial P_0}{\partial x_i} + \frac{\mu_0}{\rho_0} \frac{\partial^2 U_i}{\partial x_j \partial x_j} + g_i \qquad (1.3.3)$$

The essential characteristics of turbulent flows were first recognized by Osborne Reynolds. He noted that flows only became turbulent in nature when the dimensionless parameter $R_e = U_r L_r \rho_0/\mu_0$, known as the *Reynolds number*, exceeded some critical value, and that it was the magnitude of this parameter which determined the main features of the flow patterns. The exact value of the critical Reynolds number depends on many factors, including the choice of the reference length L_r and the reference velocity U_r. Typically, for flow in a tube or pipe, if the diameter is taken as the reference length and the mean velocity is taken for U_r, then the critical Reynolds number is about 2000. Enormous ranges of Reynolds numbers are encountered in nature, e.g., in oceanography one is generally dealing with values of many millions while for flow of air in the human lung the Reynolds numbers in the bifurcations close to the alveoli are of the order unity (Olson *et al.*, 1972).

For a turbulent flow it is convenient to separate the instantaneous velocity $U_i(t)$ at a point into the sum of a constant ensemble-averaged velocity $E[U_i]$ together with a fluctuating component $u_i(t)$, i.e.,

$$U_i = E[U_i] + u_i \tag{1.3.4}$$

and similarly for the pressure $P_0(t)$, i.e.,

$$P_0 = E[P_0] + p_0 \tag{1.3.5}$$

The functional dependence on time has been dropped for notational simplicity. For practical purposes it is usually necessary to assume the flow to be statistically stationary whereupon ensemble averages can be replaced by time averages. This approach also can frequently be applied in nonstationary conditions by assuming the flow to be quasistationary over sufficiently short periods of time. Throughout this book it will be assumed that turbulent flows are statistically stationary.

Introducing the expressions for U_i and P_0 from equations (1.3.4) and (1.3.5) into equation (1.3.3) and averaging each term yields (for steady flows)

$$\frac{\partial}{\partial x_j} E[U_i] E[U_j] + \frac{\partial}{\partial x_j} E[u_i u_j] = -\frac{1}{\rho_0} \frac{\partial E[P_0]}{\partial x_i} + \frac{\mu_0}{\rho_0} \frac{\partial^2 E[U_i]}{\partial x_j \partial x_j} + g_i \tag{1.3.6}$$

which is frequently referred to as *Reynolds' equation*. Note that in order to determine the statistically averaged flow field from equation (1.3.6) one must have a knowledge of $E[u_i u_j]$. Determination of the magnitude of this term over various regions of a flow field plays a major role in many experimental investigations. Since $\rho_0 E[u_i u_j]$ can be interpreted as an additional stress (i.e., additional to the viscous stress) produced by the turbulence, it is termed the *Reynolds stress*. As an example, for pipe flow in the x_1 direction with u_2 measured vertically upward, the $E[u_1 u_2]$ component of the Reynolds stress will be zero in the center of the pipe but negative in the region just above the lower wall. Techniques for measuring Reynolds stresses will be discussed in Section 3.2.

The Reynolds stress, although important, does not give any information about the spatial extent of turbulent eddies in the flow. Spatial variations are most readily described in terms of the Eulerian velocity correlation functions. Consider two points A and B located at different spatial positions within the flow and let $U_i(t)$ and $U'_j(t)$ be the components of the instantaneous velocity at the two points. If $\mathbf{a}$ and $\mathbf{b}$ are unit vectors drawn at A and B, respectively, defining two directions, then the velocities along these two directions will be $U_i a_i$ and $U'_j b_j$. The correlation between the velocities in these two directions is defined as

$$E[U_i a_i U'_j b_j]$$

Expressing the instantaneous velocities as the sum of mean and fluctuating parts, we obtain

$$U_i a_i = (E[U_i] + u_i)a_i = E[U_i]a_i + u_i a_i \tag{1.3.7}$$

$$U'_j b_j = (E[U'_j] + u'_j)b_j = E[U'_j]b_j + u'_j b_j \tag{1.3.8}$$

The correlation can be written

$$E[U_i a_i U'_j b_j] = E[E[U_i]a_i E[U'_j]b_j] + E[u_i a_i u'_j b_j] \tag{1.3.9}$$

since the other two products average to zero. The first term on the rhs of equation (1.3.9) can be evaluated without knowledge of the velocity fluctuations, i.e., only the last term contains statistical information on the turbulence structure. For this reason it is the covariance between the two velocity components, i.e., the last term in equation (1.3.9), which is normally measured. For theoretical analysis it is convenient to work in terms of the covariance tensor $R_{ij} = E[u_i u'_j]$:

$$E[u_i a_i u'_j b_j] = R_{ij} a_i b_j \tag{1.3.10}$$

Although R_{ij} determines the most important characteristics of the turbulence, a complete set of higher-order covariances is necessary in order to specify fully the statistics of the flow field.

Measurement of the complete covariance tensor would involve an unrealistic number of observations, and in practical situations observations are generally restricted to velocity components and separations in one or two directions. Measured covariances are most frequently displayed in normalized form. The normalized value of the covariance between velocity fluctuations in a particular direction (the a_i direction) is

$$\frac{E[u_i a_i u'_j a_j]}{\{E[u_i a_i]^2 \cdot E[u'_j a_j]^2\}^{1/2}}$$

and is termed the correlation coefficient [see equation (1.2.14)]. Clearly, as the two points approach zero, the correlation coefficient approaches unity. Correlation coefficients are most frequently recorded with the velocity components and separations either in line with or perpendicular to the mean flow direction. If the mean flow is in the positive x_1 direction and the two points of measurement lie a distance r apart along the x_1 axis, with the point A upstream of B, then the function

$$f(r) = \frac{E[u_1 u'_1]}{\{E[u_1^2] \cdot E[u_1'^2]\}^{1/2}} \tag{1.3.11}$$

is known as the *Eulerian longitudinal correlation coefficient*. If the velocity components transverse to the flow are measured at the same positions, then one obtains the *Eulerian transverse correlation coefficients*:

$$g_2(r) = \frac{E[u_2 u'_2]}{\{E[u_2^2] \cdot E[u_2'^2]\}^{1/2}}$$

$$g_3(r) = \frac{E[u_3 u'_3]}{\{E[u_3^2] \cdot E[u_3'^2]\}^{1/2}} \tag{1.3.12}$$

If one attempts to measure these longitudinal and transverse correlation coefficients directly by using two conventional measuring probes such as hot wires, then a problem immediately presents itself. Since one of the probes is located directly downstream from the other, the wake from the upstream probe interferes with its reading. An important advantage of optical anemometers is that interference problems of this type do not arise. Despite this, however, two separate systems are required if the correlation coefficients are to be measured directly. In addition, mean values of the velocity product are required at a large number of separations. Both of these complications can be avoided if the experimenter is prepared to make use of an approximation known as *Taylor's hypothesis*, which makes the assumption that the eddy structure is frozen over the distance through which correlations are to be measured. This implies that

$$u_i(x_1 - E[U_1]t, x_2, x_3, 0) = u_i(x_1, x_2, x_3, t) \tag{1.3.13}$$

A temporal record of one of the velocity components at a single point can then be considered as a spatial record in the x_1 direction, with the appropriate scaling indicated by equation (1.3.13). The autocorrelation functions computed from records at a single point are then equivalent to spatial correlation functions, where the scaling from time τ to r is given by

$$|r| = E[U_1]|\tau| \qquad (1.3.14)$$

It is important to remember that Taylor's hypothesis is only an approximation and that considerable inaccuracies can result if it is applied when turbulence levels are high.

The frequently used integral or macro scales of turbulence are defined in terms of the correlation coefficients as follows:

Eulerian Longitudinal Integral Scale:

$$\Lambda_f = \int_0^\infty f(r)\, dr \qquad (1.3.15)$$

Eulerian Transverse Integral Scales:

$$\Lambda_2 = \int_0^\infty g_2(r)\, dr$$

$$\Lambda_3 = \int_0^\infty g_3(r)\, dr \qquad (1.3.16)$$

The corresponding micro or dissipation scales λ_f, λ_2, and λ_3 are computed from the second derivatives of the correlation functions at zero displacement as follows:

Eulerian Longitudinal Micro Scale:

$$\frac{1}{\lambda_f^2} = -\frac{1}{2}\left(\frac{\partial^2 f}{\partial r^2}\right)_{r=0} \qquad (1.3.17)$$

Eulerian Transverse Micro Scales:

$$\frac{1}{\lambda_2^2} = -\frac{1}{2}\left(\frac{\partial^2 g_2}{\partial r^2}\right)_{r=0}$$

$$\frac{1}{\lambda_3^2} = -\frac{1}{2}\left(\frac{\partial^2 g_3}{\partial r^2}\right)_{r=0} \qquad (1.3.18)$$

These length scales and the so-called time scales of turbulence are related by Taylor's hypothesis: a simple scaling as indicated by equation (1.3.14) is used, e.g., $\Lambda_f = E[U_1] \cdot \Lambda_t$, where Λ_t is the Eulerian longitudinal integral time scale and $\lambda_f = E[U_1]\mathcal{T}$ ($\mathcal{T}$ is the micro time scale).

For many applications it is more convenient to work in terms of frequency and wave number spectra rather than correlations. If the two points A and B are separated by distances r_1, r_2, and r_3 in the three coordinate directions, i.e., $r^2 = r_1^2 + r_2^2 + r_3^2$, then the three-dimensional energy spectrum tensor is defined by the Fourier transform relationship

$$E_{ij} = \int\!\!\!\int\!\!\!\int_{-\infty}^{\infty} R_{ij} \exp\left[-j(k_1 r_1 + k_2 r_2 + k_3 r_3)\right] dr_1\, dr_2\, dr_3 \qquad (1.3.19)$$

k_1, k_2, and k_3 being the wave numbers in the three coordinate directions. The inverse transformation is

$$R_{ij} = \frac{1}{8\pi^3} \int\!\!\!\int\!\!\!\int_{-\infty}^{\infty} E_{ij} \exp\left[j(k_1 r_1 + k_2 r_2 + k_3 r_3)\right] dk_1\, dk_2\, dk_3 \qquad (1.3.20)$$

Usually it is one-dimensional spectra that are measured, these being simply the one-dimensional *Fourier transforms* of their correlation counterparts. As an example, the normalized longitudinal spectrum function is the Fourier transform of the longitudinal correlation coefficient, i.e.,

$$\int_{-\infty}^{\infty} f(r)\, e^{-jk_1 r}\, dr$$

Due to the extremely complex nature of turbulent flows, many theoretical derivations confine themselves to a simplified situation in which the turbulence structure is assumed homogeneous, i.e., invariant to changes in the origin of coordinates, and isotropic, i.e., invariant to rotations of the coordinate system. This enormously simplifies analysis since now the correlations in the various directions must be interrelated in order to maintain symmetry. For homogeneous isotropic turbulence the longitudinal and transverse correlation coefficients are related by the expression

$$g(r) = f(r) + \frac{r}{2} \frac{\partial f(r)}{\partial r} \qquad (1.3.21)$$

and the covariance tensor is given by

$$R_{ij} = \sigma_u^2 \left(\frac{f - g}{r^2} r_i r_j + g\delta_{ij} \right) \qquad (1.3.22)$$

σ_u being the rms value of the velocity fluctuation in any chosen direction.

From equations (1.3.21) and (1.3.22) it is seen that if Taylor's hypothesis is applied, then the complete covariance tensor can be determined from a single record of the downstream velocity component. Equation (1.3.21) also implies that

$$\Lambda_2 = \Lambda_3 = \tfrac{1}{2}\Lambda_f \qquad (1.3.23)$$

Eulerian and Lagrangian Statistics

In laser anemometry the signals are produced by the motion of small particles suspended in the fluid. Hence, the Lagrangian statistics of the turbulence become important in understanding the various systems. *Lagrangian statistics* are the statistics determined by tracking the motions of individual marker particles present in the flow. The statistics of flow records observed at fixed points in space are called the *Eulerian statistics*. For the moment we will leave the question of particle trackability and assume that the fluid motions are faithfully followed.

The essential characteristics of single-particle diffusion can be inferred directly from the Lagrangian autocorrelation functions. Suppose that the flow field is homogeneous and in time T, particles, initially at the origin of coordinates, traverse a distance x_p in the mean flow direction. Then

$$x_p(T) = \int_0^T U_1(t)\, dt \qquad (1.3.24)$$

and equation (1.2.39) can be applied directly to compute the ensemble-averaged variance of the particle displacements, i.e.,

$$E[x_p - E[x_p]]^2 = 2\sigma_u^2 T \int_0^T \left(1 - \frac{\tau}{T}\right)\rho_L(\tau)\, d\tau \qquad (1.3.25)$$

where $\rho_L(\tau)$ is the Lagrangian autocorrelation function for the downstream velocity component. Similar expressions can be written down for the diffusion transverse to the mean flow direction. With the Lagrangian integral time scale defined as

$$\Lambda = \int_0^\infty \rho_L(\tau)\, d\tau \qquad (1.3.26)$$

it is seen that when $T \ll \Lambda$, then equation (1.3.25) reduces to

$$E[x_p - E[x_p]]^2 = \sigma_u^2 T^2 \qquad (1.3.27)$$

and when $T \gg \Lambda$, then

$$E[x_p - E[x_p]]^2 = 2\sigma_u^2 T \int_0^\infty \rho_L(\tau)\, d\tau$$

$$= 2\sigma_u^2 T \Lambda \qquad (1.3.28)$$

The product $\sigma_u^2 \Lambda$ is often referred to as the diffusion coefficient.

The above expressions [equations (1.3.25), (1.3.27), and (1.3.28)] can be used directly to compute the essential characteristics of particle diffusion, provided that the Lagrangian statistics are known. However, it is the Eulerian statistics of the fluid turbulence which are generally known, since these are most readily measurable, and this raises the question of how the Eulerian and Lagrangian velocity fluctuations are related. Suppose that the Eulerian vector velocity at position $\mathbf{x}$ and time t is $\mathbf{U}(\mathbf{x}, t)$. Let the vector position of a particle initially at position $\mathbf{a}$ be $\mathbf{X}(\mathbf{a}, t)$ after time t. This is related to the Eulerian turbulence field by the expression

$$\mathbf{X}(\mathbf{a}, t) = \mathbf{a} + \int_0^t \mathbf{U}(\mathbf{X}(\mathbf{a}, \tau), \tau)\, d\tau \qquad (1.3.29)$$

Fairly obviously, it is extremely difficult to apply equation (1.3.29) to compute the statistics of $\mathbf{X}$ because $\mathbf{X}$ also occurs in the rhs of the expression. Results having any practical application have been obtained only by introducing various simplifying assumptions and approximations.

One approach used in relating Eulerian and Lagrangian statistics is to introduce the space–time correlation function. Consider the case of homogeneous turbulence where the reference axes are chosen such that the mean velocity is zero. The Eulerian space–time correlation function for the ith component of velocity is

$$R_i(\mathbf{r}, \tau) = E[u_i(\mathbf{r}_0, \tau_0) \cdot u_i(\mathbf{r}_0 + \mathbf{r}, \tau_0 + \tau)] \qquad (1.3.30)$$

where $\mathbf{r}$ is the spatial separation between the points and τ the correlation lag. It can then be reasoned (Saffman, 1963; Philip, 1967) that if the magnitude $|\mathbf{r}|$ of the displacement is large compared to the Lagrangian spatial scales, then the space–time correlation function is related to the Lagrangian autocorrelation $\rho_i(\tau)$ for the ith component of velocity by the approximate expression [if the mean flow velocity is in the x_1 direction, then $\rho_1(\tau) = \rho_L(\tau)$]

$$\sigma_u^2 \rho_i(t) = \int_{\text{all } \mathbf{r}} R_i(\mathbf{r}, t) p(\mathbf{r}; t)\, d\mathbf{r} \qquad (1.3.31)$$

Here $p(\mathbf{r}; t)$ is the probability density for a displacement $\mathbf{r}$ in time t, which is generally assumed to be Gaussian. As an example, if the turbulence is isotropic, then

$$p(\mathbf{r}; t) = (2\pi E[x_p^2])^{-3/2} \exp\left(-\frac{r^2}{2E[x_p^2]}\right) \quad (1.3.32)$$

where $r = |\mathbf{r}|$ is the radial distance traversed by the particle. With the space–time correlation function known, equations (1.3.25), (1.3.31), and (1.3.32) provide an integral relationship from which the Lagrangian autocorrelation function can be computed. Philip (1967) and Saffman (1963) have solved this integral equation numerically for specific forms of the space–time correlation function.

For many purposes a simple empirical relationship between the Eulerian correlation coefficient and the corresponding Lagrangian auto-covariance function is all that is required. A frequently used expression relating $\rho_L(t)$ to the Eulerian autocovariance $\rho_E(t)$ of the downstream component of velocity was introduced by Hay and Pasquill (1957) and Engelund (1968):

$$\rho_L\left(\frac{E[U_1]t}{\alpha_l \sigma_u}\right) = \rho_E(t) \quad (1.3.33)$$

α_l being a constant for the particular type of flow under consideration. $\rho_E(\tau)$ is related to the longitudinal correlation coefficient through Taylor's hypothesis, i.e., $\rho_E(\tau) = f(E[U_1]\tau)$. Equation (1.3.33) implies that the Lagrangian and Eulerian covariance functions have the same over-all shape but different time scales. Typically the Lagrangian time scales are an order of magnitude longer than the corresponding Eulerian scales. For homogeneous isotropic turbulence it can be shown that α_l is approximately 2.25 (Engelund, 1968; Kofoed-Hansen and Wandel, 1967). Equation (1.3.33) gives a direct indication, in a laser anemometry system, of whether or not diffusion effects across the measuring region will be significant. For example, if the rms turbulence level is 5% of the mean velocity and the Eulerian integral time scale is 0.001 sec for a mean flow speed of 10 msec^{-1}, then applying equation (1.3.33) together with Taylor's hypothesis shows that the Lagrangian integral time scale is $\Lambda \approx 8.9$ cm, so the measurement region must be very much less than 8.9 cm if diffusion effects are to be negligible.

Motion of Particles in a Fluid

So far only the motion of hypothetical marker particles has been considered. No account has been taken of any relative motion between the particle and fluid. We will now investigate the magnitude of this relative motion as a function of particle size and density in order that the reader will be in a position to assess the suitability of any particular natural or artificial seeding condition for his own application. There are a number of effects which can be distinguished and conveniently treated separately, i.e., inertial effect, gravity, Magnus effect, shear flow lifting force, spatial averaging of turbulence, Brownian motion. In order to evaluate these it will be assumed that the particles are rigid and spherical and that they move in a Newtonian incompressible fluid. More general expressions can be written for the motion of particles of arbitrary shape (Hinze, 1972), but these cannot readily be evaluated in any quantitative manner. Since the inertial effect generally predominates, it will be considered in the greatest detail.

Inertial Effects

If a particle has a density different from that of the surrounding fluid, then, because of inertia, the particle velocity will not respond instantaneously to the velocity changes in the surrounding fluid, and the result will be a damping of the high-frequency fluctuations. The most important situation to consider here occurs when the particle density is much greater than that of the surrounding fluid, as is usually the case in air flows. When the density ratio is closely matched, then particle trackability is not usually a problem. Particle sizes are generally so small that it is safe to assume that drag forces are given by Stokes' resistance law (Batchelor, 1970). For example, if a 1-μm particle is suspended in an airstream at room temperature and pressure, then for a relative velocity of 1 msec^{-1} the Reynolds number will be approximately 0.064. Stokes' resistance law is, strictly speaking, only valid when Reynolds numbers are of the order unity or less, although it still gives reasonable accuracy at $R_e = 5$. At higher Reynolds numbers the true drag is greater than that predicted by Stokes' law, so that particles will respond to changes in flow velocity better than the theory indicates. In the Stokes' flow regime the drag force D_f is proportional to the difference between the fluid velocity U and the particle velocity V in any given direction, i.e.,

$$D_f = 3\pi\mu_0 d_p(U - V) \qquad (1.3.34)$$

where d_p is the particle diameter. The equation of motion for the particle can then be written as (Hinze, 1972)

$$\frac{\pi}{6}d_p^3\rho_p\frac{dV}{dt} + \frac{\pi}{12}d_p^3\rho_0\left(\frac{dV}{dt} - \frac{dU}{dt}\right) = 3\pi\mu_0 d_p(U - V) + \frac{\pi}{6}d_p^3\rho_0\frac{dU}{dt} \qquad (1.3.35)$$

where ρ_p is the density of the particle. In the derivation of equation (1.3.35) the following assumptions have been made:

(1) The particle is spherical and small in size compared with the smallest wavelength of the fluid motion.
(2) The pathlines of the particle and the fluid coincide, i.e., no over-shooting takes place.
(3) The flow is not perturbed by the presence of the particle.

Also, the so-called Basset term, which takes account of deviations from the steady state condition, has been disregarded. The four different terms in equation (1.3.35) can be interpreted as follows:

Term (1) Force required to accelerate the particle
Term (2) Force required to accelerate the added mass (Rouse, 1959)
Term (3) Stokes' drag force
Term (4) Force due to the pressure gradient caused by the fluid acceleration

For the purpose of analyzing equation (1.3.35) it is convenient to rewrite it in the following form:

$$\frac{dV}{dt} + K_v V = K_v U + \frac{3\rho_0}{2\rho_p + \rho_0} \frac{dU}{dt} \qquad (1.3.36)$$

where

$$K_v = \frac{36\mu_0}{(2\rho_p + \rho_0)d_p^2} \qquad (1.3.37)$$

Consider ρ_p to be large compared with ρ_0; then the last term in equation (1.3.36) can be neglected [this point is considered in greater detail by Karchmer (1972)], leaving

$$\frac{dV}{dt} + K_v V = K_v U \qquad (1.3.38)$$

Solutions to equation (1.3.38) can easily be obtained for specific boundary conditions, e.g., Jonsson (1974) has considered a particle starting from rest in a constant velocity flow field, a particle in a flow having constant acceleration, and a particle in an oscillating flow. We will assume the flow velocity to be varying sinusoidally since the results for this case can be extended most easily to turbulent flows.

Let the fluid velocity be

$$U(t) = e^{j\omega_m t} \qquad (1.3.39)$$

and the corresponding particle velocity

$$V(t) = a_m e^{j\omega_m t} \qquad (1.3.40)$$

where a_m is the complex amplitude of the particle oscillation. Substitution into equation (1.3.38) gives

$$j\omega_m a_m e^{j\omega_m t} + K_v a_m e^{j\omega_m t} = K_v e^{j\omega_m t} \qquad (1.3.41)$$

Thus we have

$$a_m = \frac{K_v}{j\omega_m + K_v} = \frac{K_v^2 - K_v j\omega_m}{\omega_m^2 + K^2} \qquad (1.3.42)$$

and the required real amplitude is

$$|a_m| = (a_m a_m^*)^{1/2} = \frac{K_v}{(K_v^2 + \omega_m^2)^{1/2}} \qquad (1.3.43)$$

In a turbulent flow, equation (1.3.43) can be regarded as a transfer function relating the power spectrum $\Phi_U(\omega)$ of the fluid flow to the power spectrum $\Phi_v(\omega)$ of the particle velocity, i.e.,

$$\Phi_v(\omega) = |a_m|^2 \Phi_U(\omega) \qquad (1.3.44)$$

although it must be emphasized that this is only an approximate relationship. Note that the damping effect of the transfer function increases rapidly with frequency.

Gravity

If the particles have a density different from that of the surrounding fluid, then gravity forces will cause them to either settle downwards or drift vertically upwards, depending on whether they are heavier or lighter than the surrounding fluid. The magnitude V_v of this vertical velocity can be estimated by equating the gravitational force $\frac{1}{6}\pi d_p^3(\rho_p - \rho_0)g$ to the Stokes' drag force $3\pi d_p \mu_0 V_v$. Thus we have

$$V_v = \frac{d_p^2 g}{18\mu_0}(\rho_p - \rho_0) \qquad (1.3.45)$$

where a positive V_v indicates a downwards motion.

Magnus Effect

If a spherical particle moves relative to the surrounding fluid and also has a rotation, then a force will be exerted on the particle in a direction perpendicular to the relative velocity and the axis of rotation. This is generally referred to as the *Magnus effect* (Batchelor, 1970). Although the phenomenon is complex in nature, an order-of-magnitude estimate of the force can be obtained by considering two-dimensional potential flow around a cylinder of diameter d_p. The pressure force in the vertical direction integrated around the circumference is (Batchelor, 1970) $\frac{1}{2}\rho_0(V - U)\pi d_p^2\Omega_p$. This is the force per unit length of cylinder. Since the force F_m on a sphere of diameter d_p will be of the same order of magnitude as the force on a cylinder of length $\frac{1}{2}d_p$, we can write to a first approximation,

$$F_m = \tfrac{1}{4}\pi\rho_0(V - U)d_p^3\Omega_p \tag{1.3.46}$$

In the above expressions Ω_p is the angular velocity of rotation. The direction of the force on the particle can easily be ascertained by remembering that an undercut tennis ball tends to rise, although it must be remembered that the two phenomena do not have identical fluid dynamic interpretations due to their vastly different scales.

In the majority of laser anemometry situations the Magnus effect will be extremely small.

Shear Flow Lifting Force

Another effect that will generally be small, but that could become significant in certain extreme situations is caused by the fact that particles suspended in a shear flow experience a lifting force caused by the velocity gradient. This problem has been considered in detail by Saffman (1965). For a two-dimensional flow field with uniform velocity gradient dU/dy Saffmann estimated the lifting force as

$$F_l = 20(U - V)d_p^2\left(\mu_0\rho_0\frac{dU}{dy}\right)^{1/2} \tag{1.3.47}$$

where $(U - V)$ is the relative velocity of the particle and the surrounding fluid. In deriving equation (1.3.47) it has been assumed that the Reynolds numbers are small compared with unity.

The lifting effect can be significant in the region immediately adjacent to a boundary, where velocity gradients are generally high.

Spatial Averaging of Turbulence

If a particle of diameter d_p is carried by a turbulent flow, then, even if the particle and fluid densities are the same, the particle will not respond fully to velocity fluctuations caused by eddies of size less than d_p. Thus, there is a spatial filtering effect which causes the velocity variance of the particle to be less than the corresponding velocity variance of the surrounding fluid. There will also be a corresponding increase in the Lagrangian integral time scale. In laser anemometry it is important to ensure that there is negligible turbulent energy at wave numbers less than d_p.

Brownian Motion

When a small particle is suspended in a fluid, the molecular bombardments cause high-frequency random movements which result in the particle diffusing through the fluid. This so-called *Brownian motion* can be considered as superimposed on top of the movements caused by the macroscopic turbulent fluctuations. The Brownian motion of particles in a fluid at rest can be determined from the classical analysis due to Einstein (Kittel, 1958), under the assumption that the resistance to motion is given by Stokes' law. The mean square displacement in, say, the x direction is

$$E[x_p^2] = \frac{2k_b T_f t}{3\pi d_p \mu_0} \tag{1.3.48}$$

where T_f is the absolute temperature of the fluid in °K, k_b is Boltzmann's constant (1.4×10^{-23} J deg^{-1}), and t is the time over which the particle has diffused. Note that the mean square displacement is inversely proportional to both particle diameter and fluid viscosity. Hence, the effect tends to be greatest for small particles in gas flows.

Propagation of a Laser Beam Through a Turbulent Medium

In the analysis of the various optical systems to be described later in the book it will be assumed that the laser beams propagate through the fluid medium without distortion, the implication being that the refractive index of the fluid is constant over the region under consideration. However, in certain practical situations the effects of refractive index variations can be very significant, particularly if the propagation distances are large. Refractive index changes arise principally from temperature variations in the fluid or from varying concentrations of solvents, such as salt, in the case of liquids. In high-speed gas flows, density, and hence refractive index, gradients are also produced by the dynamic pressure fluctuations. In liquid flows this cause can be neglected. When the flow is turbulent the two main effects of refractive index changes are the following:

(i) The beam undergoes random changes in the direction of propagation, and hence it cannot be focused down onto a stationary point in the flow region.

(ii) Random phase changes occur across the wavefronts of the beam, which causes loss of spatial coherence. Since laser beams generally have very small diameters, the loss of spatial coherence tends to be of secondary importance.

The whole subject of light propagation through a turbulent medium in which there are refractive index variations is one of considerable complexity, but has been extensively covered in the literature because of its importance in optical communications. For quantitative analyses the reader is referred to the publications by Tatarski (1967) and Jonsson (1974). Typically, for a laser beam passing through a 0.5-m water channel with temperature fluctuations in the range 20–21 °C, one might expect total rms beam deflections of the order 0.1 mm according to Jonsson's analysis.

1.4. Basic Optical Components

In setting up a practical laser system for flow measurement purposes it is clear that a range of optical components will be required, these being chosen to fit the specific requirements of the experimental or industrial situation. For example, in a laser Doppler system there are a large number of ways in which the laser beam can be split, the various types of beam splitters having their individual merits. In this section we will describe some of the most important phenomena associated with coherent radiation and the optical components which are most frequently used in laser anemometry.

Analysis of Lens Systems

The majority of the phenomena associated with the passage of light through an optical system can be described by using the relationships of *Fourier transform optics*, which derive from the Fresnel and Fraunhofer diffraction theories. For a complete analysis of these theories the reader is referred to the texts of Born and Wolf (1959), Papoulis (1968), and Goodman (1968). Fraunhofer diffraction can be regarded as an approximation to

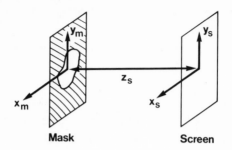

Figure 1.4.1. Axes used in diffraction theory.

Fresnel diffraction, applicable in theory only under certain limiting conditions, but giving reasonably good approximations in many practical situations. The Fresnel theory is itself an approximate method based on the concept that light propagation is a scalar phenomenon.

Figure 1.4.1 indicates an aperture S in an infinite opaque mask which is assumed to be illuminated with a plane monochromatic light field $\mathscr{E}(x_m, y_m)$, x_m and y_m being coordinates of points on the mask. If the diffracted light is observed on a screen placed parallel to the mask a distance z_s away, then the field amplitude $\mathscr{E}(x_s, y_s)$ at coordinates x_s and y_s on the screen is given by the Fresnel theory as (Goodman, 1968)

$$\mathscr{E}(x_s, y_s) = \frac{\exp(jkz_s)}{j\lambda z_s} \exp\left[\frac{jk}{2z_s}(x_s^2 + y_s^2)\right]$$

$$\times \int\limits_{-\infty}^{\infty}\!\!\int \left\{\mathscr{E}(x_m, y_m)\exp\left[\frac{jk}{2z_s}(x_m^2 + y_m^2)\right]\right\}$$

$$\times \exp\left[-\frac{2\pi j}{\lambda z_s}(x_m x_s + y_m y_s)\right] dx_m\, dy_m \qquad (1.4.1)$$

In the above relationship λ is the wavelength of the incident light and k the wave number, i.e., $k = 2\pi/\lambda$. It is assumed, in the derivation of equation (1.4.1), that the distance z_s is very much greater than the size of the aperture in the mask and also that the observation region on the screen is limited to a small area close to the axis. The exact expression for the distance between two points (x_m, y_m) and (x_s, y_s) located, respectively, on the mask and on the screen is

$$r_s = [z_s^2 + (x_s - x_m)^2 + (y_s - y_m)^2]^{1/2} \qquad (1.4.2)$$

However, in deriving the Fresnel diffraction relationship [equation (1.4.1)], this length is approximated by

$$r_s = z_s \left[1 + \frac{1}{2}\left(\frac{x_s - x_m}{z_s}\right)^2 + \frac{1}{2}\left(\frac{y_s - y_m}{z_s}\right)^2 \right] \tag{1.4.3}$$

The region where equation (1.4.3) is valid is said to be the *Fresnel diffraction region*.

Combining the factors preceding the integral in equation (1.4.1) as a single term

$$A_s = \frac{\exp(jkz_s)}{j\lambda z_s} \exp\left[\frac{jk}{2z_s}(x_s^2 + y_s^2)\right] \tag{1.4.4}$$

which is independent of the coordinates x_m and y_m, we see that the observed optical field is given by the Fourier transform relationship

$$\mathscr{E}(x_s, y_s) = A_s F\left[\mathscr{E}(x_m, y_m) \exp\left\{\frac{jk}{2z_s}(x_m^2 + y_m^2)\right\}\right] \tag{1.4.5}$$

where the Fourier transform $(F[\,])$ is evaluated at radian frequencies $2\pi x_s/(\lambda z_s)$ and $2\pi y_s/(\lambda z_s)$.

Fraunhofer makes the additional and more restrictive assumption that

$$z_s \gg \tfrac{1}{2}k(x_m^2 + y_m^2) \tag{1.4.6}$$

over the whole region of the aperture, in which case the exponential term in equation (1.4.5) becomes approximately unity. This greatly simplifies the calculation of the diffracted field, since now

$$\mathscr{E}(x_s, y_s) = A_s F[\mathscr{E}(x_m, y_m)] \tag{1.4.7}$$

Photodetectors respond to the optical intensity

$$I(x_s, y_s) = |\mathscr{E}(x_s, y_s)|^2 \tag{1.4.8}$$

rather than to the wave amplitude. As an example, let the amplitude transmittance function for the mask be given by

$$T_m(x_m, y_m) = \text{rect}\,(x_m/a)\,\text{rect}\,(y_m/c) \tag{1.4.9}$$

i.e., the aperture is rectangular with dimensions a and c in the x_m and y_m directions, respectively. If the mask is then illuminated by a plane wave of unit amplitude, the field transmitted by the mask will be equal to the transmission function. Then from equation (1.4.7) the Fraunhofer diffracted field at distance z_s from the mask is

$$\mathscr{E}(x_s, y_s) = A_s ac \,\text{sinc}\left(\frac{\pi a x_s}{\lambda z_s}\right) \text{sinc}\left(\frac{\pi c y_s}{\lambda z_s}\right) \tag{1.4.10}$$

where $\text{sinc } x = (\sin x)/x$. From equation (1.4.8) the intensity distribution on the screen is then

$$I(x_s, y_s) = \frac{a^2 c^2}{\lambda^2 z_s^2} \text{sinc}^2 \left(\frac{\pi a x_s}{\lambda z_s}\right) \text{sinc}^2 \left(\frac{\pi c y_s}{\lambda z_s}\right) \qquad (1.4.11)$$

In all practical flow measurement systems, lenses are featured as the most important optical components. (It will be assumed that lenses are spherical unless otherwise stated.) For the purpose of calculating field and intensity distributions at various locations within the system, lenses can generally be regarded as thin, in which case their only effect is to cause a phase delay in the wavefront proportional to the thickness of the lens at the position where the ray enters. If it is assumed that the lens lies perpendicular to the optical axis, with its center at the origin, the thickness at a point where the coordinates are (x_0, y_0) can be approximated by

$$\Delta_0(x_0, y_0) = \Delta_m - \frac{x_0^2 + y_0^2}{2L(n_g - 1)} \qquad (1.4.12)$$

where Δ_m is the maximum thickness of the lens, L is its focal length, and n_g is the refractive index of the glass from which it is made. This is known as the paraxial ray approximation. It follows from equation (1.4.12) that, if $\mathscr{E}_f(x_0, y_0)$ is the field in a plane immediately in front of the lens, the field $\mathscr{E}_b(x_0, y_0)$ immediately behind the lens is given by

$$\mathscr{E}_b(x_0, y_0) = P(x_0, y_0) \exp\left(jk n_g \Delta_m\right) \exp\left[\frac{-jk}{2L}(x_0^2 + y_0^2)\right] \mathscr{E}_f(x_0, y_0) \qquad (1.4.13)$$

where the pupil function $P(x_0, y_0)$, defined by

$$P(x_0, y_0) = \begin{cases} 1 & \text{inside the lens aperture} \\ 0 & \text{outside the lens aperture} \end{cases} \qquad (1.4.14)$$

has been introduced to account for the finite size of the lens aperture. The second term on the rhs of equation (1.4.13) represents simply a constant phase delay and will be disregarded from this point onwards since it does not affect the transformation properties of the lens.

Suppose now that a plane wave of unit amplitude is incident on an object having a transmittance function T_m placed immediately in front of a converging lens of focal length L (by "in front of" we mean on the side from which the light is propagating). Since the field incident on the lens will in this case be T_m, the complex wave amplitude immediately behind the lens will, from equation (1.4.13), be

$$\mathscr{E}_b(x_0, y_0) = T_m(x_0, y_0)P(x_0, y_0) \exp\left[\frac{-jk}{2L}(x_0^2 + y_0^2)\right] \quad (1.4.15)$$

The Fresnel diffraction formula [equation (1.4.1)] can then be applied to compute the field at some distance from the lens. At a distance L behind the lens for example, i.e., in the back focal plane of the lens, the field strength at coordinates (x_s, y_s) becomes

$$\mathscr{E}(x_s, y_s) = A_s F[T_m(x_0, y_0)P(x_0, y_0)] \quad (1.4.16)$$

where the Fourier transform is evaluated at radian frequencies $2\pi x_s/(\lambda L)$ and $2\pi y_s/(\lambda L)$. Notice that the Fourier transform relationship is not an exact one, due to the presence of the term A_s. Although the first term on the rhs of equation (1.4.4), which defines A_s, can be disregarded for all practical purposes since it represents a constant phase shift, the second term introduces phase curvature into the diffracted field.

Phase curvature can be completely eliminated if the object is placed in the front focal plane of the lens, i.e., at a distance L in front of the lens, rather than directly in contact with the lens. If it is assumed that the lens aperture is infinite in extent, i.e., the pupil function is everywhere unity, it can easily be verified, by using equations (1.4.1) and (1.4.13), that if an object having the transmittance function $T_m(x_m, y_m)$ is placed in the front focal plane and is illuminated with a plane wave of unit amplitude, then the field in the back focal plane (disregarding any constant phase shift terms) is

$$\mathscr{E}(x_s, y_s) = F[T_m(x_m, y_m)] \quad (1.4.17)$$

where the Fourier transform is evaluated at radian frequencies $2\pi x_s/(\lambda L)$ and $2\pi y_s/(\lambda L)$. Equation (1.4.17) shows that there is an exact Fourier transform relationship between the field amplitudes in the back and front focal planes of a lens.

The Fourier transform relationship of equation (1.4.17) is strictly valid only when the lens aperture is infinite, and of course this is not realizable in practice. Thus, a modified image arises due to the finite solid angle over which the lens is able to collect light from the object. This effect is known as *vignetting*. The errors associated with vignetting usually outweigh those caused by phase curvature. Thus, in forming a transform image, it is common practice to place the object as close to the lens as possible. For example, in the mask laser Doppler velocimeter system, to be described in Section 2.2, one would generally place the mask close to the focusing lens rather than in the front focal plane in order to form the best fringe pattern in the back focal plane.

The Fourier transform relationships just derived are not only useful for the analysis of particular systems but also helpful to the experimenter in the arrangement of the various masks and spatial filters which are generally required in a practical system. The concept of spatial filtering is clearly illustrated by the classical Abbe–Porter experiment (Goodman, 1968). In this experiment a wire mesh is placed at some distance from a converging lens and is illuminated by a collimated beam, the image being formed on a screen placed in the image plane behind the lens. By inserting masks in the back focal plane of the lens, various components of the transmitted optical spectrum can be eliminated and the results observed in the image plane. For example, if the mask contains just a horizontal slit centered on the optical axis, then the horizontal lines disappear from the image. If a small opaque stop is placed on the optical axis, then the result will be a contrast reversal in the image. Spatial filtering techniques are employed fairly extensively in flow measurement systems. For example, in the two-beam system shown in Figure 2.1.1, opaque stops are introduced to block the direct beams, thereby ensuring that only light scattered from the object, in this case the particles in the flow, can reach the photodetector. Lading (1972), Rudd (1969), and Manning (1973) are among a number of authors who have analyzed laser Doppler optical systems using the Fourier transform technique just described.

The surfaces of a spherical lens either form part of a sphere or are flat, while for cylindrical lens the curved surfaces are sections of a cylinder. Out of the six combinations of convex, concave, and flat surfaces three of these, namely, double convex, plano convex, and positive meniscus, result in lenses having positive focal lengths. The other three types of lenses, i.e., double concave, plano concave, and negative meniscus, have negative focal lengths and are sometimes referred to as negative or diverging lenses. (Meniscus lenses have one concave and one convex face; in the positive meniscus the concave face has the greater radius of curvature, and in the negative meniscus the convex face has the greater radius.) Negative lenses are sometimes used for wavefront correction purposes, as in the three-dimensional laser Doppler system indicated in Figure 2.2.8. In applying equation (1.4.13) to establish the field behind a lens, due account must be taken of the sign of L. When computing the field behind a cylindrical lens aligned, say, along the y axis, the y_0 term arising in the second exponential of equation (1.4.13) should be dropped since the lens offers only a constant phase delay to the field in the y

direction. Thus, a cylindrical lens may be treated as equivalent to a transparency with transmittance function

$$T_c(x_0, y_0) = P(x_0, y_0) \exp(-jkx_0^2/2L) \qquad (1.4.18)$$

Since cylindrical lenses tend to focus a laser beam to a narrow strip rather than to a spot, they can frequently be used to advantage where elongated measuring regions are required.

In any lens system it is impossible to eliminate completely aberrations (image defects), but these can be reduced to a minimum by employing only high-quality components and using only the central regions of lenses as far as possible. The principal types of aberration, i.e., spherical, coma, astigmatism, curvature of field, and distortion, are discussed in most elementary texts on geometric optics. Many lenses are of the doublet type, i.e., made of two different glasses cemented together or, alternatively, of the apochromatic type, i.e., made from a combination of three glasses. The object here is to correct for chromatic aberration caused by the fact that the refractive index of glass is a function of the optical wavelength. With laser sources, however, there is no need to use lenses corrected for chromatic aberration since there is only a single wavelength.

Thin-Film Coatings

In laser anemometry thin-film optical coatings are used extensively for two purposes: (a) antireflection coating of optical surfaces and (b) production of semireflecting surfaces for beam splitters.

Light that is reflected from the various optical surfaces and reaches the photodetector can prove to be a major source of noise in a system. High signal-to-noise ratios can generally be maintained only if the intensity of background radiation reaching the detector is small in comparison with the intensity of scattered radiation. The long coherence lengths associated with laser sources allow the reflected rays to set up multiple interference patterns which pass through the system onto the detector. To minimize this effect it is desirable that all optical surfaces be coated with antireflection films. The most commonly used material for antireflection coatings is magnesium fluoride, which has a refractive index of 1.38. If the substrate is glass, with refractive index 1.5, then it is clear that since incident light falling onto the front surface of the component will be propagating into a medium of increasing refractive index at both surfaces of the coating, then the rays reflected from both front and back surfaces of the coating will undergo 180°

phase changes (Leaver and Chapman, 1971). For minimum reflectance these rays should be 180° out of phase. Clearly, then, the coating thickness should be an integral multiple of $(\lambda/4)/1.38$, under the assumption that the radiation is incident normal to the surface. By "reflectance" we mean the ratio of the intensity of reflected light to the intensity of transmitted light. Theoretically, it is possible to reduce the reflectance to essentially zero, but only when the refractive index of the coating is equal to the square root of the substrate refractive index. Since in practice only certain materials are suitable for coating optical components, the reflectance generally cannot be reduced very dramatically with a single coating. For example, at an uncoated air–glass interface the reflectance is of the order of 4%, which can be reduced to about 1.3% with a single coating of magnesium fluoride. More significant reductions can be achieved by using a number of coatings of differing refractive index, and it is common practice in preparing optical components to use three or four thin-film layers of varying refractive index. For a detailed discussion the reader is referred to the texts of Maissel and Glang (1970) and Holland (1956). The side walls of laboratory flow rigs are frequently constructed from Perspex (polymethyl methacrylate), and this can easily be thin-film-coated in the same way as glass although it will be found that the coating tends to be easily damaged on continual handling. Perspex has a refractive index of approximately 1.49, and although a single coat of magnesium fluoride will give a significant reduction in reflectivity, multiple coatings are generally to be preferred.

Beam splitters, to be described later in this section, often employ partially silvered mirrors, i.e., surfaces which are coated with a very thin film of reflecting material, so thin that a significant proportion of the incident light is transmitted directly through the film. Aluminum is the most commonly used material for this purpose. By varying the thickness of the coating it is possible to form virtually any ratio of transmittance to reflectance. It is important to note that since reflectance and transmittance are functions of the optical wavelength, generally speaking a beam splitter employing a partially silvered surface will only operate satisfactorily at a given wavelength.

Vacuum deposition by evaporation is the most commonly employed technique for producing optical coatings. The apparatus required for this is quite simple and is available in many university and industrial research laboratories. The material to be deposited is heated inside a vacuum chamber in which the substrate is placed. At very low pressures evaporation takes place, and the mean free paths are such that molecules from the evaporated source impinge directly onto the substrate, thus building up the thin-film layer. A light source and detector are generally used to monitor continuously reflectance and transmittance.

Properties of Laser Sources

It is not generally necessary that the user fully understand the working of various laser sources in order that he be able to apply them in anemometry. We will concern ourselves only with the main characteristics that affect the quality of the signal. The most important property of radiation from a laser is its degree of coherence which can be described in general terms by a three-dimensional coherence function in which the monochromaticity describes the phase coherence in the direction of propagation, sometimes referred to as temporal coherence, and the spatial coherence describes the phase correlation across the wavefront. Laser manufacturers generally specify the coherence length, which is equal to the velocity of light times the coherence time. This is more useful in practice since it gives the distance along the beam over which phase correlation is lost. If, for example, a single beam is split and the two components are recombined to form a fringe pattern, then the path difference along the beams should be significantly less than the coherence length. Otherwise, clear fringes would not be formed. As the path difference is increased the fringe visibility gradually approaches zero. For anemometry purposes lasers with nominally plane wavefronts are used. Because of the high degree of spatial coherence, the shape of the wavefront can be defined precisely, unlike a thermal source, where there is a degree of uncertainty caused by the finite spatial extent of the source. For this reason it is possible to focus down the laser beam to a very intense spot, much smaller than the spot obtainable with an incoherent source. For practical purposes the spot size can be considered as only diffraction-limited; i.e., it is limited only by the laws of diffraction outlined earlier in this section and not by the coherence properties of the laser. The method of calculating the diffraction-limited spot size will be considered in Section 2.3.

For flow measurement systems continuous wave (cw) gas lasers are most generally used, and in the remainder of the book it will be assumed that all sources are of this type. However, it is worth noting that pulsed lasers have been employed extensively in high-speed photography and undoubtedly have anemometry applications. The central component in a laser is the resonator cavity, which has highly reflecting mirrors at each end and is filled with low-pressure gas. This is excited by an electrical discharge, which, under certain conditions, results in stimulated emission that acts as an amplifier for radiation traversing back and forth between the end mirrors. A certain amount of light passes through the end mirrors in the form of an intense and highly coherent beam. In most lasers, the mirrors are external to the tube, and the ends of the cavity are fitted with *Brewster windows*, i.e., glass windows tilted at the Brewster angle of incidence (approximately 56°). These transmit components polarized parallel to the plane of incidence, with nominally 100% transmittance. Hence, the resulting beam is highly polarized in this direction. The components perpendicular to the plane of incidence are only partially transmitted and so are essentially damped out after many traversals between the mirrors. In other lasers the mirrors are fitted internally in the resonator cavity. A single internal Brewster window is then sometimes incorporated in order to produce a linearly polarized beam. However, in the cheaper low-power lasers there is frequently no Brewster window, in which case the resulting beam is unpolarized since the stimulated emissions are random in nature and the mirrors do not reflect with any preferred direction of polarization. It is essential that the user check carefully the polarization specifications of the laser to be employed and bear in mind that beams polarized at right angles do not form an interference pattern. Generally speaking, lasers giving linearly polarized beams are most suitable for anemometry applications. For some of the systems described in Section 2.2 a plane-polarized beam is essential.

In comparing different lasers for a specific application it is also important to consider the noise characteristics in relationship to the total power. For a detailed analysis of the various noise sources the reader is referred to the article by Bloom (1965). The primary sources of noise are spontaneous emission, plasma, and mode interference. The first two take the form of white-noise-like fluctuations in intensity, but their magnitudes are not usually sufficiently large in comparison with the over-all intensity to cause any significant effect on the output to the complete system. The effects of mode interference, on the other hand, can be substantial. Most lasers are multimode, i.e., they have a multiple-frequency output, the exact locations of these frequencies being highly sensitive to changes in gain, resonator length, and other uncontrollable factors and hence being very unstable. The various modes tend to interfere, which causes random beating effects that give rise to low-frequency fluctuations in intensity, rather than to noise as in the accepted sense of white noise. Multimode operation also causes an effective reduction in the coherence length of the beam. The longitudinal spacing f_m between the modes is generally specified by the manufacturer and is typically of the order a few hundred megahertz for a low-power HeNe laser. Alternatively, if it is not specified, it can be calculated from the relationship

$$f_m = U_c/2L_c \tag{1.4.19}$$

where U_c is the speed of light and L_c is the cavity length. The number of modes N_m can then be calculated from the relationship $N_m \approx f_D/f_m$, where f_D is the linewidth of the atomic transition (full width at half-amplitude points). Foreman (1967) gives data quantifying the loss of signal in a laser Doppler velocimeter system caused by various path differences between the two beams as a function of the number of longitudinal modes.

Multimode HeNe and argon–ion are the most commonly used lasers in anemometry, since they both offer a high degree of reliability and low cost in relation to power output. It is possible to obtain single-mode lasers, but these generally are much lower in power and higher in cost. Bloom (1966) quotes the linewidth for HeNe operating at 6328 Å as approximately 1700 mHz and the corresponding linewidth for argon–ion as 3500 mHz. Applying equation (1.4.19), we can see that a typical value for the longitudinal-mode spacing in a 1-mW HeNe laser would be 550 mHz. Argon–ion lasers can provide very much greater power outputs than HeNe lasers, typically a few watts as compared with a few milliwatts. This advantage, however, is partly offset by their poorer noise characteristics. For a laser Doppler system (to be described in Section 2.2), where one is relying on interference effects to produce the signal, it is usually necessary to incorporate an etalon when operating with an argon–ion source, in order to increase the coherence length. HeNe lasers have adequate coherence lengths, but it should be noted that higher power outputs are associated with greater noise levels.

Photodetectors

Intuitively, one feels that since high-power lasers are expensive in addition to being bulky and dangerous to operate, a low-power laser should be employed, the reduction in power being compensated for by having a more sensitive detector. However, there are fundamental considerations which place lower limits on the laser power required and affect the choice of both light source and detector. The role of the detector in relation to the source and the optical system as a whole can only be understood by considering the quantum nature of electromagnetic radiation.

The current obtained from a photodetector is dependent upon the number of photons incident on the surface per unit time and also on the *quantum efficiency* α', defined as the number of photoelectrons emitted from the photodetector surface per incident photon. The quantum efficiency is a function of wavelength, among other factors, and might typically be of the order 10%. From Einstein's law the energy of a photon is $h_c U_c / \lambda$, where h_c is Planck's constant $(6.62 \times 10^{-34}$ J sec), U_c is the velocity of light $(3 \times 10^8$ m/sec), and λ is the wavelength of the radiation. Hence, if the incident power is P_c watts, the number of photons per second will be

$$n_p = P_c \lambda / h_c U_c \tag{1.4.20}$$

and the number of photoelectrons per second will be $\alpha' n_p$, where n_p is given by the above expression. The incident power is determined by integrating the optical intensity over the surface of the detector, the intensity being found for a particular optical system and seeding condition by the methods described in Sections 2.1–2.3. If the detector signal is to be analyzed by analog techniques, then a continuous signal is required. This is obtained by amplifying the resulting current with a circuit having a finite bandwidth. However, since there are only a finite number of photoelectron emissions per second, this signal always exhibits high-frequency fluctuations, termed *shot noise*. This is generally the factor which limits the choice of laser power, since if the shot noise is to be filtered out, by use of a low-pass filter preceding the analog-analyzing system, then clearly the photoelectron emission rate should be very much greater than the highest frequency to be analyzed. When considering continuous signals it is convenient to define the *sensitivity* of the detector, sometimes referred to as the radiant sensitivity. The sensitivity η is equal to the ratio of the photocurrent to the incident power of the radiation. Thus, from equation (1.4.20) we have

$$\eta = \frac{\alpha' e_0 n_p}{P_c} = \frac{\alpha' e_0 \lambda}{h_c U_c} \tag{1.4.21}$$

where η is measured in A/W and e_0 is the electron charge $(1.6 \times 10^{-19}$ C).

For quantitative predictions of the shot-noise magnitude it can be assumed that the number of arrivals in a given time interval displays a Poisson probability density. This of course is only a rough approximation, as in general the Poisson rate parameter will itself be a random variable, but it will suffice for estimation of noise levels. For a Poisson point process the variance of the number of arrivals in a given time interval is equal to the mean number of arrivals. It follows that if the mean current is i_0, the expected number of photoelectrons in a sample time of T sec is $i_0 T / e_0$. The rms shot noise is then

$$i_{rms} = (2e_0 i_0 \, \Delta f)^{1/2} \qquad (1.4.22)$$

where we have replaced T by $1/(2\Delta f)$, Δf being the bandwidth of the photo-detector amplifier.

In the measurement of high-speed gas flows and in certain other situations it sometimes turns out that an analog signal would be completely dominated by shot noise. In this situation the only approach is to employ a photon-counting technique and to analyze the resulting data by digital methods. This technique, which will be described in detail in Chapter 4, allows one to achieve optimum sensitivity and often to operate at low laser powers even in unseeded gas flow.

Two types of detectors are commonly used, photodiodes (photoconductive solid state detectors) and photomultipliers, although other types of detectors, e.g., channel electron multipliers, may have advantages in certain circumstances. It is generally accepted (Buchhave, 1973) that at high light levels and small bandwidths photodiode detectors are the most satisfactory. Under these conditions, which pertain to most liquid flow measuring situations, high signal-to-noise ratios can usually be achieved without difficulty.

Photodiodes have the advantage of being small in size and relatively inexpensive; further, they do not require any high-voltage power supply as do photomultiplier tubes. They are invariably incorporated into an ac preamplifier circuit. Thus the output signal is insensitive to the background light level. It is common practice to operate photodiodes under daylight conditions without any optical screening.

At low light levels and wide bandwidths, which occur in high-speed gas-flow-measuring situations, photomultipliers are superior (Melchoir *et al.*, 1970). In a photomultiplier, amplification of the photocurrent is obtained by employing a dynode chain. A potential gradient is maintained across the various dynode stages by means of a high-voltage supply. Photoelectrons emitted from the cathode impinge on the first dynode and emit secondary electrons which in turn are accelerated onto the second dynode by the potential gradient, and so forth. It should be remembered that the amplification process is itself statistical in nature and results in additional shot noise. Thus equation (1.4.22) represents only a lower limit to the noise that can be expected. The reader is referred to the articles by Robben (1971) and Anderson and McMurtry (1966) for details.

When photon counting techniques are used, photomultipliers fitted with discriminator units are employed so that the photoelectron emissions at the cathode result in unit height pulses at the output. It is then convenient to consider the detector as having an overall quantum efficiency α, which we will define as the ratio of the number of output pulses to the number of incident photons. This will clearly be dependent upon the setting of the discriminator level as well as the exact characteristics of the tube. Associated with the discriminator will be a "dead time," which is normally introduced by including a delay time into the circuitry. This inhibits the formation of two pulses in very rapid succession and is necessary because of the ringing (or overshoot) effects associated with the signal that reaches the discriminator. Dead times are typically of the order of 50 nsec and result in a reduced correlation between counts at delay times of this order. This does not generally cause any serious problems, but sometimes means that the first point on a count correlation has to be ignored.

The two primary sources of noise other than shot noise that degrade the output from a photodetector are dark current and Johnson noise. Dark current arises because even in complete darkness electrons are emitted from a detector surface due to agencies other than incident photons. Johnson noise is caused by the spontaneous emission of electrons in the resistive loads following a detector. With a photomultiplier the current is highly amplified before it passes through the resistive load connected across the output, so Johnson noise effects tend to be insignificant and the dominant noise contribution is from dark current. For high-quality tubes the so-called dark count, i.e., the number of photoelectron emissions per second, is typically as low as 100 and can therefore be disregarded in all but the most sensitive photon counting experiments. To obtain the minimum dark count tubes should be kept in the dark when not in operation and should be maintained at the minimum possible temperature when operating. With photodiode detectors Johnson noise is important since it is amplified through all the various stages of the preamplifier circuit. However, as indicated earlier in this section, photodiodes are only used where light levels are high, and in this situation noise is not a major problem.

The sensitivity of a photodetector is in general a function of the optical wavelength, and spectral response curves are invariably specified by the manufacturer. Most detectors have their maximum sensitivity in the blue–green range rather than in the red, which tends to be inconvenient since HeNe are the most commonly available lasers and these give a red beam.

Beam Splitters

The majority of the velocity-measuring systems to be described in Chapter 2 require some form of beam splitter to separate the incident laser beam into two components. Frequently the two beams are required to be as nearly as possible the same intensity, and in other cases, e.g., in heterodyne laser Doppler velocimeter systems, two beams of widely differing intensities are required. We will describe only some of the simplest and most frequently used beam splitters, and it will become immediately obvious to the reader that there is an almost limitless number of modified arrangements which can be devised.

In its simplest form a beam splitter can be a thin plate of glass, or optical flat, aligned at an angle to the incident laser beam. This results in transmitted and reflected rays of widely differing intensities, so its application is rather limited. The intensity ratio can be varied, however, by coating one of the surfaces with a thin metallic film by using the vacuum deposition technique described earlier in this section. Frequently a glass plate is semisilvered on one surface and then a plane plate is cemented on top so that the metallic film is sandwiched between the two plates. The resulting component is less easily damaged on handling than a front-silvered mirror. Semireflecting mirrors of this type can be readily purchased off the shelf since they are used extensively in various types of interferometers and spectrometers (James and Sternberg, 1969). The most frequent requirement in laser anemometry is for two parallel beams originating from the same source. This can easily be arranged, as indicated in Figure 1.4.2a, by placing the semisilvered mirror at 45° to the incident beam and using an additional front-silvered mirror to realign the reflected ray in a direction parallel to the incident beam. This scheme has the advantages that large beam separations can easily be obtained and that light losses are relatively low. However, set against this are two serious disadvantages. First, it tends to be difficult to align the mirrors so that the emerging beams are exactly parallel. This means in practice that both mirrors need to be mounted into a rigid integrated unit incorporating fine screw adjustments. Second, there is a path difference between the two beams which can cause serious problems in laser Doppler anemometry if the coherence length of the laser is not considerably longer than the separation between the mirrors. Equalization of path lengths can be achieved by inserting a glass block or, alternatively, a suitable combination of mirrors, into the path of the shorter beam although use of either of these techniques will introduce light losses and make alignment more difficult. Figure 1.4.2a

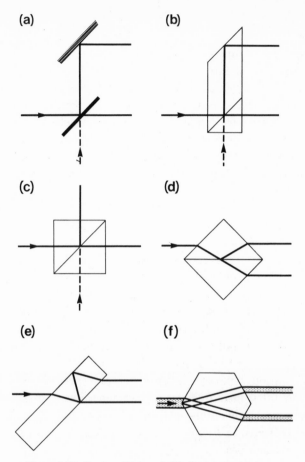

Figure 1.4.2. Beam splitters suitable for laser anemometry.

also indicates (by the broken line) that the incident beam can be perpendicular to the transmitted beams. This is sometimes convenient where space is severely restricted.

There are various adaptations of the two-mirror arrangement which employ prisms and are more convenient to use since the complete beam splitter can be constructed as a single component and consequently alignment problems do not arise after manufacture (Bedi and Thew, 1972; Blake, 1972b). With prisms the light losses tend to be greater at large beam separations because of the lengths of glass through which the beams travel. Also, the same difficulties arise due to the path difference between the beams. In Figure 1.4.2b a construction employing two prisms is indicated, but arrangements making use of three right-angle prisms (Bedi, 1971) or three right-angle prisms and a square block are also possible. As indicated in the figure, the incident beam can be either perpendicular or parallel to the transmitted beams.

A very simple form of beam splitter, commonly used in interferometry, is comprised of a thin-film metallic coating sandwiched between the hypotenuse sides of two 45°–90° prisms, the complete beam splitter being in the form of a cube. With the incident beam perpendicular to one of the faces, as illustrated in Figure 1.4.2c, the two beams emerge at right angles and the beam splitter simply acts as a replacement for the semisilvered mirror indicated in Figure 1.4.2a. Alternatively, the incident beam can be aligned at 45° to the face, as indicated in Figure 1.4.2d, in which case the two beams emerge parallel. This arrangement has the advantage that path length differences are not introduced. Also different separations can be obtained by varying the position at which the incident beam strikes the face. Various angular separations between the emerging beams can be achieved by rotating the prism.

Plane blocks of glass are frequently used for beam splitting (Brayton and Goethert, 1971; Vasilenko et al., 1972a). Figure 1.4.2e indicates the principle. The block is tilted at an angle to the incident beam, and at the back face the transmitted beam emerges slightly displaced. The reflected rays undergo a second reflection at the front face and eventually emerge parallel to the original transmitted beam. With an unsilvered glass block the two beams will have widely differing intensities, but if the surface regions where the refractions take place are suitably silvered (i.e., semisilvered on the back face and completely silvered on the front face), any desired intensity ratio can be obtained. Features of this type of splitter are that the beams always emerge parallel and that varying beam separations can be achieved by rotating the block. By using two similar blocks aligned at opposite directions of incidence, the path differences between the two beams can be eliminated (Brayton and Goethert, 1971).

Notice the similarity between the five different methods of beam splitting just described. In all of these optical arrangements the result is an amplitude splitting of the beam, i.e., the two beams which emerge have an intensity profile the same shape as the incident beam. It is fairly clear that one of the major problems in making a beam splitter of this type is in obtaining a coating which gives the required ratio between the intensities of the transmitted beams. Sometimes it is convenient to make adjustments in intensity by introducing a neutral density filter into one of the beams, although this procedure should be avoided where possible since it results in an overall loss of laser power. When using any of these beam-splitting arrangements it is important to check the polarization of the beams at various stages, since reflected rays tend to be highly polarized in a direction parallel to the reflecting surface. If the beams are to be recombined to form an interference pattern, then it is desirable that the incident beam be plane-polarized in a direction parallel to the plane of the reflecting surfaces, for if an unpolarized beam is used, the components polarized parallel and per-pendicular to the plane of incidence will be unequally reflected, resulting in a loss of fringe contrast. If the beam splitter is to be rotated relative to the laser in order to achieve a rotation of the fringe pattern, then the incident beam should be passed through a half-wave plate which is rotated by an amount equal to half the angular rotation of the beam splitter, in order that the correct direction of polarization be maintained.

Figure 1.4.2f shows a simple method of wavefront splitting a laser beam. This technique is particularly convenient if a low-power unpolarized laser beam is used since problems of matching intensity and planes of polarization are virtually eliminated. The beam splitter is a hexagonal, or possibly diamond-shaped, prism having one sharp edge which is positioned half-way across the incident beam, which gives two parallel D-shaped beams. The main disadvantage of this method is that if a mask is not used to aperture the two transmitted beams, then their unusual shape tends to be inconvenient, especially for theoretical analysis. Matching the intensities of the two beams proves to be no problem, however, provided that the prism is mounted on a screw-adjusted traverse.

The beam-splitting techniques described above are the most commonly used in laser anemometry although there are many other possibilities, e.g., a Kosters prism (Thompson, 1968) or simply a block of calcite. Sometimes a beam splitter is followed by a combination of mirrors or prisms which increases the range of possible beam separations. Where two parallel beams from the splitter are to be focused to form a fringe pattern another useful measure is to employ a combination of two lenses rather than a single lens for focusing. This allows one to adjust the position at which the fringe pattern is formed by simply altering the distance between the two lenses.

Diffraction Gratings

An alternative way of producing two or more beams originating from the same source is to use a diffraction grating. The optical efficiency with which a grating splits a beam is generally low compared with the beam splitters illustrated in Figure 1.4.2 although the grating has the great advantage that the transmitted beams can be shifted in frequency by the simple procedure of physically moving the grating relative to the incident beam. This technique will be described in detail in Section 2.2.

Both transmission and reflection gratings can be used for beam splitting in laser anemometry although the transmission type are generally more convenient. The most readily available transmission gratings are in the form of plastic sheets on which there are a large number of parallel, equally spaced, indentations. These gratings are replicas produced by molding the plastic material around a drum on which a continuous scratch has been produced in the form of a very fine screw thread. The primary disadvantage with this type of component is that most of the incident light passes straight through, only a small proportion of the laser power being diffracted into the various orders. This problem can be partially overcome by using a blazed grating on which the shape of the indentations resembles a series of steps whose angle of inclination is chosen in such a way that a major part of the incident light is deflected into one order.

For laser anemometry applications the spacing between grating lines is sometimes required to be of the order 0.1 mm, i.e., very large in comparison to the spacings normally used in spectrometry applications. At this scale gratings are frequently made by depositing strips of metal onto a glass plate. Radial gratings constructed in this manner can readily be purchased. These are the most convenient gratings to use when optical frequency shifting techniques are to be employed.

Acousto-optic and Electro-optic cells

For certain laser anemometry applications it is necessary to incorporate either electro-optic or acousto-optic cells into the system. The three commonly used components are referred to as Bragg cells (acousto-optic), Pockels cells, and Kerr cells (electro-optic), and these can all be obtained commercially, complete with electrical drive units.

Bragg cells are either in the form of a block of solid transparent material or a small cell filled with liquid, the principle of operation being the same in either case. Along one side of the cell is a piezoelectric transducer coupled to a high-frequency electrical supply. This produces a train of plane acoustic waves which move across the cell at the speed of sound and are absorbed at the far end by some damping material. Since the sound waves cause variations in the refractive index of the medium, the effect is that of a three-dimensional moving diffraction grating. At a certain angle of incidence, the Bragg angle, nearly all of the incident light is diffracted into the first order, the beam which emerges being frequency shifted by an amount equal to the frequency of the sound wave. The cell needs to be wide enough for the light to traverse at least one full wavelength of the ultrasonic wave. Gordon (1966) gives a detailed review of the properties of Bragg cells.

Electro-optic cells are used in essence to produce a controllable rotation in the planes of polarization of an incident beam and are extensively employed as light shutters and optical modulators. The Kerr cell is a transparent container filled with liquid, usually nitrobenzene, and has plates on either side across which a potential can be applied. If the incident beam is plane-polarized, then when a potential is applied across the plates, the direction of polarization will rotate as the beam passes through the cell. Since the amount of rotation is dependent on the applied potential, the cell can be used as an optical shutter or intensity modulator if a polaroid sheet or other analyzer is placed across the exit. Pockels cells operate in a similar manner but are made from solid crystals, usually ammonium dihydrogen phosphate (ADP) or potassium dihydrogen phosphate (KDP). For a detailed comparison of various types of electro-optic cells the reader is referred to the articles by Chenoweth *et al.* (1966) and Kaminow and Turner (1966).

Ways in which acousto-optic and electro-optic cells are employed in velocity-measuring systems are described in Section 2.2.

Chapter 2

OPTICAL CONFIGURATIONS

In this chapter we describe the optical configurations which are most commonly used for the measurement of flow velocity. A large number of optical arrangements have been proposed in current literature. While most of these are quite novel and have merits in particular practical situations, they are essentially variations on a set of basic optical geometries. We will confine our attentions to what we consider to be the fundamental arrangements, and describe only very briefly some of the diversifications. Laser Doppler velocimeters (LDV) form by far the largest class of instruments and hence will be treated in greatest detail. In the first few sections we will be concerned primarily with the practical aspects associated with the various optical designs rather than with the mathematical analysis of the systems. This will be covered in detail in Section 2.6 and in subsequent chapters of the book.

In all the optical configurations, a laser beam is focused onto a specified observation point in the flow. Laser light is scattered by small particles, present (or seeded) in the flow, as they pass across this point. These particles are often referred to as scattering centers. They should ideally be of microscopic size and have densities close to the density of the surrounding fluid. Otherwise, they will not faithfully follow the flow, and the exact flow characteristics will not be portrayed. For ordinary tap water that has been filtered by passing through a fine gauze there is generally an abundance of minute scattering particles which can safely be assumed to follow precisely the flow, their densities being of the same order as the water. The signal under these conditions is a continuous one since there will always be a number of particles passing through the beam at any given instant. In air, however, the situation is different since the concentration of naturally occurring dust particles is generally very much lower. In this case the signal appears as a series of discrete pulses, each pulse corresponding to the passage of a single particle across the observation region. Discontinuous signals are generally more difficult to analyze than continuous ones, and it is primarily for this reason that LDV systems have found their greatest application in the measurement of liquid flows. We will see later, however, that photon correlation methods of analysis can quite readily cope with the air flow situation.

One way of increasing the strength of signals is to artificially seed the flow with particles. One then has, in theory, complete control over the nature of the scattering medium and can quantitatively calculate the errors caused by differences in velocity between the fluid medium and the scattering centers. Various types of apparatus for seeding air flows have been described in the literature (Melling and Whitelaw, 1973). Liquid flows are most commonly seeded by adding small quantities (about 1 : 100,000 concentration) of polystyrene spheres of diameter something less than 1 μm. These have a specific gravity very close to that of water (about 1.04) and can readily be obtained in suspension. Although seeding is commonly used for air flows, because of the low particle concentrations, it is generally unnecessary with liquids.

2.1. Two-Beam Systems

Given that in air flow naturally occurring dust particles appear sparsely and for most practical purposes can be assumed to faithfully follow the fluid motions, it is not surprising that some of the earliest attempts at employing optical techniques to flow measurement were directed toward measuring the transit times of scattering centers across two light beams focused in the flow. One such system has been described by Thompson (1968).

The main components of his system are shown in Figure 2.1.1a. A laser beam is spread by a cylindrical lens, and a second cylindrical lens is used to focus the light into the flow region. Following the second lens is a beam

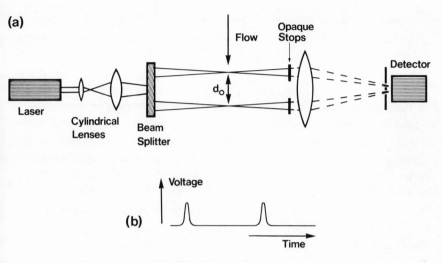

Figure 2.1.1. Modified version of two-beam system proposed by Thompson: (a) optical layout; (b) pulses produced by a single particle.

splitter, so that there are two separate beams brought to a focus in the focal plane of this lens. This produces two narrow strips of light in the flow, separated by a short distance d_0. On the collection side, these strips are imaged onto the surface of a single detector with a further lens, a mask containing two slit apertures being placed in front of the detector. The direct beams are blanked off with opaque stops so that effectively only light scattered from the focal region reaches the detector. To examine this point further it is necessary to consider the scattering of light by particles in the flow.

Suppose that the scattering particles are spherical and of radius r_p, which is greater than the wavelength of the incident laser light. According to the Mie scattering theory the scattered intensity will then be approximately the same as the intensity distribution produced by an opaque disc of the same radius. This approximation is only strictly valid when $r_p \gg \lambda$, but suffices for our purpose. Most particles in room air will be of the order 1–2 μm, whereas, for example, a HeNe laser has a wavelength of 0.63 μm. The diffraction pattern takes the form of a series of concentric rings. The position of the first intensity minimum subtends an angle of

$$\theta_s = 3.83\lambda/(2\pi r_p)$$

with the axis of the incident beam (Van de Hulst, 1957). If $\Delta\theta/2$ is the half-angle of convergence of the incident beams, then, for the direct light to be blocked completely, the field stops must have a width at least equal to

$l_p \, \Delta\theta$, where l_p is the distance of the stops from the focus of the transmitting lens. Also, for a significant amount of light to be incident on the detector surface $\theta_s > \Delta\theta/2$. It can easily be seen that this latter condition is nearly always fulfilled in a practical situation. The method of blocking the illuminating beam and observing only the scattered light is the same as used in the so-called dark background microscope. This type of instrument is often used for observing very small objects lying on a transparent plate where it is important that the eye is not swamped by the intensity of the background illumination, which may reduce its sensitivity. Ideally in a velocity-measuring system light should fall onto the detector only when scattering particles are present. If the patches are removed, the system can still work satisfactorily but the signal-to-noise ratio decreases due to the fact that fluctuations in the laser power pass directly to the detector. With no patches, the signal is essentially a constant dc level which decreases suddenly as a particle traverses and blocks one of the beams. With the patches present, the signal level increases with the passage of a particle, as indicated in Figure 2.1.1b. In the system described by Thompson, the transit times are recorded for individual particles with an oscilloscope. The pulse due to a particle traversing the beam is used to trigger the oscilloscope, the transit time being obtained by visually observing the position of the second pulse on the screen (Figure 2.1.1b). In the optical system, if the line passing the centers of the focal spots is in the flow direction, then for a transit time (ξ) and a beam spacing (d_0) the velocity is simply $U = d_0/\xi$. For a turbulent flow it is theoretically possible to obtain a complete probability density of flow velocity by recording the instantaneous velocities from a large number of particles. This procedure would be very tedious since a great many samples would be required to obtain a good statistical average.

In two-beam systems of the type just described the necessity for recording each particle velocity individually can be eliminated if a correlator is used for analyzing the detector signal. It is generally preferable to have two separate detectors, one for each beam and to cross-correlate the outputs rather than to autocorrelate the output from a single detector on which both beams are imaged. The cross-correlation function, with the signal from the upstream detector delayed by an amount τ, will have a peak at a value of τ corresponding to the mean passage time across the beams, and the rms width of this peak will be a measure of the turbulent intensity. The same peak is obtained by correlating the output of the single detector, but additional terms are produced which are generally unwanted. This point will be discussed more fully in Chapter 5. The accuracy of measurement is limited by the finite size of the diffraction-limited beam spots. If the beam widths are

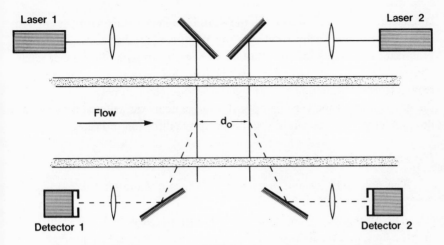

Figure 2.1.2. Two-beam system suitable for photon cross-correlation analysis.

not extremely small compared to the beam separation, then even for a constant velocity flow a broad cross-correlation peak is produced.

Lading (1973) has described a two-beam cross-correlation anemometer. His optical configuration is similar to that of Thompson except that two separate detectors are used to collect the scattered light. He reduces the number of optical components by passing the laser beam directly through a beam splitter which forms two diverging beams. These are focused down to two spots in the flow by a single lens, and a single lens is used for collection.

The two-beam method becomes extremely powerful when used in conjunction with a photon correlator. A suitable optical geometry is shown in Figure 2.1.2 (Durrani and Greated, 1975). Because of the sensitivity of the detectors it is desirable that incident light from the lasers does not fall directly on them. Hence scattered light is collected at an angle to the incident beams in preference to using opaque stops. By using two separate lasers, interference effects between the beams are eliminated and, further, the beams can be adjusted to any desired separation by moving the mirrors. A single right angle prism with silvered faces can conveniently be used to replace the two mirrors which focus the incident beams when small separations are required.

2.2. LDV Optical Configurations

Most optical systems used for measuring flow velocities employ one of the so-called laser Doppler configurations. There has always been considerable debate as to whether the word Doppler can justifiably be applied to all of the various geometries, but this point is of academic, rather than of practical interest. More important are the relative merits of the heterodyne and real fringe systems to be described in this section, particularly with regard to ease of alignment and signal-to-noise characteristics. To simplify the description of the various optical arrangements we will assume that the flow velocity to be measured is constant in the direction indicated.

Heterodyne Systems

The first LDV system described by Yeh and Cummins (1964) was of the heterodyne type and is sometimes described as a true Doppler anemometer. The principle of its operation is quite simple. A laser beam is directed into the flow, and the light scattered by particles in the fluid is observed with a photodetector at an angle to the original direction of propagation of the beam. The Doppler principle tells us that the frequency of the scattered light will be shifted by an amount proportional to the flow velocity, but clearly in most practical situations the frequency shift is going to be extremely small compared with the optical frequencies involved. However, the shift can easily be observed if the scattered light is mixed (or heterodyned) with light from the laser which is unshifted in frequency. The photodetector signal then contains a beat frequency equal to the Doppler shift frequency proportional to the flow velocity.

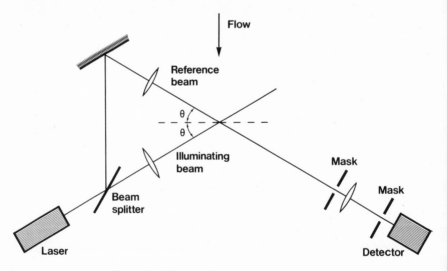

Figure 2.2.1. Forward-scatter heterodyne system.

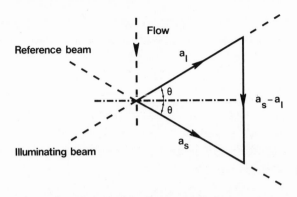

Figure 2.2.2. Vector diagram illustrating the principle of
the heterodyne system shown in Figure 2.2.1.

Figure 2.2.1 shows a practical and commonly used geometry for the heterodyne system. The laser beam is split, usually with a glass plate, and the two resulting beams focused into the flow with lenses, each beam subtending the same angle θ with the normal to the flow direction. The lower beam (illuminating beam) is generally much more intense than the other beam (reference beam) which is used for heterodyning with the scattered light. The photodetector is aligned with the reference beam on the other side of the flow region. In the most general case the flow region from which scattered light is collected (observation volume) can be adjusted by means of two apertures in front of the detector. A lens is often used for collection, as indicated, but is not essential. To obtain the maximum beat signal the reference beam should have an intensity of the same order as that of the scattered light falling onto the detector, which in practical terms means that the illuminating beam should be about ten or more times intense than the reference beam. The optimum ratio is normally found by attenuating the reference beam, e.g., with crossed polaroids, and adjusting the attenuation for maximum signal.

The relationship between the velocity and beat frequency can be seen more easily if we refer to Figure 2.2.2. Suppose that the wave vectors associated with the illuminating beam and scattered light falling onto the detector are, respectively,

$$\mathbf{k}_I = (2\pi/\lambda_I)\mathbf{a}_I \tag{2.2.1}$$

$$\mathbf{k}_s = (2\pi/\lambda_s)\mathbf{a}_s \tag{2.2.2}$$

where $\mathbf{a}_I$ and $\mathbf{a}_s$ are unit vectors in the direction of the illuminating beam and the direction of the scattered light observed by the detector, i.e., in the direction of the reference beam; λ_I and λ_s are, respectively, the wavelengths of the illuminating and scattered beams. If $\mathbf{U}$ is the velocity vector of the scattering centers, then by the Doppler relationship, the frequency shift is

$$\omega_0 = (\mathbf{k}_s - \mathbf{k}_I) \cdot \mathbf{U} \tag{2.2.3}$$

In nearly all practical situations $|\mathbf{k}_s| \approx |\mathbf{k}_I|$ to a very close approximation as the frequency shift is small compared with the optical frequencies. Therefore, with a negligible error, we can write

$$\omega_0 = |\mathbf{k}_I|(\mathbf{a}_s - \mathbf{a}_I) \cdot \mathbf{U} \tag{2.2.4}$$

The vector term in the brackets is indicated in Figure 2.2.2. It is a vector in the direction of the flow, having a magnitude of $2 \sin \theta$, where θ is the half-angle between the illuminating and reference beams. The scalar relationship for the frequency is therefore

$$\omega_0 = 4\pi U \sin \theta n_f / \lambda \tag{2.2.5}$$

where n_f is the refractive index of the flow medium, U is the magnitude of the velocity, and λ denotes the wavelength of the illuminating laser light in free space. The frequency in Hertz is

$$f_0 = 2U \sin \theta n_f / \lambda \tag{2.2.6}$$

For measurements in air n_f can be taken, for all practical purposes, to be unity. When measuring in liquids, the total effect caused by the beams propagating from air to a medium of greater refractive index and back again must be taken into account. This point will be raised later, but it turns out that the Doppler frequency can be calculated from equation (2.2.6), with n_f equal to unity for flat and uniformly thick walls.

The heterodyne system just described is simple in principle, but obtaining good signal-to-noise ratios can prove quite difficult in a practical situation. The reason for this is that in essence there are three different optical units: illuminating, reference, and collection units, and these three have to be kept in exact alignment for the proper operation of the system. Our experience is that the system is very satisfactory for small-scale experiments where the complete set of components can be mounted on a single optical table. In this situation vibration effects can be almost entirely eliminated, and it often turns out that the problem of scanning across

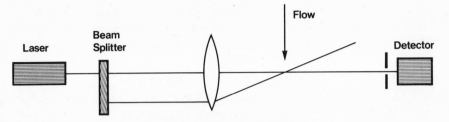

Figure 2.2.3. Single-lens heterodyne system.

different regions of the flow can be dealt with by moving the actual flow section through the beams rather than attempting to move the optics and risking misalignment.

Although convenient for the purpose of alignment, there is no fundamental reason why the reference beam should pass through the measuring region at all. The laser beam can be split and directed round the outside of the flow region with a series of mirrors, to be recombined with the scattered light on the other side. The original system of Yeh and Cummins was of this type, and versions of their scheme have been described by a number of other authors (Angus *et al.*, 1969; Rizzo, 1972). Generally speaking, because of the resulting increase in the number of optical components one has to be even more careful to insulate against vibrations. However, there are circumstances in which physical restraints make it convenient to have only one beam passing through the flow.

The simplest way of overcoming the alignment problem is to use a single lens for focusing the incident and reference beams. A number of investigators have described heterodyne systems of this type (Eliasson and Dandliker, 1974; Lading, 1972), probably the simplest and most practical being that due to Bedi (1971). Figure 2.2.3 shows schematically the geometry proposed by Bedi. The beam splitter should be of a type which allows part of the laser beam to pass directly through without deflection, thus allowing a straight through path from the laser to the detector. This aids alignment, particularly in measurement in circular ducts and it also allows the measuring direction to be rotated without the observation volume being moved. It can be seen that the path lengths of the incident and reference beams from the laser to the observation volume are generally different. This can cause a reduction, or even a complete loss, of the signal if the coherence length of the laser is not sufficiently great. This can be overcome by inserting a path length compensator, usually in the form of a block of glass, into the reference beam, between the beam splitter and the observation volume. With a HeNe laser this is usually unnecessary. A disadvantage of this optics is that one is actually measuring the velocity component in a direction perpendicular to the bisector of the angle between the illuminating and reference beams rather than perpendicular to the reference beam itself, this latter direction normally being the direction of the flow which one wants to measure. The difference between the velocity values in these two directions becomes very small as the angle between the beams is made small. The problem here is that a small beam angle gives a poor spatial resolution, as we will see later. The system therefore has practical advantages but is limited particularly in its application to turbulence measurement.

Real Fringe Systems

It was pointed out by Rudd (1969) that by focusing two parallel beams in the flow with a single lens one was in fact producing Young's interference fringes. Rudd's paper was fundamental to the development and understanding of LDV systems, and since its publication there have been numerous developments and modifications of the real fringe system.

A modified version of the original system used by Rudd is shown schematically in Figure 2.2.4. The transmitting optics is essentially the same as that used in the classical Young's fringes experiment. The laser beam is diverged and collimated to produce a parallel beam of a few centimeters diameter, which passes through a mask in which there are two parallel slits. The two resulting beams are refocused to form the interference pattern in the flow region, and finally the two beams emerging from the other side of

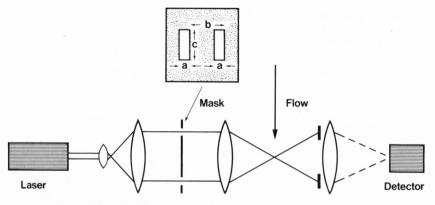

Figure 2.2.4. Modified version of the optical system proposed by Rudd.

the flow region are brought to a focus on the surface of a photodetector. The main features of the Rudd optics are its conceptual simplicity and the ease with which the precise nature of the Doppler signal can be calculated. If the mask has apertures of width a and depth c placed at a distance b apart, then the light intensity in the back focal plane, i.e., a plane through the center of the observation volume, is

$$I(x, y) = \frac{\sin^2 (k_1 x)}{(k_1 x)^2} \frac{\sin^2 (k_2 y)}{(k_2 y)^2} \cos^2 (bk_1 x/a) \qquad (2.2.7)$$

where x and y are the coordinates relative to the center of the fringe pattern, $k_1 = \pi a n_f/(\lambda L)$ and $k_2 = \pi c n_f/(\lambda L)$, L being the focal length of the focusing lens and λ the wavelength of the laser light. We have assumed here that the refractive index of the medium is unity throughout and have normalized to unit intensity at the center of the fringe pattern. As the fringe pattern is simply imaged onto the detector surface, a single scattering particle will cut off a varying amount of light as it passes across the pattern, the greatest amount of light being cut off as it passes a bright fringe. From equation (2.2.7) the fringe spacing is $\lambda L/bn_f$, so for a velocity U along the x axis the signal frequency in Hertz is $f_0 = bUn_f/(\lambda L)$. If the angle between the two beams is small, then the sine of the half-angle θ between the beams is $\sin \theta = b/(2L)$, so $f_0 = 2U \sin \theta n_f/\lambda$, i.e., the same expression that was obtained for the heterodyne system [equation (2.2.6)].

It will be seen later that the finite number of fringes within the observation volume places limitations on the accuracy of measurement, the smaller the number of fringes through which the scattering centers pass, the greater the inaccuracies introduced. In this respect the Rudd optics with two narrow slits in the mask is not optimum for the measurement of turbulent flows. Figure 2.2.5 illustrates this point. The photographs were taken by replacing the photodetector with a short focal length lens whose position along the optical axis was adjusted so that the magnified fringe patterns were projected onto photographic plates. With two slits in the mask, i.e., with $c/a \gg 1$, the fringe pattern is elongated in the direction of the flow (Figure 2.2.5a). In situations where the flow is highly turbulent or where the fringe pattern is rotated relative to the flow direction this is undesirable since particles will tend to traverse only a few fringes in the pattern. This situation is improved, however, if the two slits are replaced by square apertures. The resulting fringe pattern is shown in Figure 2.2.5b. A major disadvantage with the Rudd system is that the unscattered laser light falls directly onto the photodetector, with the result that small fluctuations in the

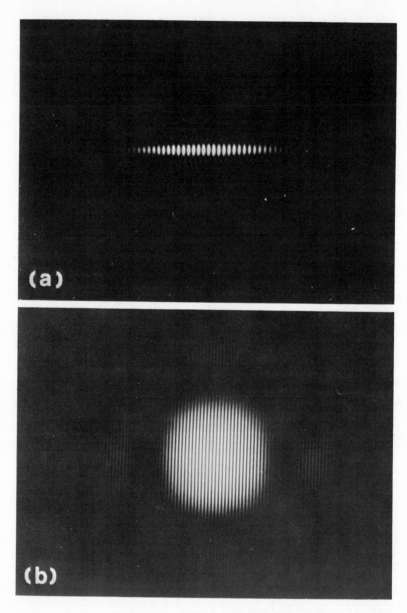

Figure 2.2.5. Fringe patterns produced in the back focal plane of the focusing lens with the modified Rudd system. Mask geometries: (a) $c/a \gg 1$, i.e., narrow slits; (b) $c = a$, i.e., square apertures.

laser output show up as noise on top of the signal. It is possible to record the laser output with a separate detector and subtract the noise electronically (Watrasiewicz, 1970), but a much simpler way of effecting the same result is to mask off the direct laser beams on the detection side so that only scattered light falls onto the detector (Greated, 1971*a*). Sometimes two lenses are used on the detection side, and their position is adjusted so that the beams are parallel between them. Two opaque patches of exactly the same size as the mask apertures can then be placed between the lenses to block the direct beams. With this method the beams can in theory be blocked completely without loss of scattered light (Greated, 1971*b*).

It is possible, in theory at least, to obtain signals from the Rudd system with the mask placed on the collection side instead of on the transmission side, i.e., the laser beam is expanded and then focused directly into the flow without attenuation, the scattered light having to pass through the mask before being focused onto the detector. The mask can either be placed close up to a single lens on the collection side, as indicated by Rudd, or alternatively two lenses can be used for collection, the first one being adjusted so that the measuring point is in its front focal plane. The mask is then placed between the two lenses. One can conveniently think of a virtual fringe pattern being formed in the flow in this situation.

The efficiency of the Rudd system can be improved very significantly by replacing the first two lenses and the mask with a beam splitter as shown in Figure 2.2.6. This is now the most commonly used LDV configuration. We have shown the scattered light being collected at an angle to the axis of the transmitting optics. This results in a reduction in signal level but a considerable improvement in spatial resolution if a suitably chosen pinhole is

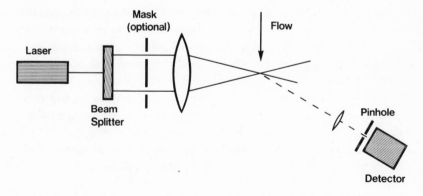

Figure 2.2.6. The most commonly used forward-scatter real fringe system.

placed in front of the detector. For most liquid flow situations and when the photon correlation method is being employed, signals are generally strong enough to allow collection in this way. When signals are too weak, the transmission and detection optics are aligned on the same axis. The configuration shown in Figure 2.2.6, which is generally referred to as "forward-scatter real fringe" can be used with or without the mask. The use of a mask causes a loss of light but has advantages in certain situations. For example, it allows easy adjustment of the number of fringes when the beam spacing is fixed, which can be particularly useful in small-scale experiments. Also, setting the mask dimensions exactly makes for easy calibration of the system. Since the fringe spacing is dependent only on the angle between the beams, the Doppler frequency in the real fringe systems is independent of the angle at which scattered light is collected.

The main advantage of the real fringe configurations, as compared to heterodyning, is that they are quite simple to align and are not as sensitive to small vibrations. Also, there is no need for adjusting the relative intensities of an incident and reference beam, since fairly obviously, the maximum fringe contrast and hence the maximum signal level are obtained when the two beams forming the fringe pattern are of equal intensity.

With the cosine term in equation (2.2.7) written as

$$\tfrac{1}{2}(1 + \cos 2bk_1x/a) \tag{2.2.8}$$

it can be seen that as a single particle passes across the fringe pattern the signal produced has both a low-frequency component (centered about zero frequency) and a high-frequency component (centered about the Doppler frequency). In direct analog signal analysis, this low-frequency component is generally either filtered out or ignored whereas in the photon correlation method both high- and low-frequency components are retained. In either case, however, when there is a continuous stream of scattering centers passing the fringe pattern the overall signal is the superposition of a large number of pulses at random phase orientation (this point will be discussed in greater detail in Chapter 3). This results in fluctuations on top of a dc level which is dependent on the over-all intensity of the scattered light. Only the fluctuations can be used in the flow measurement process, and the rms value of these can tend to zero for a very high density of infinitely small scattering particles. This point is intuitively obvious if one thinks of a cloud of uniform density passing the fringes. More precisely, the rms value of the electrical signal fluctuations is proportional to the square root of the number of scatterers by analogy with the random walk. It has been shown by a number of authors (Drain, 1972; Manning, 1973; Wang, 1972; Wang and Snyder, 1974) both theoretically and experimentally, that when the concentration of scattering centers is low (i.e., the number per unit volume), then the real fringe systems give considerably better signal-to-noise ratios than the heterodyne systems. For very high concentrations the heterodyne systems appear to have the better signal-to-noise characteristics, though a number of published theoretical predictions on this point give contradictory results. A practical point worth noting is that with the real fringe systems, signal levels can be increased by having a large collection angle so it is advantageous to use a collecting lens with as small an f number as possible.

Backscattering Geometries

To employ any of the systems so far described it is essential that there be visible access to both sides of the flow region. By observing the backscattered rather than the forward-scattered light, however, it is possible to make a system which can be used when there is only access to one side of the flow region. In general, to operate in the backscattering mode greater laser power is required since the scattering intensities are much less. As the intensities tend to be greatest near to the optical axis, it is both efficient and convenient to use the same lens for transmission and collection.

Figure 2.2.7 shows a backscattering version of the real fringe system which is simple to construct and has high optical efficiency. The laser beam is split in the usual way and the two resulting beams are passed through apertures in a mirror tilted at 45° to the optical axis. A mask M_1 can be used if required. Lens L_1 brings the two beams to a focus at the measuring point and light scattered in the backwards direction is collected back through the same lens and deflected by the mirror. A second lens L_2 images the fringe pattern onto the photodetector. A pinhole in a mask M_2 can be used in front of the detector to limit the observation volume. One great advantage with a geometry of this type is that it can be carefully aligned on construction and need never be realigned in use, even when the beams propagate through a change in refractive index. Despite this, the system can be made quite versatile by making the mask M_1 and the focusing lens interchangeable. The alignment procedure is simple. A piece of plain white paper or other similar material is placed at the focus of lens L_1 and the components are adjusted until a clear image is formed on the detector.

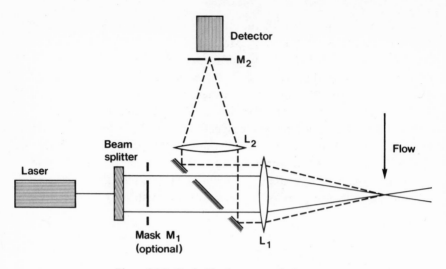

Figure 2.2.7. Typical backscatter optical system.

A number of novel variations on the geometry shown in Figure 2.2.7 have been proposed. Blake (1972*a*, *b*), for example, eliminates the necessity for a mirror by having both lenses centered on the same axis. The lens nearest the laser is drilled with two holes through which the two beams emerging from the beam splitter pass. The second lens alone is used to focus the beams, but the backscattered light passes through both lenses and is brought to a focus on the detector which is placed near the beam splitter between the two beams. To make this possible a photodiode of quite small dimensions is required. Heterodyne systems working in the backscattered mode have also been similarly devised (Huffaker, 1970), but in general the practical difficulties associated with their operation tend to be greater. For example, in the system proposed by Huffaker feedback of the scattered signal into the laser cavity has to be carefully minimized.

We have indicated that the real fringe forward-scatter geometry is the most generally useful, but nevertheless there are others which have merits in particular situations. It seems natural then to devise an optical unit which can be used in any of the four modes: (a) real fringe forward scatter, (b) real fringe back scatter, (c) heterodyne forward scatter, or (d) heterodyne back scatter. Such a unit is described by Durst and Whitelaw (1973), and a number of commercial organizations have produced similar universal integrated optical units.

Systems Employing Gratings

One of the earliest remote optical anemometers, developed by Gaster (1964), did not employ a laser source at all. A narrow strip of light was formed in the flow using a 250-W mercury vapor lamp with a condenser lens and suitable masks. This illuminated scattering particles in the flow whose images were formed on the surface of a square wave transmission grating by means of a separate optical system aligned at right angles to the transmission optics. The detector, in this case a photomultiplier, was placed just behind the grating so that a periodic signal was produced as the images of the particles moved across the grating lines. A most useful feature of this arrangement was that the frequency of the signal could be shifted up or down at will if a rotating radial grating was used. This point will be discussed in greater detail further on in this section.

More recently a number of authors have described rather more sophisticated systems employing laser sources with gratings in various configurations. As with the original system described by Gaster, their principal merit lies in the fact that the frequencies can be shifted by simple mechanical means. There are a number of ways in which a diffraction grating can be used. It can be included in the detection optics in the manner just described or it can be simply imaged into the flow, with a single lens and with the collection of the scattered light done in the same way as with the real fringe systems. With either of these two methods, unwanted higher harmonics are produced in addition to the fundamental signal frequency if a square wave transmission grating is used. Suppose that a laser beam of radius r_u impinged on a grating whose rulings are distance d_g apart, $d_g - a_g$ being the effective width of the rulings. The intensity distribution just behind the grating will be

$$I(x, y) = \sum_k \exp\left(-\frac{x^2 + y^2}{r_u^2}\right) \operatorname{rect}\left(\frac{x - kd_g - \phi_g}{a_g}\right), \qquad k = 0, \pm 1, \pm 2, \dots$$

$$(2.2.9)$$

ϕ_g being the displacement of the center of the laser beam relative to the center of one of the gaps between two successive rulings. If this is imaged into the flow with a single lens, then the distribution in the back focal plane will have the same form but will be magnified (or reduced) in size by the magnification factor l_I/l_0, l_I and l_0 being, respectively, the distance of the image and the object (the grating) from the lens. The temporal variation in intensity, observed by a particle moving along the x axis with a constant velocity U will have a definite periodicity. The frequency of this will be, say,

f_0 Hz, corresponding to the Doppler frequency in the real fringe and hetero-dyne systems. There will also be a low-frequency component due to the exponential term in equation (2.2.9), but the important point to note is that in this case higher harmonics of frequency $3f_0, 5f_0, \ldots$, etc. will also be present. Fortunately, because these are well separated from the fundamental frequency, they can be filtered off without difficulty.

In the measuring region the distance between fringes will be $d_g l_I / l_0$, so for the fringes perpendicular to the flow direction the signal frequency (corresponding to the Doppler frequency) is

$$f_0 = \frac{U}{d_g} \frac{l_0}{l_I} \tag{2.2.10}$$

A generally better way of using the grating is to block off all the emerging orders except the two first-order beams. A fixed grating is then really being used as a beam splitter. A single lens is then used to bring the beams to a focus in the flow exactly as with the previously described imaging system. The advantage now is that the higher-order-frequency components are eliminated, although this is at the expense of a reduction in intensity since the zero-order beam usually contains most of the power. As the half-angle between the two first-order beams emerging from the grating is $\sin^{-1}(\lambda/d_g)$, they will subtend an angle of $[\sin^{-1}(\lambda/d_g)]l_0/l_I$ with the optical axis at the point of measurement. Thus the Doppler frequency is approximately

$$f_0 = \frac{2U}{d_g} \frac{l_0}{l_I}$$

Note that this is twice the frequency one obtains with the imaging system. In practice, this is the most satisfactory system to use, except in situations where only a low-power laser is available.

If the grating is used as a beam splitter, then one can of course work equally well in the heterodyne mode or, alternatively, utilize one of the many variations on the real fringe geometry which can be devised. Some possibilities are described by Wang (1974). He shows that it is quite feasible to use a grating system with an only partially coherent source, i.e., when a laser is not available.

Measurement of Velocities in More Than One Direction

An important characteristic of all the LDV's described is that they measure directly a single component of velocity. This is not the case with, for example, a hot-wire anemometer. If a hot wire is aligned, say along the z axis, then it will respond to velocity fluctuations in both the x and y directions. This indicates that LDV systems are well suited to the measurement of three components of velocity simultaneously. In fact, a number of authors have described instruments having this capability. The details of these are rather complicated, and we will not attempt to describe them but rather just indicate briefly the underlying ideas.

The heterodyne configurations seem most easily adaptable to three-dimensional measurements. A typical system is described by Huffaker (1970), who developed an instrument capable of performing measurements in high-speed gas flows. The laser beam is focused directly into the flow and is split on the receiver side of the flow region into effectively three reference beams. Scattered light is observed with three separate detectors located at 120° spacings on the arc of a circle whose center lies on the original laser beam axis. The reference beams are mixed with the three scattered rays in the same way as with a one-component system. The algebraic relationships, given by Huffaker, between the three frequency shifts and the three velocity components are somewhat lengthy, In practice, an on-line computer facility is required to extract meaningful information from the outputs of the three channels. A very similar optical configuration and details of possible variations are described by Lennert *et al.* (1970).

Another very versatile instrument has been designed by Rizzo (1972). The main components of this are shown in Figure 2.2.8. The laser beam is split into two equal-intensity components, one of which is directed into the flow. The other beam (reference beam) passes around the outside of the flow rig and impinges on a static scattering plate. Scattered light is then collected at three different angles, from both the stationary plate and the moving particles, the scattered rays from these two sources being mixed together on the surfaces of the three detectors. With this configuration the rays scattered by the plate have a longer distance to travel to the detectors than the rays scattered by the particles, so the curvatures of the spherical wavefronts would be different if no correction was made and the signal quality would be spoilt. Wavefront correction is accomplished by inserting negative lenses in the reference beam channels as indicated. The whole instrument is mounted on a framework which allows the illuminating beam to be rotated relative to the flow, the collection optics remaining fixed. This means that the Doppler frequency and the size of the measuring region are adjustable parameters. Systems of this type are particularly suitable for use with large-scale flow rigs such as wind tunnels.

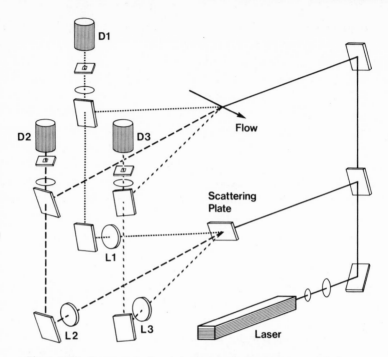

Figure 2.2.8. Arrangement for measuring three velocity components simultaneously. L1, L2, and L3 are negative lenses and D1, D2, and D3 are photodetectors.

Nearly all instruments designed for the simultaneous measurement of three components of velocity employ three separate detectors. It is possible, however, to make an instrument which uses only a single detector, providing, of course, that the angles between the beams are chosen so that the ranges of Doppler frequencies associated with the three separate velocity components are different. Separation of the three-component signals is then achieved by electronic filtering. Such a velocimeter has been designed by Hallermeier (1973) for measuring underwater waves.

There are many laboratory situations in which one only requires two components of velocity, e.g., in Reynolds stress investigations, in which the variation of the cross product $E(u_1u_2)$ is to be measured. In this case the optics becomes much simpler. Bourke *et al.* (1971) have used a two-component heterodyne system for measuring Reynolds stresses. By making use of the fact that two beams linearly polarized at right angles do not interfere, one can devise a two-component real fringe instrument which has two sets of orthogonally polarized interference fringes within the measuring volume. Various ways have been proposed for implementing this idea (Brayton *et al.*, 1973; Blake, 1972*b*; Bossel *et al.*, 1972*b*). The laser beam can be split into three components which are polarized in directions 0°, 45°, and 90°, and all three beams can be brought to a focus in the flow with a single lens. This produces two patterns plane-polarized in directions 0° and 90°, and the beam splitting is generally arranged so that these are orientated at right angles. The two signals produced by the passage of scattering particles are separated by polaroids in front of the two detectors so that each detector effectively observes only one fringe pattern. The method relies on the fact that the scattered light will be plane-polarized in the same direction as the incident radiation, which does not strictly apply. Also side walls and the characteristics of the flowing fluid can affect the polarization. This means that there is a tendency for the two optical channels to interfere. Blake (1972*a*) has suggested that a simple means of overcoming this problem is the use of two separate colors rather than beams polarized in different directions. The two colors can be emitted simultaneously from, for example, an argon–ion laser and separated using optical filters.

Effect of Side Walls

It was stated earlier that laser anemometers have been most successful in the measurement of liquid flows. The laser beams then have to pass from air through the side walls of the container into the flowing liquid, thus undergoing refraction due to the change in refractive index. On detection, the refraction process will effectively be reversed. To save unnecessary complication in the descriptions of the various optical geometries we have assumed that the instruments were being used in air. We now ask the question: How is the Doppler frequency affected by a change in refractive index?

The situation is depicted in Figure 2.2.9. Typically the side walls will be flat and of uniform thickness, with a refractive index greater than the liquid. For example $n_{\text{air}} \simeq 1$, $n_{\text{glass}} \simeq 1.5$, $n_{\text{water}} \simeq 1.3$. For a given velocity, the Doppler frequency in both the heterodyne and real fringe systems is determined by the half-angle θ between the beams at their point of intersection, the refractive index n_f of the fluid, and the free-space wavelength λ, this last term being constant for a given light source. If the angle between each beam and the optical axis is θ_a in air, then, taking $n_{\text{air}} = 1$, we obtain $\sin \theta = \sin \theta_a / n_f$, irrespective of the refractive index of the side wall. Thus, the Doppler

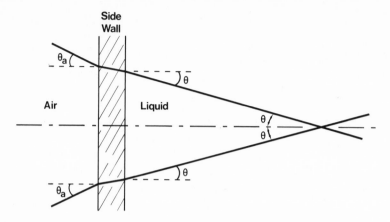

Figure 2.2.9. Schematic representation of the refraction of beams as they pass from air into a liquid, through the side walls of the container.

frequency can be written as

$$f_0 = (2U \sin \theta_a)/\lambda \tag{2.2.11}$$

and we end up with the convenient result that the Doppler frequency will be independent of the refractive index of both the side walls and the fluid. In more complex situations this result might not apply, particularly if the side walls are not of uniform thickness, in which case there will be a lens effect.

An important consideration in laser anemometry, to be dealt with more fully later, is that of spatial resolution. Normally, one would like the observation volume to be as small as possible. In general the size of the observation volume in the direction of the optical axis is greater for small intersection angles, so an increase in the refractive index of the liquid leads to a poorer spatial resolution.

Frequency Shifting

There are numerous important flow situations in which the velocities are continuously reversing in direction between positive and negative values. Water waves and flow behind a step are but two examples. All the systems described so far produce signals with the same Doppler frequency regardless of whether the scattering particles are moving in the forward or reverse direction and are thus unable to resolve this sign ambiguity. This point can most easily be visualized by considering a real fringe system. With $y = 0$ in equation (2.2.7), for example, one obtains the same temporal variation in intensity when $x = Ut$ as when $x = -Ut$, the pattern being symmetric about the y axis. It is sometimes possible to incorporate facilities in the electronic processing system for dealing with this situation, but these generally work satisfactorily only when the velocity variations are more or less periodic. A system devised for measuring under periodic water waves will be described in Chapter 6. For a versatile instrument which will resolve sign ambiguity it is necessary to include some form of frequency shifting device into the optics. Three methods for performing this will be described below.

The most readily available frequency shifters are Bragg cells. The principles on which these work have already been described in Chapter 1. If the laser beam is incident on the Bragg cell at an angle θ_I equal to the Bragg angle θ_B, then it is possible to diffract nearly all (up to 90% in the most favorable conditions) of the light into a first-order mode. The diffracted ray emerges at the same angle to the normal and is shifted in frequency by an amount ω_s, the frequency of the acoustic wave. Typically for a water cell ω_s is of the order 20 mHz, which is at the top of the range of most signal analyzing systems, so generally some method of reducing the frequency is needed. This can be done in one of two ways. Either a single Bragg cell is used in the optics and the resulting electronic signal shifted down by mixing with a VCO (*voltage-controlled oscillators*) or, alternatively, two cells can be used.

Single Bragg cell configurations have been described by a number of authors, e.g., Mazumder (1970); Lanz *et al.* (1971). In a real fringe configuration the cell is placed in one beam, as indicated in Figure 2.2.10. Some type of mask is needed to allow only the first-order beam to pass. In order to maintain symmetry it is desirable that both beams pass through equal size apertures. A mirror is required for realigning the beam which emerges from the cell. For optimum efficiency the beam splitter should be adjusted to give beams of equal intensity incident on the mask. The frequency shift which is superimposed on the Doppler frequency is simply equal to ω_s, i.e., it is

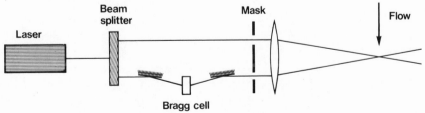

Figure 2.2.10. A real fringe geometry employing Bragg cell frequency shifting.

independent of the angle θ at which the focused beams converge. This also applies when a Bragg cell is used with a heterodyne configuration. In this case the cell can most conveniently be placed in the reference beam since this usually has to be attenuated in any case.

A simple way of reducing the frequencies and of introducing greater flexibility at the same time is to employ two Bragg cells, one in each beam. The driving frequencies are adjusted to slightly different values, the observed shift being equal to the difference between these two frequencies. Typically the driving frequencies might be 20 and 20.1 mHz, giving a 100-kHz shift. Generally the relative spectral width of a shifted beam will be extremely small and any resulting errors can be neglected. For example, Cummins *et al.* (1963) have produced frequency shifts with a spectral width of the order 4 kHz for a drive frequency of 25 mHz.

Probably the simplest and certainly the cheapest way of frequency shifting in an efficient manner is to use a rotating diffraction grating. Figure 2.2.11 shows the configuration which has generally been found most satisfactory. The laser beam is directed straight through a radial grating which rotates at constant angular velocity. All the emerging light is blocked except for the $+1$ and -1 orders which are focused into the measuring volume. If the direction of rotation is from the -1 to the $+1$ order as indicated, then the $+1$ order will be raised in frequency by an amount ω_s and the -1 order lowered in frequency by the same amount. From the Doppler principle, if V_g is the velocity at which the grating passes the beam, then

$$\omega_s = (V_g \sin \alpha_g)/\lambda$$

where α_g is the angle between the zero and $+1$ orders and λ the wavelength of the incident laser light. The difference in frequency between the $+1$ and -1 orders will be $2\omega_s$. Now α_g is set by the spacing d_g of the grating lines;

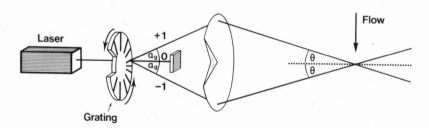

Figure 2.2.11. Frequency shifting using a rotating diffraction grating.

$\sin \alpha_g \, v \, \lambda/d_g$. The frequency difference will then be

$$2\omega_s = 2V_g/d_g \qquad (2.2.12)$$

and the Doppler frequency will be

$$\omega_0 = \frac{2V_g}{d_g} + \frac{2U \sin \theta}{\lambda} \qquad (2.2.13)$$

Notice that the frequency shift only depends on the rate at which the grating lines pass the beam.

There are several variations of the system shown in Figure 2.2.11. For example, the grating can be imaged directly into the flow, retaining all the orders, or, alternatively, only the zero and $+1$ (or -1) orders may be used. In either of these two cases note that the frequency ω_0 is half that given by equation (2.2.13). Also, of course, a rotating grating can be used in the heterodyne mode. Mazumder (1970) describes a system which uses a reflection grating fitted around the perimeter of a rotating disc. This acts essentially in the same way as the transmission grating and can be easily made by bending an ordinary grating replica. The method introduces practical difficulties though. First, the grating replica has to be joined at some point around the perimeter; it is not easy to do this without introducing a phase jump in the periodicity of the grating lines. Second, the amount of light reflected back into the laser cavity can be high enough to produce undesirable resonance effects and to affect the coherence properties of the beam.

When using a radial diffraction grating one must remember that the finite radius of the grating disc will result in a spread of the Doppler frequency. This is because the rulings are closer at points nearer the center of the grating, and hence the Doppler frequency is higher for a given flow velocity. As the beam must extend over a finite distance in the radial direction there will be different Doppler frequencies associated with different regions of the beam. This effect is minimized by making the ratio R_g/r_u as large as possible, R_g being the distance between the beam center and the center of the grating and r_u, the beam radius. This means in practice that radial gratings of quite large diameter are needed, typically 15 or 20 cm. The frequency shift, on the other hand, only depends on the number of rulings that pass the beam per second. This depends only on the angular velocity of rotation and the total number of rulings on the grating, i.e., it is independent of the radius.

Another way of mechanically producing a frequency shift is to use a rotating scattering plate. In the three-component arrangement shown in Figure 2.2.8, for example, the static scattering plate can simply be replaced by a ground glass disc rotated by a synchronous motor. One is then directly comparing the velocities of the particles in the flow with the constant velocity of the disc at the point of scattering. Normally the disc is aligned so that velocity at the point where the reference beam is scattered is in the same direction as the mean flow velocity. A rather simpler geometry operating on the same principle is described by Hiller and Meier (1972). Their arrangement eliminates the need for a beam splitter. The laser beam is focused directly onto the scattering disc, which takes the form of a disc of thin Plexiglas or polyethylene foil. This is such that the main part of the beam penetrates without deflection, only a small proportion being scattered by the inhomogeneities. Both main beam and scattered light together are then brought to a focus in the flow with a second lens. Light scattered from the focal spot in the flow is now already mixed with light scattered from the rotating disc. Three detectors are used to observe the component Doppler frequencies, and the frequency shifts are adjusted by altering the speed of rotation of the disc.

The main practical difficulty in both the radial grating and rotating scattering disc arrangements is in producing an absolutely constant speed of rotation. Any slight unsteadiness or vibration will show up on the Doppler signal and will introduce measurement inaccuracies. One can often avoid the necessity for delicate balancing of the mechanism by arranging for rotation to be in the horizontal rather than the vertical plane although this is not generally convenient from the point of view of optical layout.

Electro-optic cells, either liquid Kerr cells or certain electro-optic crystals, can be used for frequency shifting. As with the acousto-optic Bragg cell, no moving parts are involved, so potentially there are advantages over the rotating grating although as yet it appears that not all of the practical difficulties have been overcome. Some possible schemes are described by Drain and Moss (1972). In these a rotating electric field is generated either in one or in a series of cells by applying sinusoidal electric potentials with appropriate phase relationship. A plane-polarized laser beam is converted to circular polarization with a quarter-wave plate before passing through the electro-optic cell configuration and is either upshifted or downshifted in frequency depending upon whether the two fields have the same or opposite sense of rotation. The frequency shift is equal to twice the rotational frequency of the applied field. Electro-optic cells have the advantage that they can be made to work approximately in the range 1 kHz to 100 mHz, which is convenient for most LDV systems. On the other hand, they tend to give a much broader frequency spectrum than Bragg cells, which is undesirable. Efficiency is higher than with a diffraction grating and of course the absence of any mechanical moving parts allows easy adjustment of the frequency shift.

An electro-optic technique for frequency shifting which appears simpler to implement has been proposed by Foord *et al.* (1974). This can be described more correctly as phase shifting although the overall effect is the same as with the other methods. With a real fringe system incorporating a frequency shifter one can picture the fringes as moving continuously across the measuring region with a constant translation velocity. The frequency shift corresponds to the number of fringes per second passing a fixed spatial position and is an upwards shift in frequency if the fringes move in the reverse direction to the flow and a downward shift if they move with the flow. With phase shifting, on the other hand, the fringes are made to move in a cyclical manner over a distance of one fringe spacing. The motion in the forward direction is at constant velocity and the flyback time to the initial position is made as short as possible. This motion is indicated diagrammatically in Figure 2.2.12; d_f being the distance between two consecutive fringes, f_s the frequency shift, and T_f the flyback time. In a real fringe system the motion is implemented by using two electro-optic crystals, one in each beam, driven in opposite phase sense by a sawtooth electrical potential. The correct value of the peak voltage to be applied can easily be found by expanding the fringe pattern by using a short-focal-length lens and observing this visually on a screen. When the voltage is correct the image will appear uniformly bright.

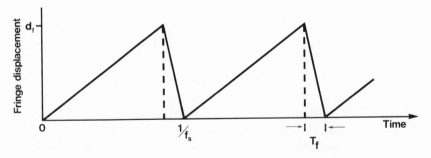

Figure 2.2.12. Sawtooth waveform of the fringe motion when optical phase shifting is employed.

Low-Frequency Suppression

If no frequency shifting is used, the low-frequency components in LDV signals can have a range which overlaps and distorts the Doppler signal, so hindering analysis. Generally speaking this arises either when there is a very high turbulence level or when there are only a few fringes in the measuring volume. The situation is discussed in greater detail in Section 3.2. At constant velocity or low turbulence level the unwanted low-frequency components are well separated from the Doppler frequencies and can be filtered off electronically. This is not possible though when the turbulence level becomes very high.

Using polarized beams makes it possible to eliminate the low-frequency component within the optics. Suitable optical arrangements have been described by Bossel et al. (1972a) and Vasilenko et al. (1972b). The two beams focused down to the measuring point are polarized at right angles, i.e., at 0° and 90°. The +45° and −45° components of these two beams interfere to form effectively two interference patterns which can be observed independently by using polarization filters aligned at either +45° or −45°. These two patterns are 180° out of phase, so by using two separate photodetectors preceded by polarization filters aligned at +45° and −45°, two signals are observed that have the same amplitude but are 180° out of phase. The low-frequency component is eliminated by subtracting the two signals with a difference amplifier.

Systems giving low-frequency suppression can conveniently be set up by a Wollaston prism for beam splitting. As with the two velocity component schemes which employ polarized light beams, the method relies on the assumption that the planes of polarization are unchanged by the scattering process.

2.3. Fabry–Perot Method

An alternative approach to laser Doppler anemometry is to measure the frequency shift of the scattered laser light directly by optical means. This method is only applicable to very-high-velocity flows since the shifts are otherwise excessively small compared with the optical frequencies. Jackson and Paul (1970 and 1971) have described experiments using an optical configuration essentially the same as the one depicted in Figure 2.2.1, the main difference being that the detector is replaced by a *confocal Fabry–Perot interferometer.* In this case the reference beam acts simply as a zero-frequency masker from which the Doppler shift in the radiation scattered from the illuminating beam is measured. As the axis of the Fabry–Perot coincides with the reference beam axis the angle 2θ between the two beams defines the frequency-to-velocity conversion constant. The factor which limits application to the measurement of low velocities is the finite spectral resolution of the interferometer. Typically one might have a frequency shift of 500 mHz at supersonic velocities, which would require an instrumental band width of the order 5 mHz, which corresponds to a very-high-resolution instrument. Conventional plane Fabry–Perots have resolutions of the order 100 mHz. Even this is difficult to maintain except under carefully controlled conditions. On the other hand, confocal systems can be obtained with resolutions of the order 1 mHz.

The Fabry–Perot acts essentially as a narrow-band optical filter whose center frequency can be altered by changing the spacing between the mirrors. The filter frequency is controlled by the sawtooth waveform from an oscilloscope which also controls the X axis of the display, the Y display being the output from the detector in the interferometer. A complete arrangement for signal collection is shown in Figure 2.3.1. The display gives a peak at the Doppler frequency as the Fabry–Perot is scanned across the range in the

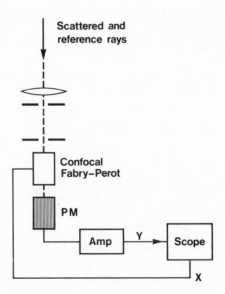

Figure 2.3.1. Signal collection using a Fabry–Perot interferometer (PM is a photomultiplier).

same manner as the wave analyzer display in a real fringe or heterodyne LDV.

The method of signal detection makes it an advantage to have the Doppler frequency as high as possible. Increasing the angle between the beams (Figure 2.2.1) has the effect of raising the frequency and at the same time improving the spatial resolution. For this reason spatial resolution can generally be made very high in a Fabry–Perot system. Another advantage is that there is no directional ambiguity, thus the need for frequency shifting devices is eliminated.

It is possible, at least in theory, to make a Fabry–Perot system which produces a continuous trace of the instantaneous velocity. The interferometer is made to scan rapidly across the spectrum so that the velocity fluctuations show up as fluctuations in the position of the spectrum peak. Two different mechanisms for producing such rapid scans have been proposed. Cooper and Greig (1963) have constructed an etalon which is driven at resonance by an applied oscillatory voltage. Their system was of the plane etalon type but could be adapted to a confocal arrangement. Another rather simpler scheme employing a rotating shutter has been described by Paul and Jackson (1971), who indicate that their instrument should be capable of tracking velocity fluctuations of frequency up to 1 mHz. For continuous velocity measurement a voltage output is required which is proportional to the frequency at which the spectrum has a peak. This is best obtained by first differentiating the spectrum display signal so that a zero crossing in the differentiated signal corresponds to the spectrum peak, regardless of the height in the spectral peak. This is then converted to a signal proportional to the frequency at which the zero crossing occurs, by means of a zero-crossing discriminator.

2.4. *Comparison of Systems*

The optical setups which have been described all have their own particular merits and shortcomings, and there are numerous variations which could be devised to meet specific requirements. The question is, how does one decide on the most suitable arrangement for a given experimental situation? In this section we will summarize some of the most important practical features on which a comparison can be based. The choice will be dependent on the method of signal analysis and the type of photodetector to be used. If photon correlation methods are to be used for signal processing (these will be discussed in detail in Chapter 4) photomultipliers are required, adjusted for single photon response. This results in extreme sensitivity and means that the optical efficiency of the system becomes of less importance, e.g., loss of intensity through beam splitters and other components can be tolerated. If analogue processing methods are to be used, then one can have either a photodiode or photomultiplier as detector, the latter generally being the more sensitive. In this case the electrical signal must dominate over the shot noise. Thus, producing a high signal level becomes one of the major objectives.

For photon correlation analysis the two-beam optical configurations give outputs which are more easy to interpret. Generally speaking, they are more robust in operation and are insensitive to vibrations or changes in scattering particle characteristics. Thus they are particularly well suited to many industrial situations or, more generally, to measurements in hostile environments. The strongest signals appear to be obtained with two circular spots of light in the flow rather than with two narrow slits, but unfortunately the former geometry raises problems of alignment. If, for example, the turbulence level is very high or the line joining the two spots is rotated relative to the mean flow direction, then only a small proportion of the particles passing the first beam will also pass through the second, so the signal will be lost. It seems, however, that the full potentials of the two-beam methods have not yet been fully realized. Lading (1973), for example, has shown that it is possible to separate out the velocities of different size particles in a flow and it will also be shown in Chapter 4 that information on Lagrangian time scales of turbulence can be obtained.

Of the LDV schemes, the real fringe geometries seem to offer the most advantages and hence have become the most popular. In nearly all practical situations they provide a better signal-to-noise ratio at the output than do the heterodyne schemes and also offer ease of alignment in that the transmission and detection units are essentially independent. On the other hand, the heterodyne method allows for greater flexibility in the optical layout, e.g., only one beam need pass through the flow. Also by using two separate focusing lenses and a sharp angle of beam intersection it is possible to obtain a higher spatial resolution in the direction of flow. Actually if the very highest spatial resolution is required, the most satisfactory method is to use a real fringe method with the scattered light collected at an angle to the axis of the transmission optics. This reduces the size of the measuring volume along the axis which is normally much greater than the size in the flow direction. Backscattering with a single lens for transmission and collection is intuitively the most attractive scheme since no alignment is required once the instrument has been made. The only major disadvantage here seems to be that very high laser powers are required. To give some idea of powers, it is quite common when measuring with a forward-scatter system in unseeded tap water to use a 1-mW HeNe laser with a photodiode detector. This power is also sufficient in low-speed unseeded air flow if photon correlation is used. For supersonic air flow in backscatter one would typically require a 1-W laser power with the photon correlation method. Analogue methods of analysis would be impractical in this extreme situation.

An LDV becomes a very much more flexible instrument if a frequency shift facility is incorporated. In reversing-flow situations an upward shift of sufficient value is used to ensure that the Doppler frequencies never become negative. In high-turbulence flows upward frequency shifting has the effect of reducing the relative size of the frequency fluctuations as compared with the mean frequency. This makes frequency tracking easier. In very-high-speed flows a downward shift is sometimes required to bring the frequencies within the range of the signal analyzing equipment. The two Bragg cell method probably produces the best quality signals and is now wisely used. It is expensive, however, and also difficult to align since the cells must be oriented exactly at the Bragg angle for maximum efficiency. Optical efficiency is high, of the order of 75%. The rotating grating method is the cheapest and produces very good quality signals if only small shifts are needed, say, of the order 100 kHz. Optical efficiency tends to be low, of the order 20% if only the $+1$ and -1 orders are used. Alignment, on the other hand, causes no difficulties. Electro-optic cells potentially offer a very powerful means of frequency shifting but are less popular than rotating gratings or acousto-optic cells primarily because they are expensive and tend to give inferior signal quality. Efficiency lies somewhere between the other two methods. Electro-optic cells are most easily used in a phase shifting mode.

With a Fabry–Perot interferometer the velocity range at the upper end becomes virtually unlimited, but the scheme becomes impractical for velocities below about 500 msec^{-1} because of the poor spectral resolution. The system is also expensive and cumbersome, so arranging for scanning of the flow volume can be a problem.

2.5. Long-Range and Microscopic Measurements

Although the vast majority of practical applications have been concerned with the study of velocities in flow regions of the order of 1 cm to

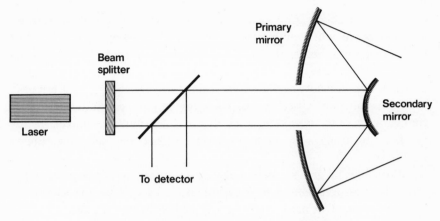

Figure 2.5.1. Mirror arrangement for a long-range LDV.

1 m in size, special-purpose LDV systems have been developed also for measuring at long ranges in the atmosphere and for measuring on microscopic scales. The principles involved are the same, but at these scales many new practical difficulties arise.

Considering the problems of long-range measurement first, obviously some of the major difficulties arise because of the large sizes of the optical components. Generally the beams are projected more or less vertically into the atmosphere from a ground station and operate in backscatter mode. Lenses of impractical size are avoided by using a concave mirror both for focusing the beams and also for collecting the scattered light. Various schemes are possible, but usually the laser beam is split and passed through an opening in the center of the mirror. A small secondary mirror then deflects the beams onto the large primary mirror as indicated in Figure 2.5.1. This is essentially an adaptation of the Cassegrain telescope, and one could in fact equally well devise an adaptation of a Newtonian telescope (Born and Wolf, 1959). In Figure 2.5.1 we have indicated only one means of collecting the scattered light. There are a number of other possibilities, e.g., a plane mirror with two apertures can be used, as in the scheme depicted in Figure 2.2.7. Farmer and Brayton (1971) and Hughes *et al.* (1972) both describe complete systems, and the latter authors give results of measurements recorded at a range of 50 m. These compare very well with measurements taken with a conventional propeller anemometer located at the same place. Obviously at these ranges very high laser powers are needed, e.g., Hughes *et al.* used a 5-W CO_2 laser for their measurements.

When the observation volume is formed by focusing two laser beams into the flow region, then the size of the measuring region is determined by the diffraction-limited spot size of the focused beams. At great distances this can be excessively large if a beam expander is not employed before focusing. This difficulty can be overcome by forming the fringe pattern from two nonparallel unfocused beams. These can be produced either by using a configuration of the type indicated in Figure 1.4.2a (with the mirror slightly tilted) or by using a prism beam splitter of the type shown in Figure 1.4.2d.

Probably the greatest potential of laser anemometry lies in its application to measurements in biology because it has the unique features of being noncontact in nature and also adaptable to the microscopic scales involved in this area of fluid dynamics. A major problem in this situation is the correct alignment of the probing volume within the flow region. An approach for dealing with this has been described by Mishina and Asakura (1974); they refer to their instrument as a laser Doppler microscope. In essence an ordinary microscope with white light illumination is combined with a real fringe LDV operating in backscatter, which allows the operator visually to align the probing position on the specimen. The authors succeeded in measuring a velocity profile across a flow cell of only 1-mm section.

2.6. *Analysis of Optical Configurations*

In this section we shall present a rigorous analysis for the signal generation in specified LDV configurations. In particular we shall derive expressions for the optical field distributions, size of observation volume, and finally the photocurrent amplitude arising in the heterodyne and real fringe systems.

We shall first briefly discuss some preliminaries on the scattering of light by small particles and on the intensity profile of a focused laser beam. These are necessary for establishing later results. Throughout this section we shall consider the refractive index of any medium through which light propagates for the LDV to be unity. Any other value of the refractive index may be easily included, as shown in Section 2.2.

As stated in Section 2.1, if a stationary (spherical) particle is placed in a planar optical field $\mathscr{E}(\mathbf{r})$, where $\mathbf{r}$ denotes the position of the particle, then the far-field scattered radiation at any other point $(\mathbf{r}_1)$ can be determined from Mie scattering theory (Van de Hulst, 1957; Kerker 1969). To a first approximation

$$\mathscr{E}(\mathbf{r}_1) = \frac{\sigma \mathscr{E}(\mathbf{r})}{jk|\mathbf{r}_1 - \mathbf{r}|} e^{jk|\mathbf{r}_1 - r|} \tag{2.6.1}$$

where $\lambda = 2\pi/k$ is the wavelength of incident radiation and σ denotes the (scattering) *amplitude function* of the particle and is a dimensionless factor. The exact expression for σ consists of a series of Legendre polynomials, which are too complicated to be included here. Suffice it to say that σ is a function of the wavelength λ and the diameter of the scattering particle. Effects of scattering on the polarization of the field at $\mathbf{r}_1$ are considered in detail by Eliasson and Dandliker (1974).

In the following analysis equation (2.6.1) will be freely employed under the assumption that the scattering centers present in the flow for a laser velocimeter setup are, though random in size, approximately spherical. This is accurate for most seeded flows, and largely true for unseeded gas flows. For an ensemble of scattering particles σ will obviously be a random variable.

When an unapertured laser beam is brought to a focus, it converges to a diffraction-limited spot, such that, to a close approximation, the radiation wavefronts in the vicinity of the focus may be considered as plane and parallel. The intensity distribution near the focal point is Gaussian, and can be expressed as (Kogelnik, 1965)

$$I(x, y, z) = I_0 \exp \left\{ -\frac{x^2 + y^2}{r_0^2[1 + (\lambda z/\pi r_0^2)^2]} \right\} \tag{2.6.2}$$

$$\simeq I_0 \exp \left(-\frac{x^2 + y^2}{r_0^2} \right) \tag{2.6.3}$$

where the focal point is at the origin of the coordinate system, and I_0 represents the (maximum) intensity there. The waist radius r_0 of the beam at focus is

$$r_0 = 2\lambda/\pi\Delta\theta = (\lambda/\pi)(f/2r_u) \tag{2.6.4}$$

where $2r_0$ is the diffraction-limited beam diameter at $1/e$ points of the intensity distribution; f is the focal length of the beam-focusing lens; $2r_u$ is the unfocused beam diameter at $1/e$ points of the intensity distribution (i.e., the radius of the beam in the front focal plane of the lens), and is $1/\sqrt{2}$ times the radius at $1/e^2$ points; $\Delta\theta$ is the far-field convergence angle of the beam.

Then the field distribution of a focused laser beam may be expressed as

$$\mathscr{E}(x, y, z) = \mathscr{E}_0 \exp \left(jkz - \frac{x^2 + y^2}{2r_0^2} \right) \tag{2.6.5}$$

with

$$\mathscr{E}_0 = I_0^{1/2} \, e^{-j2\pi vt}$$

and v is the optical frequency of laser light. In the following analysis the $e^{-j2\pi vt}$ term will be omitted since it does not make any significant contribution.

Real Fringe Systems

Figure 2.6.1 is a simplified diagram for a real fringe optical configuration. Two (identically) plane-polarized and coherent beams are brought to a focus at F_0, where they cross the optical axis (z) at an angle θ. The wavefronts of the beams, considered as planar near F_0, interfere to form parallel planes of adjacent bright and dark illumination or interference fringes. Thus a bright fringe plane is produced by two wave crests that propagate in phase, while a dark fringe is created by two out-of-phase wavefronts.

For a real fringe system the (two) beam intensities are identical. The flow is considered as being along the x axis, with the y axis normal to the plane of paper; (x_1, y_1, z_1) and (x_2, y_2, z_2) are coordinates referred to the directions of propagation of the beams. Transformation of the coordinates of any point between the three orientations is as follows:

$$x_1 = x \cos\theta - z \sin\theta$$
$$z_1 = z \cos\theta + x \sin\theta$$
$$x_2 = x \cos\theta + z \sin\theta \qquad (2.6.6)$$
$$z_2 = z \cos\theta - x \sin\theta$$
$$y_1 = y_2 = y$$

The receiving optics consists of a converging lens which images the beam crossover region (observation volume) on to the detector. As stated in Section 2.2, the direct light from the laser beams is generally blocked off on the detection side of the observation volume so that only scattered radiation reaches the photodetector. We shall consider the receiving optics to be aligned with the optical axis. Identical results are obtained when scattered radiation is collected at an angle to the optical axis such as in Figure 2.2.6, provided the angle (2θ) between the beams is small.

Consider a stationary scattering particle located at $P(x, y, z)$ (Figure 2.6.1), whose amplitude (scattering) function is σ. Let $\mathscr{E}_1(x_1, y_1, z_1)$ and

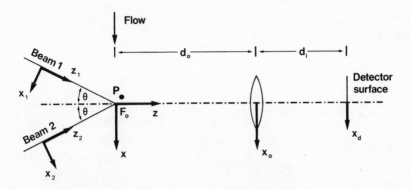

Figure 2.6.1. Notation used for a real fringe optical system.

$\mathscr{E}_2(x_2, y_2, z_2)$ be the radiation incident on the particle due to beams 1 and 2, respectively, where (x_1, y_1, z_1) and (x_2, y_2, z_2) are the coordinates of P in terms of two-coordinate systems, which are related through equation (2.6.6). Then at any point $Q(x_0, y_0)$ on the plane incident on the converging lens, the field scattered by the particle due to incident radiation $\mathscr{E}_1$ is given by

$$\mathscr{E}_{1s}(x_0, y_0) = \frac{\sigma \mathscr{E}_1(x_1, y_1, z_1)\, e^{jks_0}}{jkd_0} \qquad (2.6.7)$$

where

$$s_0 = d_0 + \frac{1}{2d_0}(x - x_0)^2 + \frac{1}{2d_0}(y - y_0)^2$$

Immediately behind the lens, the scattered field due to $\mathscr{E}_1$ is

$$\mathscr{E}'_{1s}(x_0, y_0) = \mathscr{E}_{1s}(x_0, y_0)P(x_0, y_0) \exp\left[-j\frac{k}{2f}(x_0^2 + y_0^2)\right] \qquad (2.6.8)$$

where $P(x_0, y_0)$ denotes the lens pupil function and f its focal length. For our analysis, we consider the lens aperture as large compared to the beam intersection region, thus $P(x_0, y_0) = 1, \forall (x_0, y_0)$.

From equation (2.6.7) the scattered field due to $\mathscr{E}_1$ on any point (x', y') on the detector surface is

$$\mathscr{E}_{1s}(x', y') = \int\int_{-\infty}^{\infty} \frac{\mathscr{E}'_{1s}(x_0, y_0)\, e^{jks'}}{j\lambda d_i}\, dx_0\, dy_0 \qquad (2.6.9)$$

when

$$s' = d_i + \frac{1}{2d_i}(x' - x_0)^2 + \frac{1}{2d_i}(y' - y_0)^2$$

Substituting equations (2.6.7) and (2.6.8) into (2.6.9) and performing the desired integrations, we have

$$\mathscr{E}_{1s}(x', y') = -2\pi \frac{\sigma}{k^2} \frac{d_i}{d_0} \mathscr{E}_1(x_1, y_1, z_1)$$

$$\times \exp\left[jk(d_i + d_0) + j\frac{k}{2d_i}\left(x'^2 + x^2\frac{d_i}{d_0}\right) + j\frac{k}{2d_i}\left(y'^2 + y^2\frac{d_i}{d_0}\right) \right]$$

$$\times \delta\left(x' + \frac{xd_i}{d_0}, y' + \frac{yd_i}{d_0}\right) \qquad (2.6.10)$$

where $\delta(x, y)$ denotes a delta function. To derive equation (2.6.10) we use the fact that $1/d_i + 1/d_0 = 1/f$.

Conducting an analysis similar to the above, we find that the scattered radiation incident at any point on the photodetector due to light scattered by the particle from beam 2 is given by

$$\mathscr{E}_{2s}(x', y') = -2\pi \frac{\sigma}{k^2}\left(\frac{d_i}{d_0}\right) \mathscr{E}_2(x_2, y_2, z_2)$$

$$\times \exp\left[jk(d_i + d_0) + j\frac{k}{2d_i}\left(x'^2 + x^2\frac{d_i}{d_0}\right) + j\frac{k}{2d_i}\left(y'^2 + y^2\frac{d_i}{d_0}\right) \right]$$

$$\times \delta\left(x' + \frac{xd_i}{d_0}, y' + \frac{yd_i}{d_0}\right) \qquad (2.6.11)$$

In the real fringe geometry, *only* scattered radiation is collected by the receiving optics, and all the incident radiation is blocked off. As such, the field at any point (x', y') on the photodetector surface is given by equations (2.6.10) and (2.6.11) as

$$\mathscr{E}_D(x', y') = \mathscr{E}_{1s}(x', y') + \mathscr{E}_{2s}(x', y') \qquad (2.6.12)$$

The integrated intensity over the detector surface is

$$\int_s |\mathscr{E}_D|^2 \, dA$$

and the photocurrent generated by this field is

$$i_F = \eta \int_s |\mathscr{E}_D|^2 \, dA$$

where η is the sensitivity of the photodetector, which is usually a function of the wavelength of the incident radiation, and S is the surface area of the detector, which in general is much larger than the image of the beam inter-section region. (It is common practice to place a pinhole in front of the detector to make its effective area just greater than the image size. Less of the light originating from outside the observation volume can then fall onto the detector surface.) Hence

$$i_F = \eta \int\limits_{-\infty}^{\infty}\int |\mathscr{E}_{1s}(x', y') + \mathscr{E}_{2s}(x', y')|^2 \, dx' \, dy'$$

Substituting equations (2.6.10) and (2.6.11) into the above equation, we have

$$i_F = \eta\left(2\pi\frac{M\sigma}{k^2}\right)^2 [|\mathscr{E}_1(x_1, y_1, z_1)|^2 + |\mathscr{E}_2(x_2, y_2, z_2)|^2$$
$$+ 2\,\text{Re}\,[\mathscr{E}_1(x_1, y_1, z_1)\mathscr{E}_2^*(x_2, y_2, z_2)]]$$

where * denotes complex conjugate and $M\ (=d_i/d_0)$ is the magnification factor of the receiving optics.

According to Mie scattering theory, for small values of θ and for spherical scattering particles, we have

$$\lambda^2\sigma/\pi = C_{sc} \qquad (2.6.13)$$

where C_{sc} is called the *scattering cross section* of the particle (Kerker, 1969). Hence

$$i_F = \eta(\tfrac{1}{2}MC_{sc})^2[|\mathscr{E}_1(x_1, y_1, z_1)|^2 + |\mathscr{E}_2(x_2, y_2, z_2)|^2$$
$$+ 2\,\text{Re}\,[\mathscr{E}_1(x_1, y_1, z_1)\mathscr{E}_2^*(x_2, y_2, z_2)]] \qquad (2.6.14)$$

It is worth stating that identical results hold for the photocurrent if fringes are formed at the observation point without the aid of a focusing lens (as indicated in Section 2.2), provided the wavefronts in the interference region are planar.

Heterodyne Systems

A simplified layout for a heterodyne system is given in Figure 2.6.2. We will assume that there is no converging lens on the receiving side (unlike the real fringe systems), and the reference beam is directly incident on the photodetector surface. Two unapertured laser beams called the reference and illuminating beams are brought to focus at F_0 either with two separate lenses as shown in Figure 2.2.1 or with a single lens (Figure 2.2.3). At F_0 they cross the optical axis z at an angle θ. Near F_0 the wavefronts of the two

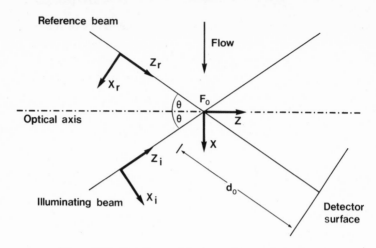

Figure 2.6.2. Notation used for heterodyne configuration.

beams are planar, and they meet to form an interference pattern. The intensity of the reference beam is considerably less than that of the illuminating beam.

As shown the photodetector is aligned with the reference beam axis (z_r) (Figures 2.2.1 and 2.6.2). The flow takes place along the x axis, while the y axis appears normal to the plane of the paper. (x_i, y_i, z_i) and (x_r, y_r, z_r) represent the orientation of the coordinate systems for the illuminating and reference beams. They are related to the coordinate system of the flow through a set of equations identical to equation (2.6.6), where r replaces 1 and i replaces 2.

Presence of a scattering particle in the vicinity of the beam cross section leads to scattered radiation which is collected by the photodetector. Thus if $\mathscr{E}_i$ and $\mathscr{E}_r$ represents the fields incident on the particle due to the illuminating and reference beams, then the scattered field at any point (x', y') on the photodetector surface consists of

$$\mathscr{E}_{is}(x', y') = \frac{\sigma}{jkd_0} \mathscr{E}_i \, e^{jks_1} \tag{2.6.15}$$

and

$$\mathscr{E}_{rs}(x', y') = \frac{\sigma}{jkd_0} \mathscr{E}_r \, e^{jks_1} \tag{2.6.16}$$

where

$$s_1 = d_0 + \frac{1}{2d_0}(x_r - x')^2 + \frac{1}{2d_0}(y_r - y')^2$$

and σ is the amplitude (scattering) function of the particle located at (x_r, y_r, z_r) in terms of the reference beam coordinate system. It is worth noting that (x', y', d_0) refer to coordinates of any point on the photodetector in terms of the reference beam coordinate system.

The total field incident at any point on the photodetector is

$$\mathscr{E}_D(x', y') = \mathscr{E}_r(x', y') + \mathscr{E}_{is}(x', y') + \mathscr{E}_{rs}(x', y')$$

where $\mathscr{E}_r(x', y')$ is the direct field due to the reference beam. Thus the photocurrent is given by the surface integral

$$i_T = \eta \int_s |\mathscr{E}_D|^2 \, dA$$

$$= \eta \int_s (|\mathscr{E}_r|^2 + |\mathscr{E}_{is}|^2 + |\mathscr{E}_{rs}|^2) \, dA + \eta \int_s (\mathscr{E}_r \mathscr{E}_{rs}^* + \mathscr{E}_r^* \mathscr{E}_{rs}) \, dA$$

$$+ \eta \int_s (\mathscr{E}_{rs} \mathscr{E}_{is}^* + \mathscr{E}_{rs}^* \mathscr{E}_{is}) \, dA + \eta \int_s (\mathscr{E}_r \mathscr{E}_{is}^* + \mathscr{E}_r^* \mathscr{E}_{is}) \, dA$$

$$= i_0 + i_{RH} + i_F + i_{DH} \tag{2.6.17}$$

where i_0 represents the contribution of the individual fields to the photocurrent, i_{RH} represents the current produced by the mixing (or heterodyning) of the reference beam with the light scattered from the reference beam (this term is not present if the reference beam passes round the outside of the flow region), i_F is the fringe current due to the heterodyning of the two scattered radiations, and i_{DH} is the so-called Doppler heterodyne current which arises from the mixing of the reference beam with the scattered field from the illuminating beam (Adrian and Goldstein, 1971).

Of these four contributions to the total current, only the Doppler heterodyne and fringe currents are of significance, since the other two contributions do not contain the Doppler frequency information. In all practical situations the intensity of the illuminating beam is far greater than that of the reference beam, which gives a very poor fringe contrast. Thus the amplitude of i_F is very small compared with the amplitude of i_{DH}, and for this reason the fringe current can be neglected. Considering the detector surface as large in comparison with the image of the beam intersection area, we have from equation (2.6.15)

$$\int_s \mathscr{E}_r \mathscr{E}_{is}^* \, dA = \int\int_{-\infty}^{\infty} \mathscr{E}_r(x', y') \mathscr{E}_{is}^*(x', y') \, dx' \, dy'$$

$$= \frac{2\pi\sigma}{k^2} \mathscr{E}_i^* \int\int_{-\infty}^{\infty} \frac{\mathscr{E}_r(x', y')}{-j\lambda d_0} e^{-jks_1} \, dx' \, dy' \qquad (2.6.18)$$

However, the integral represents the inverse propagation convolution (Mayo, 1970) of the reference field incident at any point (x', y') on the detector surface to the reference field incident on the particle at (x_r, y_r, z_r). Hence

$$\int_s \mathscr{E}_r \mathscr{E}_{is}^* \, dA = \frac{2\pi\sigma}{k^2} \mathscr{E}_i^*(x_i, y_i, z_i) \mathscr{E}_r(x_r, y_r, z_r) \qquad (2.6.19)$$

The Doppler heterodyne current is thus given by

$$i_{DH} = \frac{4\pi\sigma\eta}{k^2} \operatorname{Re} \left[\mathscr{E}_r(x_r, y_r, z_r) \mathscr{E}_i^*(x_i, y_i, z_i) \right]$$

where $\mathscr{E}_i(x_i, y_i, z_i)$ represents the illuminating field incident on the particle and $\mathscr{E}_r(x_r, y_r, z_r)$ is the reference beam field incident on the particle.

Employing the scattering cross section of the particle as defined in equation (2.6.13), we may write i_{DH} as

$$i_{DH} = \eta C_{sc} \operatorname{Re} \left[\mathscr{E}_r(x_r, y_r, z_r) \mathscr{E}_i^*(x_i, y_i, z_i) \right] \qquad (2.6.20)$$

Observation Volume

From the earlier analysis of this section it is possible to determine the interference volume for specific configurations and to derive expressions for the time-varying photocurrent when the scattering particle is considered as moving with the same velocity as the flow.

The interference volume or probe volume may be defined as the beam crossover region within which a scattering center would produce an appreciable photocurrent due to collective scattering from the two interfering beams.

Heterodyne System

In the heterodyne system two unapertured laser beams intersect at F_0 (Figure 2.6.2), and their field distribution in the vicinity of this focus is given by equation (2.6.5). Thus the field incident on a particle located at (x, y, z) due to the illuminating beam may be expressed as

$$\mathscr{E}_i(x_i, y_i, z_i) = \mathscr{E}_I \exp\left(-\frac{x_i^2 + y_i^2}{2r_0^2} + jkz_i\right) \qquad (2.6.21)$$

while the contribution to the incident field on the particle arising from the reference beam is given by

$$\mathscr{E}_r(x_r, y_r, z_r) = \mathscr{E}_R \exp\left(-\frac{x_r^2 + y_r^2}{2r_0^2} + jkz_r\right) \qquad (2.6.22)$$

where $\mathscr{E}_I^2$ and $\mathscr{E}_R^2$ are the intensity of the two beams at F_0. We have assumed here that both focal spots have the same radius r_0 at their point of intersection. Obviously (x_i, y_i, z_i) and (x_r, y_r, z_r) represent the coordinates of the particle location in terms of the axes of coordinates of the two beams such that

$$x_i = x \cos \theta + z \sin \theta \qquad x_r = x \cos \theta - z \sin \theta$$

$$z_i = z \cos \theta - x \sin \theta \qquad z_r = z \cos \theta + x \sin \theta \qquad (2.6.23)$$

$$y_i = y_r = y$$

From equation (2.6.20) the dual-scatter photocurrent caused by the presence of a single stationary particle near the beam crossover region is given by

$$i_{DH} = \eta C_{sc} \mathscr{E}_R \mathscr{E}_I \exp\left(-\frac{x_i^2 + y_i^2 + x_r^2 + y_r^2}{2r_0^2}\right) \cos k(z_i - z_r)$$

Substitution of equation (2.6.23) leads to

$$i_{DH} = \eta C_{sc} \exp\left(-\frac{x^2 \cos^2 \theta + z^2 \sin^2 \theta + y^2}{r_0^2}\right)[\mathscr{E}_R \mathscr{E}_I \cos(2kx \sin \theta)] \quad (2.6.24)$$

It may be seen from equation (2.6.24) that the heterodyne photocurrent is a maximum if the scattering particle is located at the focus $(0, 0, 0)$, and that it decays to approximately $1/e$ of its peak value if the scattering particle is located on the ellipsoid

$$x^2 \cos^2 \theta + z^2 \sin^2 \theta + y^2 = r_0^2 \qquad (2.6.25)$$

This ellipsoid defines the boundaries of the probe volume. Figure 2.6.3 illustrates a cross section of the probe volume in the beam crossover region. It also indicates the generation of the interference pattern. Figure 2.6.4 is the envelope of the probe volume defined by equation (2.6.25). The ellipsoid has

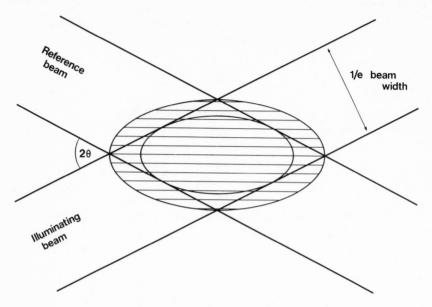

Figure 2.6.3. Beam intersection region in the heterodyne system. The inner ellipse represents equation (2.6.25) and the outer ellipse is the locus of points at which the signal falls to e^{-2} of its maximum value.

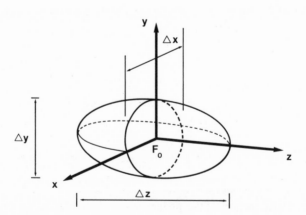

Figure 2.6.4. Envelope of probe volume in the heterodyne system, as defined by equation (2.6.25).

dimensions

$$\Delta x = 2r_0/\cos\theta$$

$$\Delta y = 2r_0 \qquad\qquad (2.6.26)$$

$$\Delta z = 2r_0/\sin\theta$$

(Note that some authors define the fringe volume as the region in which the photocurrent decays to $1/e^2$ of its maximum value.)

As an example, consider a system where a HeNe laser beam ($\lambda = 632.8$ nm) of radius $r_u = 0.5$ mm is split to form the illuminating and reference beams, which are both brought to a focus at F_0 with lenses of focal length 10 cm, the half-angle of their intersection being $\theta = \tan^{-1} 0.2$.

From equation (2.6.4), the radii of the diffraction-limited spots will be $r_0 = 0.0403$ mm. From equation (2.6.26), the dimensions of the measuring region will then be

$$\Delta x = 0.082 \text{ mm}, \qquad \Delta y = 0.081 \text{ mm}, \qquad \Delta z = 0.41 \text{ mm}$$

Real Fringe Systems

In a real fringe system, the two laser beams that are brought to focus at the observation point to produce a fringe pattern may be either unapertured laser beams (Figure 2.2.6) or, as in the case of mask systems, may have been transmitted through apertures with specified geometries (Figure 2.2.4). In real fringe systems a single lens is normally used for focusing the two beams, as indicated in Figure 2.6.5.

We shall study both the *Gaussian beam* (unapertured laser beam) and *mask* systems. As stated in Section 2.2, the mask invariably takes the form of two rectangular apertures, i.e., modification of Young's slit configuration. In later chapters we will refer to this as *the* mask system. However, for

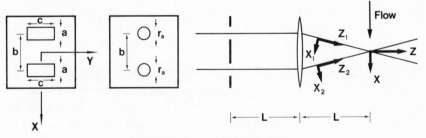

Figure 2.6.5. Mask configurations.

completeness in this section, we will also derive expressions for the photo-current when the mask consists of a pair of circular apertures. These expressions involve Bessel functions which are fairly cumbersome to handle and difficult to manipulate for extracting information on the flow parameters —hence the lack of popularity of this setup. On the other hand, masks with circular apertures are extremely simple to construct and this partly offsets the theoretical disadvantages.

In the mask systems, either a beam splitter is used to produce two collimated beams which are incident on the mask apertures (Figure 2.2.6) or, alternatively, the laser beam is expanded and collimated without a beam splitter (Figure 2.2.4) to produce a single beam incident on the mask. In either case, since each mask aperture is small compared to the diameter of the incident beam, the light amplitude across the apertures can be assumed constant to a good approximation. It will also be assumed that the wavefronts incident on the mask are plane. From elementary Fourier optics it is then simple to show that the field distribution of each beam at F_0 is essentially the spatial Fourier transform of the aperture through which it passes (Goodman, 1968, see also p. 57).

(i) Rectangular-Aperture Mask

For a rectangular aperture in the mask (Figure 2.6.5), the field distribution of beam 1 near focus is

$$\mathscr{E}_1(x_1, y_1, z_1) = \mathscr{E}_0 \, e^{jkz_1} \operatorname{sinc}\left(\frac{kx_1 a}{2L}\right) \operatorname{sinc}\left(\frac{ky_1 c}{2L}\right) \qquad (2.6.27)$$

where $\operatorname{sinc}(x) = (\sin x)/x$; a and c are dimensions of the aperture; L is the focal length of the focusing lens, and $\mathscr{E}_0^2$ is the intensity of beam 1 at F_0.
Similarly the field distribution of beam 2 near F_0 is

$$\mathscr{E}_2(x_2, y_2, z_2) = \mathscr{E}_0 \, e^{jkz_2} \operatorname{sinc}\left(\frac{kx_2 a}{2L}\right) \operatorname{sinc}\left(\frac{ky_2 c}{2L}\right) \qquad (2.6.28)$$

equations (2.6.27) and (2.6.28) may be substituted into equation (2.6.14) to yield the fringe current at the output of the photodetector, due to the presence of a particle near F_0. Since (x_1, y_1, z_1), (x_2, y_2, z_2), and (x, y, z) refer to the location of the particle in the three-coordinate systems, equation (2.6.6) may be employed to relate them.

From the optical geometry of Figure 2.6.5, equation (2.6.6) may be recast into

$$x_1 = x - \frac{zb}{2L}, \qquad z_1 = z + \frac{xb}{2L}$$

$$x_2 = x + \frac{zb}{2L}, \qquad z_2 = z - \frac{xb}{2L} \qquad (2.6.29)$$

$$y_1 = y_2 = y$$

Thus for a rectangular aperture mask system equation (2.6.14) yields the fringe photocurrent as

$$i_F = \eta(\tfrac{1}{2}MC_{sc})^2 \mathscr{E}_0^2 \operatorname{sinc}^2 \left(\frac{\pi yc}{\lambda L}\right)$$

$$\times \left[\operatorname{sinc}^2 \beta_1 + \operatorname{sinc}^2 \beta_2 + 2 \operatorname{sinc} \beta_1 \operatorname{sinc} \beta_2 \cos \left(\frac{2\pi xb}{\lambda L}\right) \right] \qquad (2.6.30)$$

where

$$\beta_1 = \frac{\pi a}{\lambda L}\left(x - \frac{zb}{2L}\right), \qquad \beta_2 = \frac{\pi a}{\lambda L}\left(x + \frac{zb}{2L}\right)$$

It is obvious from equation (2.6.30) that the photocurrent has a maximum value if the scattering center is located at F_0 and that it decays to negligible values if the particle is located beyond the first zeros of any of the sinc terms. This allows the fringe volume to be determined, and Figure 2.6.6a lllustrates the envelope of the volume. It is diamond-shaped, rather like two wedges stuck together back to back. The dimensions of the fringe volume from equation (2.6.30) are

$$\Delta x = \frac{2\lambda L}{a}, \qquad \Delta y = \frac{2\lambda L}{c}, \qquad \Delta z = \frac{4\lambda L^2}{ab} \qquad (2.6.31)$$

The cosine term indicates the fringe spacing

$$\Delta x_F = \lambda L/b \qquad (2.6.32)$$

and the number of fringes

$$N_F = \Delta x/\Delta x_F = 2b/a \qquad (2.6.33)$$

As an example, let $\lambda = 632.8$ nm, i.e., the wavelength of a HeNe laser, $L = 10$ cm, $a = c = 1$ mm and $b = 2$ cm (it is worth noting here that it is seldom practical to have a lens with an F number less than 2, which restricts the maximum value of b/L to 0.25 if it is assumed that the beam spacing is one half of the lens diameter).

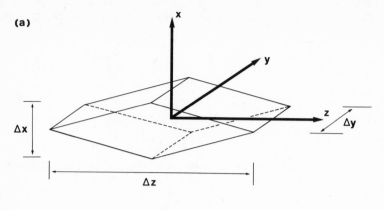

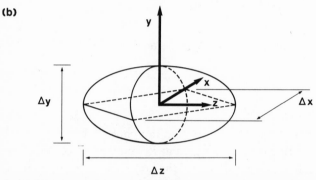

Figure 2.6.6. Fringe volume for mask systems with (a) rectangular apertures;
(b) circular apertures.

From equation (2.6.31) the dimensions of the observation volume are

$$\Delta x = \Delta y = 0.127 \text{ mm}, \qquad \Delta z = 1.27 \text{ mm}$$

and from equation (2.6.33) the number of fringes is

$$N_F = 40$$

(ii) *Circular-Aperture Mask*

If instead of a rectangular aperture in the mask, a circular aperture is employed, then the field distribution of beam 1 near focus is

$$\mathscr{E}_1(x_1, y_1, z_1) = \mathscr{E}_0\, e^{jkz_1} J_1(w_1)/w_1 \qquad (2.6.34)$$

where J_1 is the first-order Bessel function, $w_1 = (kr_a/L)(x_1^2 + y_1^2)^{1/2}$, r_a is the radius of the circular aperture, and L the focal length of the focusing lens in Figure 2.6.5. $\mathscr{E}_0^2$ is the intensity of beam 1 at F_0.

Similarly, the field distribution of beam 2 near focus is

$$\mathscr{E}_2(x_2, y_2, z_2) = \mathscr{E}_0 \, e^{jkz_2} J_1(w_2)/w_2 \qquad (2.6.35)$$

where $w_2 = (kr_a/L)(x_2^2 + y_2^2)^{1/2}$. Substitution of equations (2.6.34) and (2.6.35) into (2.6.14), and use of (2.6.29) to obtain the fringe photocurrent due to a particle located at (x, y, z), yields

$$i_F = \eta(\tfrac{1}{2}MC_{sc})^2 \mathscr{E}_0^2 \left[\frac{J_1^2(\beta_3)}{\beta_3^2} + \frac{J_1^2(\beta_4)}{\beta_4^2} + 2\frac{J_1(\beta_3)J_1(\beta_4)}{\beta_3\beta_4} \cos\left(\frac{kxb}{L}\right) \right] \qquad (2.6.36)$$

where

$$\beta_3 = \frac{2\pi r_a}{\lambda L}\left[\left(x - \frac{zb}{2L}\right)^2 + y^2\right]^{1/2}$$

$$\beta_4 = \frac{2\pi r_a}{\lambda L}\left[\left(x + \frac{zb}{2L}\right)^2 + y^2\right]^{1/2} \qquad (2.6.37)$$

From equations (2.6.36) and (2.6.37) the fringe volume can be determined. Its boundaries are established by the location of the particle which leads to the zeros of the Bessel function. Figure 2.6.6b illustrates this volume. The sections of the volume on the three planes are

$$z = 0: \qquad x^2 + y^2 = \left(0.61\frac{\lambda L}{r_a}\right)^2 \qquad \text{circular}$$

$$y = 0: \qquad x \pm \frac{zb}{2L} = 0.61\frac{\lambda L}{r_a} \qquad \text{rectangular}$$

$$x = 0: \qquad y^2 + \left(\frac{zb}{2L}\right)^2 = \left(0.61\frac{\lambda L}{r_a}\right)^2 \qquad \text{elliptic}$$

where $J_1(x)$ has its first zero at $x = 1.22\pi$.

The volume is conical on either side of the x-y plane. Its maximum dimensions are

$$\Delta x = \Delta y = 1.22\frac{\lambda L}{r_a}, \qquad \Delta z = 2.44\frac{\lambda L^2}{br_a} \qquad (2.6.38)$$

While the fringe spacing is the same as that for the rectangular-aperture mask system; i.e., $\Delta x_F = \lambda L/b$, for the number of fringes within the observation volume we have

$$N_F = \frac{\Delta x}{\Delta x_F} \approx 1.22\frac{b}{r_a} \qquad (2.6.39)$$

For example, if $\lambda = 632.8$ nm, $L = 10$ cm, $b = 2$ cm, and $r_a = 0.5$ mm, then the number of fringes, from equation (2.6.39) is $N_F \approx 49$, and the dimensions of the fringe volume [from equation (2.6.38)] are

$$\Delta x = \Delta y = 0.154 \text{ mm}, \qquad \Delta z = 1.54 \text{ mm}$$

Comparing equations (2.6.31) and (2.6.38) for $a = c = 2r_a$, with identical focusing lens, the fringe volume for the rectangular-aperture mask system is slightly smaller than for the circular-aperture mask system.

(iii) Gaussian Beam System

For a real fringe optical system if two unapertured beams are brought to focus at the observation point, then the field incident on a particle located at (x, y, z) due to beam 1 is given by

$$\mathscr{E}_1(x_1, y_1, z_1) = \mathscr{E}_0 \exp\left(-\frac{x_1^2 + y_1^2}{2r_0^2} + jkz_1\right) \tag{2.6.40}$$

while the contribution of the field incident on the particle due to beam 2 may be expressed as

$$\mathscr{E}_2(x_2, y_2, z_2) = \mathscr{E}_0 \exp\left(-\frac{x_2^2 + y_2^2}{2r_0^2} + jkz_2\right) \tag{2.6.41}$$

where $\mathscr{E}_0^2$ is the intensity of the two beams at the focal point. Employing equation (2.6.14) and converting the coordinate system to the (x, y, z) frame of reference, we obtain the photodetector fringe current as

$$i_F = 2(\tfrac{1}{2}MC_{sc})^2 \mathscr{E}_0^2 \exp\left(-\frac{x^2 \cos^2\theta + y^2 + z^2 \sin^2\theta}{r_0^2}\right)$$

$$\times \left[\cosh\left(\frac{xz}{r_0^2}\sin 2\theta\right) + \cos\left(\frac{4\pi}{\lambda}x\sin\theta\right)\right] \tag{2.6.42}$$

Obviously the photodetector current is maximum when the particle is at the origin of the coordinate system, i.e., at the focus. Similar to heterodyne optical configurations, the photocurrent drops to $1/e$ of its peak value if the particle is located on the ellipsoid

$$x^2 \cos^2 \theta + y^2 + z^2 \sin^2 \theta = r_0^2 \tag{2.6.43}$$

This ellipsoid is identical to that of equation (2.6.25), and its dimensions are given by equation (2.6.26). For an illustration see Figure 2.6.4.

The last cosine term in equation (2.6.42) indicates the spacing between fringes to be

$$\Delta x_F = \lambda/(2 \sin \theta) \tag{2.6.44}$$

such that the total number of fringes within the observation volume is [cf. equation (2.6.4)]

$$N_F = \frac{\Delta x}{\Delta x_F} = \frac{4r_0}{\lambda} \tan \theta = \frac{8}{\pi \Delta \theta} \tan \theta \tag{2.6.45}$$

As an Illustration, consider that $\lambda = 632.8$ nm and that a single lens of focal length 10 cm is used to focus the two parallel beams into the measuring volume. Let the beam radii be $r_u = 0.5$ mm and their separation just in front of the transmission lens 2 cm.

From equation (2.6.4), $r_0 = 0.0403$ mm, and for this value of r_0 the number of fringes [from equation (2.6.45)] is $N_F \approx 25$. From equation (2.6.44), the spacing between fringes is $\Delta x_F = 0.00318$ mm.

Photocurrent Due to Moving Scatterers

So far in this section expressions have been derived for the photocurrent generated by light scattered off a stationary particle present in the vicinity of the interference volume of a velocimeter. However in a flow situation, a scattering particle travels with the velocity of the flow. Thus it generates a time-varying photocurrent as it passes across the region of the beam intersection.

For a uniform flow velocity U in the x direction at any time instant t the coordinates of a scattering particle may be defined as $(Ut + x_0, y_0, z_0)$. This would produce an instantaneous photocurrent for the four cases discussed above (for convenience we assume $x_0 = 0$, i.e., the particle is at $(0, y_0, z_0)$ at time $t = 0$ and has zero velocity in the other two directions. It is mathematically trivial to extend the following expressions to include the cases of particle velocity in other directions). We also assume that a difference in wavelength between incident and scattered radiation off a moving particle is negligibly small. This is true for particle velocities well below that of the incident radiation. Hence the earlier results lead to the following.

Heterodyne Systems

From equation (2.6.24) for $\mathscr{E}_R \ll \mathscr{E}_I$, we have

$$i_{DH}(t) = \eta C_{sc}\mathscr{E}_R\mathscr{E}_I \exp\left(-\frac{U^2 t^2 \cos^2\theta + y_0^2 + z_0^2 \sin^2\theta}{r_0^2}\right)$$

$$\times \cos\left(\frac{4\pi}{\lambda} Ut \sin\theta\right) \tag{2.6.46}$$

Real Fringe Systems

(i) *Rectangular-Aperture Mask System.* From equation (2.6.30) we have

$$i_F(t) = \eta(\tfrac{1}{2}MC_{sc})^2\mathscr{E}_0^2 \operatorname{sinc}^2\left(\frac{\pi y_0 c}{\lambda L}\right)\left\{\operatorname{sinc}^2\left[\frac{\pi a}{\lambda L}\left(Ut + \frac{z_0 b}{2L}\right)\right]\right.$$

$$+ \operatorname{sinc}^2\left[\frac{\pi a}{\lambda L}\left(Ut - \frac{z_0 b}{2L}\right)\right] + 2\operatorname{sinc}\left[\frac{\pi a}{\lambda L}\left(Ut + \frac{z_0 b}{2L}\right)\right]$$

$$\times \operatorname{sinc}\left[\frac{\pi a}{\lambda L}\left(Ut - \frac{z_0 b}{2L}\right)\right]\cos\left(\frac{2\pi}{\lambda} bUt\right)\right\} \tag{2.6.47}$$

To generate a finite photocurrent, z_0 should be within the observation volume, hence $z_0 b/2L \simeq 0$, and, similarly, $y_0 \le \Delta y$ [of equation (2.6.31)]; hence

$$i_F(t) = 2\eta(\tfrac{1}{2}MC_{sc})^2\mathscr{E}_0^2 \operatorname{sinc}^2\left(\frac{\pi y_0 c}{\lambda L}\right)\operatorname{sinc}^2\left(\frac{\pi a}{\lambda L}Ut\right)\left[1 + \cos\left(\frac{2\pi b}{\lambda L}Ut\right)\right] \tag{2.6.48}$$

(ii) *Circular-Aperture-Mask System*

$$i_F(t) = 2\eta(\tfrac{1}{2}MC_{sc})^2\mathscr{E}_0^2\left[\frac{J_1(w)}{w}\right]^2\left[1 + \cos\left(\frac{2\pi}{\lambda L}bUt\right)\right]$$

where $w = (2\pi r_a/\lambda L)(U^2 t^2 + y_0^2)^{1/2}$. The above simplification arises since for a finite photocurrent $z_0 \le \Delta z$, and, similarly, $y_0 \le \Delta y$ of equation (2.6.38). Hence

$$i_F = 2\eta(\tfrac{1}{2}MC_{sc})^2\mathscr{E}_0^2\left[\frac{J_1((2\pi r_a/\lambda L)Ut)}{(2\pi r_a/\lambda L)Ut}\right]^2\left[1 + \cos\left(\frac{2\pi}{\lambda L}bUt\right)\right] \tag{2.6.49}$$

(iii) *Gaussian Beam System*

$$i_F(t) = 2\eta(\tfrac{1}{2}MC_{sc})^2 \mathscr{E}_0^2 \exp\left(-\frac{U^2t^2\cos^2\theta + y_0^2 + z_0^2\sin^2\theta}{r_0^2}\right)$$

$$\times\left[\cosh\left(\frac{z_0Ut}{r_0}\sin 2\theta\right) + \cos\left(\frac{4\pi}{\lambda}Ut\sin\theta\right)\right]$$

$$\simeq 2\eta(\tfrac{1}{2}MC_{sc})^2 \mathscr{E}_0^2 \exp\left(-\frac{U^2t^2\cos^2\theta + y_0^2 + z_0^2\sin^2\theta}{r_0^2}\right)$$

$$\times\left[1 + \cos\left(\frac{4\pi}{\lambda}Ut\sin\theta\right)\right] \tag{2.6.50}$$

In all cases the maximum amplitude of the photocurrent is obtained (at time $t = 0$), when the scattering particle crosses the center (origin) of the observation volume.

In general, the photocurrent generated by the passage of a single pth particle across the observation volume can be conveniently expressed as

$$i_{DH}(t) = \kappa K_p W(t)\cos 2\pi f_0 t \tag{2.6.51}$$

$$i_F(t) = \kappa K_p W(t)(1 + \cos 2\pi f_0 t) \tag{2.6.52}$$

where κK_p is a time-independent term and denotes the amplitude of photocurrent as the pth scattering particle crosses the center of the observation volume. For an ensemble of scattering particles, K_p is a random variable which varies with the size of the scattering particles, i.e., with the scattering cross section C_{sc} of the particles; κ is a constant determined from the optical geometry, laser power, and efficiency of the detection system. The quantity $W(t)$ is a low-frequency term which depends upon the intensity profile within the measuring volume and on the instantaneous flow velocity at the observation volume. It is usually referred to as the *weighting function* of the Doppler photocurrent. Thus,

$$W(t) = \exp\left(-\frac{U^2t^2\cos^2\theta}{r_0^2}\right) \qquad \text{heterodyne and Gaussian beam systems}$$

$$= \text{sinc}^2\left(\frac{\pi a}{\lambda L}Ut\right) \qquad \text{rectangular-aperture mask system}$$

$$= \left[\frac{J_1((2\pi r_a/\lambda L)Ut)}{(2\pi r_a/\lambda L)Ut}\right]^2 \qquad \text{circular-aperture mask system} \tag{2.6.53}$$

The cosine term denotes the high-frequency component of the current, and it represents the Doppler shift in the optical frequency of laser light introduced by particle motion. Hence the name "Doppler photocurrent," and the name "Doppler signal" for the subsequent signal generated. The frequency f_0 is a precise measure of the instantaneous (Eulerian) flow velocity. Thus

$$f_0 = \frac{2U}{\lambda} \sin \theta \qquad \text{Gaussian beam systems}$$

$$= \frac{b}{\lambda L} U \qquad \text{mask systems} \qquad (2.6.54)$$

as indicated earlier in equation (2.2.6).

Further, employing Δx, the width of the interference volume in the direction of flow, the mean passage time of a particle across the interference pattern may be determined as, say,

$$\Delta t = \frac{\Delta x}{U} = \frac{2r_0}{U \cos \theta} = 8^{1/2} \rho \qquad \text{Gaussian beam systems}$$

$$= \frac{2\lambda L}{aU} = \frac{2\pi}{\mu} \qquad \text{rectangular mask system}$$

$$= 1.22 \frac{\lambda L}{Ur_a} = 2.44 \frac{\pi}{\gamma} \qquad \text{circular mask system} \qquad (2.6.55)$$

The three definitions (ρ, μ, γ) allow $W(t)$ of equation (2.6.53) to be rewritten conveniently as

$$W(t) = e^{-t^2/2\rho^2}$$

$$= \text{sinc}^2 \mu t$$

$$= \left[\frac{J_1(\gamma t)}{(\gamma t)} \right]^2 \qquad (2.6.56)$$

It follows from equations (2.6.54) and (2.6.55) that

$$2^{1/2} \rho f_0 = (2r_0/\lambda) \tan \theta, \qquad \mu = \omega_0/(2b/a), \qquad \gamma = \omega_0/(b/r_a)$$

where $\omega_0 = 2\pi f_0$.

From now on, the expressions for $W(t)$ of equation (2.6.56) rather than the cumbersome expressions of equation (2.6.53) will be used throughout the book.

Usually there is a large number of scattering particles present within the vicinity of the observation volume. The photodetector current is then the sum of individual contributions arising from light scattered by each particle present. At any time instant these individual contributions are a function of the position of each particle with reference to the center of the observation volume at that instant. The total photocurrent is therefore

$$i(t) = \sum_{p=-\infty}^{\infty} i_p(t - t_p) \qquad (2.6.57)$$

where t_p is the time of arrival of the pth particle at the center of the scattering volume, and $i_p(t)$ is the photocurrent contribution of the pth particle, as given by equations (2.6.51) and (2.6.52). Here $\{t_p\}$ is a random sequence, which represents the random arrival times of the scattering particles at the observation volume. Further, as the amplitude of $\{i_p(t)\}$ varies from particle to particle with the variation of particle scattering cross section, $\{i(t)\}$ is a time-varying function with random amplitude and phase. Note the similarity between $\{i(t)\}$ and shot noise.

The summation of equation (2.6.57) is taken over infinity, since, in theory the observation volume extends indefinitely in either direction from the optical axis, and all particles that lie in the observation volume contribute to the photocurrent. The dimensions of the observation volume proposed earlier are only specified by the region where the light intensity decays to some arbitrarily small value.

Finally, it is important to note that the photocurrent model of equation (2.6.57) is strictly valid for the case of the LDV system operating on a uniform flow, or, for the case of fluid turbulence when the particle velocity does not change significantly as it crosses the region of beam intersection where it can scatter an appreciable intensity of radiation, e.g., within the boundaries of the observation volume defined earlier. For an exact model of the photocurrent it is necessary to relate the instantaneous position and velocity of each scattering particle to the consequent contribution it would make to the overall photocurrent. This would lead to

$$i(t) = \sum_{p=-\infty}^{\infty} i_p(x_p(t)) \qquad (2.6.58)$$

where

$$x_p(t) = \int_{t_p}^{t} V_p(\tau) \, d\tau \qquad \text{for all } p \qquad (2.6.59)$$

$x_p(t)$ represents the position of (any) pth particle at time t, i.e., its displacement from the center of the observation volume; $V_p(t)$ refers to the velocity of the same particle at that time; and t_p may be considered as the time instant when the pth particle crosses the center of the observation volume, i.e., the $x = 0$ plane.

Thus the photocurrent for the real fringe system may be expressed as

$$i_p(x_p(t)) = \kappa K_p \left\{ \exp \left[-\frac{x_p^2(t) \cos^2 \theta}{r_0^2} \right] \right\}$$

$$\times \left\{ 1 + \cos \left[\frac{4\pi}{\lambda} x_p(t) \sin \theta \right] \right\} \qquad \text{Gaussian beam system} \qquad (2.6.60)$$

and

$$i_p(x_p(t)) = \kappa K_p \, \text{sinc}^2 \left[\frac{\pi a}{\lambda L} x_p(t) \right] \left\{ 1 + \cos \left[\frac{2\pi b}{\lambda L} x_p(t) \right] \right\} \qquad \begin{array}{l} \text{rectangular} \\ \text{mask system} \end{array}$$

$$(2.6.61)$$

where κ, K_p are as defined by equations (2.6.51) and (2.6.52). Similar expressions hold for the circular mask and the heterodyne systems. It is easy to verify that equations (2.6.60) and (2.6.61) reduce to (2.6.52) when the flow is uniform [i.e., $V_p(t) = U$ for all p and t].

From equations (2.6.60) and (2.6.61) the weighting function of (2.6.53) can be alternatively expressed in terms of the position of the particles, and the overall photocurrent may be represented by

$$i_F(t) = \kappa \sum_p K_p W(\beta x_p(t))[1 + \cos D x_p(t)] \qquad (2.6.62)$$

and

$$i_{DH}(t) = \kappa \sum_p K_p W(\beta x(t)) \cos D x_p(t) \qquad (2.6.63)$$

where

$$D = \frac{2\pi b}{\lambda L} \qquad \text{or} \qquad \frac{4\pi}{\lambda} \sin \theta$$

and it follows from equation (2.6.53) that

$$W(\beta x_p(t)) = \exp \left[-x_p^2(t) \frac{\cos^2 \theta}{r_0^2} \right] \qquad \text{heterodyne and Gaussian beam system}$$

$$= \text{sinc}^2 \left[\frac{\pi a}{\lambda L} x_p(t) \right] \qquad \text{rectangular-aperture mask system}$$

$$= \left[\frac{J_1(\bar{w})}{\bar{w}} \right]^2 \qquad \text{circular-aperture mask system} \qquad (2.6.64)$$

where $\bar{w} = (2\pi r_a / \lambda L) x_p(t)$.

The signal-processing hardware associated with a velocimeter estimates the flow velocity from a record of the photocurrent $i(t)$ or its related voltage by the use of various techniques to be described in the following chapters.

Chapter 3

SIGNAL ANALYSIS FOR LASER DOPPLER SYSTEMS

This chapter is concerned with the analysis of the time-varying signal generated in an LDV system when uniform and turbulent flows are studied. In particular, relationships are developed between the parameters of the optical setup, the flow conditions, and the statistical properties of the ensuing Doppler-shifted photocurrent. These facilitate estimation of the flow characteristics from a record of the Doppler signal.

In Section 3.1 the main characteristics of the Doppler signal are analyzed, and in Sections 3.2 and 3.3 we concern ourselves with relationships between the signal statistics and the fluid flow parameters. Two methods of signal analysis are commonly employed. (1) *frequency domain* techniques, and (2) *frequency tracking*.

In the frequency domain method, Doppler signals are analyzed by direct spectral analysis. Characteristics of the signal spectrum will be considered in Section 3.2. Frequency tracking involves the detection of the instantaneous signal frequency by means of a tracking instrument, e.g., a phase locked loop. This latter technique is generally regarded as more accurate. We shall address ourselves in Section 3.3 to deriving in detail the statistics of the instantaneous frequency of the LDV signal arising in turbulent flows. Hardware aspects of frequency trackers will be covered in Chapter 6.

3.1. Statistics of Laser Doppler Signals

It was shown in Section 2.6 that the photocurrent generated by the radiation scattered by moving scattering centers present in a *uniform* flow is given by equation (2.6.57) as

$$i(t) = \sum_{p=-\infty}^{\infty} i_p(t - t_p) \qquad (3.1.1)$$

where $i_p(t)$ is the photocurrent contribution of the pth particle in the vicinity of the observation volume, and t_p is its arrival time at the center of the scattering volume. For specific optical configurations of the LDV, from equations (2.6.51) and (2.6.52) we have

$$i_{DH}(t) = \kappa \sum_{p=-\infty}^{\infty} K_p W(t - t_p) \cos 2\pi f_0(t - t_p) \qquad (3.1.2)$$

$$i_F(t) = \kappa \sum_{p=-\infty}^{\infty} K_p W(t - t_p)[1 + \cos 2\pi f_0(t - t_p)] \qquad (3.1.3)$$

where κ is a constant determined from the optical geometry and associated hardware of the LDV setup, and K_p is a random variable which is related to the scattering cross section of the particles and varies with particle size. $\{W(t)\}$ is the weighting function, and f_0 is related to the mean flow velocity U through equation (2.2.6).

In general, the photocurrent $\{i(t)\}$ or its associated Doppler signal voltage $\{x(t)\}$ takes two different forms, depending upon the concentration of scattering centers within the flow. For low particle concentration, such as in gaseous flows, the Doppler signal $\{x(t)\}$ consists of a sequence of randomly occurring nonoverlapping pulses of random amplitude (Figure 3.1.1a). These pulses appear whenever a scattering particle crosses the beam intersection, and their amplitude depends upon the size of the particle. When the particle concentration is high, the pulses overlap to yield a continuous signal which is essentially a superposition of the independent pulses [Figure 3.1.1b].

The photocurrent $\{i(t)\}$ represents a process similar to the conventional shot-noise process (Rice, 1944; Middleton, 1960). The derivation of its probability density function is too cumbersome to be included here. Suffice it to say that, for high particle concentrations, as $\{i(t)\}$ is the sum of a large number of statistically independent random variables, the central limit theorem leads to a Gaussian distribution. It is well-known that shot-noise-type processes approach a Gaussian probability density function (Rice,

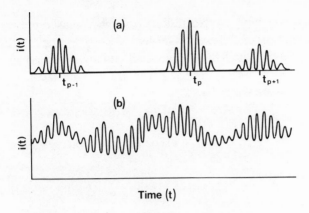

Figure 3.1.1. Doppler photocurrent (or signal) with (a) low scattering-center concentration; (b) high scattering-center concentration.

1944). Figure 3.1.2 gives an experimental verification for the Doppler signal obtained from a mask system.

The statistics of $\{i(t)\}$ may be determined in a number of ways: for low particle concentration, Campbell's theorem may be employed (see pp. 35–36);

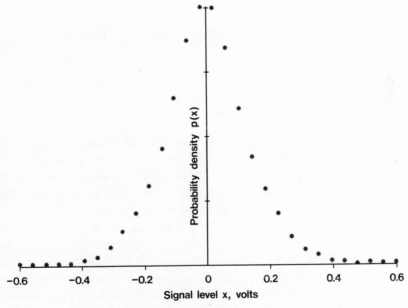

Figure 3.1.2. Experimentally measured probability density function of the Doppler signal.

alternatively, for high concentrations, as the signal represents a continuous random process, its second-order statistics may be determined from a continuous signal model. Here we shall employ a general model which would cover both cases of particle concentration and facilitate derivation of the signal statistics.

Equations (3.1.2) and (3.1.3) may be rewritten as

$$i_{DH}(t) = \kappa \sum_{p=-\infty}^{\infty} K_p \int_{-\infty}^{\infty} W(t - t') \cos 2\pi f_0(t - t') \delta(t' - t_p) \, dt'$$

$$= \int_{-\infty}^{\infty} W(t - t') \cos 2\pi f_0(t - t') \left[\kappa \sum_{p=-\infty}^{\infty} K_p \delta(t' - t_p) \, dt' \right] \qquad (3.1.4)$$

where the artifact of a δ function is used to remove the dependence on $\{t_p\}$ of the weighting function $\{W(t)\}$ and its associated carrier $\cos 2\pi f_0 t$.

As shown in Section 1.2, since the term within the curly brackets in equation (3.1.4) represents the increment in a jump process in the interval $(t', t' + dt')$, we have from equation (1.2.57)

$$dN(t') = \kappa \sum_{p=-\infty}^{\infty} K_p \delta(t' - t_p) \, dt' \qquad (3.1.5)$$

This allows equation (3.1.4) to be recast as

$$i_{DH}(t) = \int_{-\infty}^{\infty} W(t - t') \cos 2\pi f_0(t - t') \, dN(t') \qquad (3.1.6)$$

Similarly, the photocurrent output for a real fringe LDV system is

$$i_F(t) = \int_{-\infty}^{\infty} W(t - t')[1 + \cos 2\pi f_0(t - t')] \, dN(t') \qquad (3.1.7)$$

To analyze the statistics of the Doppler current, it is necessary to determine the statistical properties of the incremental process $\{dN(t)\}$.

Since the scattering centers are considered to be moving with the fluid, it is intuitively obvious that the mean number of particles crossing the optical axis plane, at the observation volume, per unit time is directly proportional to the flow velocity. For a given particle concentration, the higher the flow velocity, the larger the mean rate of particles crossing the observation volume. Similarly for low-flow velocities the mean rate of particles crossing the observation volume is low.

Thus if g is the mean (number) particle concentration per unit volume within the fluid, then to a first approximation the mean number of particles crossing the observation volume per unit time is $g(\Delta y \, \Delta z)U = N_p$, say, where Δy, Δz are the dimensions of the observation volume as defined in Section 2.6, and the flow is considered to take place in the x direction with velocity U. Let $g(\Delta y \, \Delta z) = g_0$. Then we have from Section 1.2, pp. 33–36,

$$E[dN \, (t')] = \kappa E[K_p]g_0 U \, dt'$$
$$= \kappa E[K_p]N_p \, dt'$$

and

$$\text{cov}\,[dN \, (t') \, dN \, (t'')] = \begin{cases} \left. \begin{array}{c} \kappa^2 E[K_p^2]g_0 U \, dt' \\ \kappa^2 E[K_p^2]N_p \, dt' \end{array} \right\} & t' = t'' \\ 0, & \text{otherwise} \end{cases} \tag{3.1.8}$$

The above relationships are valid since $\{K_p\}$ is independent of the occurrence times $\{t_p\}$ of the particles. $E[K_p]$ is related to the mean value of the scattering cross section, and $E[K_p^2]$ to the mean square scattering cross section of the particles present in the flow. This is strictly true for the heterodyne LDV setup, while for the real fringe systems, $E[K_p]$ and $E[K_p^2]$ are related to the higher-order statistical moments of the scattering cross section.

Denoting $E[K_p] = C_0$, $E[K_p^2] = C_1$, and a scaling factor

$$A^2 = g_0 U \kappa^2 C_1 = N_p \kappa^2 C_1 \tag{3.1.9}$$

we have from equation (3.1.6)

$$E[i_{DH}(t)] = \kappa C_0 N_p \int_{-\infty}^{\infty} W(t) \cos 2\pi f_0 t \, dt \tag{3.1.10}$$

$$\text{var}\,[i_{DH}(t)] = \frac{A^2}{2} \int_{-\infty}^{\infty} W^2(t) \, dt$$

The latter is obtained by disregarding the high-frequency term in $2f_0$, which usually integrates to zero provided the spectrum of $\{W(t)\}$ is narrow-band as compared to f_0, as is the case in practice.

Similarly it may be shown, by employing equation (3.1.8) in equation (3.1.6), that the autocovariance function for the Doppler photocurrent is

$$\text{cov}\,[i_{DH}(t)i_{DH}(t + \tau)] = \frac{A^2}{2}\left[\int_{-\infty}^{\infty} W(t)W(t + \tau) \, dt\right] \cos 2\pi f_0 \tau \tag{3.1.11}$$

In a similar manner, the statistics for the Doppler current in a real fringe system may be derived as

$$E[i_F(t)] = \kappa C_0 N_p \int_{-\infty}^{\infty} W(t)(1 + \cos 2\pi f_0 t)\, dt$$

$$\text{var}\,[i_F(t)] = \tfrac{3}{2} A^2 \int_{-\infty}^{\infty} W^2(t)\, dt \tag{3.1.12}$$

$$\text{cov}\,[i_F(t) i_F(t + \tau)] = A^2 (1 + \tfrac{1}{2} \cos 2\pi f_0 \tau) \int_{-\infty}^{\infty} W(t) W(t + \tau)\, dt$$

Prior to any sophisticated signal processing, it is usual to remove the mean value of the Doppler current and to pass it through a high-pass filter to eliminate any low-frequency noise contributions arising from the photodetection process. The high-pass signal so obtained has identical character-

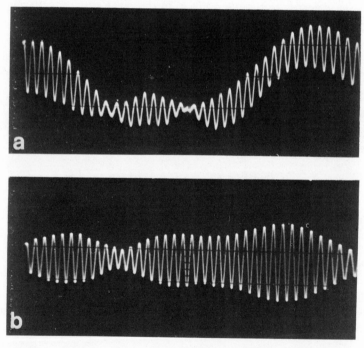

Figure 3.1.3. Doppler signal recorded from a mask LDV system with $b/a = 10$; (a) unfiltered; (b) high-pass filtered.

istics for any LDV setup (either real fringe or heterodyne).

Defining the autocorrelation of the weighting function as

$$R_w(\tau) = \int_{-\infty}^{\infty} W(t)W(t + \tau) \, dt \qquad (3.1.13)$$

we have for the Doppler current (or signal) characteristics, after high-pass filtering,

$$E[i(t)] = 0$$

$$\text{var}\,[i(t)] = \tfrac{1}{2}A^2 R_w(0) \qquad (3.1.14)$$

$$\text{cov}\,[i(t)i(t + \tau)] = \tfrac{1}{2}A^2 R_w(\tau) \cos 2\pi f_0 \tau$$

As the autocovariance function for $i(t)$, $i_{DH}(t)$, or $i_F(t)$ depends only on the lag interval τ, the photocurrent represents a stationary random process. The stationarity condition is strictly true for uniform flow studies.

Figure 3.1.3a shows the Doppler signal arising in a real fringe mask system. Notice the high-frequency content (representing the Doppler frequency shift of light) riding on a low-frequency signal. The low-frequency signal represents only the superposition of the weighting functions in equation (3.1.3). Figure 3.1.3b is a high-pass-filtered version of the signal in Figure 3.1.3a. It is the instantaneous frequency of this signal that is related to the instantaneous flow velocity.

Narrow-Band Representation

In this section we shall refer to the Doppler signal as the voltage $\{x(t)\}$ produced by passing $i(t)$ through a unit resistor. Then, by employing equations (3.1.6) or (3.1.7) the filtered Doppler signal after mean removal may be expressed as

$$x(t) = \int_{-\infty}^{\infty} W(t - t') \cos 2\pi f_0(t - t') \, dN\,(t') \qquad (3.1.15)$$

where

$$E[dN\,(t)] = 0 \qquad \text{for all } t$$

$$\text{cov}\,[dN\,(t_1)\,dN\,(t_2)] = \begin{cases} A^2 \, dt_1 & t_1 = t_2 \\ 0 & \text{otherwise} \end{cases} \qquad (3.1.16)$$

The cumbersome representation of equation (3.1.14) may be recast into

$$x(t) = a(t) \cos 2\pi f_0 t + b(t) \sin 2\pi f_0 t$$
$$= H(t) \cos [2\pi f_0 t - \phi(t)]$$
$$= H(t) \cos \theta(t) \qquad\qquad (3.1.17)$$

where

$$a(t) = \int_{-\infty}^{\infty} W(t - t') \cos 2\pi f_0 t' \, dN(t')$$
$$\qquad\qquad (3.1.18)$$
$$b(t) = \int_{-\infty}^{\infty} W(t - t') \sin 2\pi f_0 t' \, dN(t')$$

$$H^2(t) = a^2(t) + b^2(t), \qquad \phi(t) = \tan^{-1}[b(t)/a(t)] \qquad (3.1.19)$$

Here $\{a(t)\}$, $\{b(t)\}$ are random processes, and their statistics may be determined from equation (3.1.16):

$$E[a(t)] = E[b(t)] = 0 \qquad \text{for all } t$$

$$E[a^2(t)] = E[b^2(t)] = \frac{A^2}{2} \int_{-\infty}^{\infty} W^2(t) \, dt$$

$$E[a(t_1)b(t_2)] = 0 \qquad \text{for all } t_1, t_2 \qquad\qquad (3.1.20)$$

$$E[a(t)a(t + \tau)] = E[b(t)b(t + \tau)] = \frac{A^2}{2} \int_{-\infty}^{\infty} W(t)W(t + \tau) \, dt$$

$$= \tfrac{1}{2} A^2 R_w(\tau)$$

disregarding second-order harmonic terms.

Hence $\{a(t)\}$ and $\{b(t)\}$ may be considered as orthogonal components of the envelope $\{H(t)\}$ of the random process $\{x(t)\}$. Further, as the weighting function $W(t)$ is narrow-band as compared to the Doppler frequency f_0 (see Section 2.6), the preceding analysis indicates that the Doppler signal detected at the photodetector output of the velocimeter leads to a narrow-band random process after filtering. Equation (3.1.17) conforms to the well-known representation of such a process.

Since $\{x(t)\}$ or $\{i(t)\}$ is Gaussian, its orthogonal components $\{a(t)\}$, $\{b(t)\}$ are also Gaussian, with zero mean and variance as given by equation (3.1.20). Also, it follows that the envelope $\{H(t)\}$ has a Rayleigh distribution, and the random phase $\{\phi(t)\}$ is uniformly distributed over the interval $(0, 2\pi)$. From equation (3.1.17) it may be seen that the effect of the random amplitudes of the individual photocurrent contributions from particles crossing the observation volume at random, is reflected as the random amplitude $\{H(t)\}$ and an associated random phase $\{\phi(t)\}$ of the filtered Doppler signal.

For a constant flow velocity, the instantaneous frequency of the Doppler signal is given by

$$\omega_i(t) = \frac{d\theta}{dt} = 2\pi f_0 - \frac{d\phi(t)}{dt}\,\text{rad/sec} \tag{3.1.21}$$

from equation (3.1.17). This indicates that the flow velocity can be obtained by processing the Doppler signal through an ideal frequency-to-voltage converter, which would yield its instantaneous signal frequency. From equation (3.1.21), the frequency-voltage converter output would consist of a constant value $2\pi f_0$, which represents the flow velocity, and a random component $\{d\phi(t)/dt\}$ due to the effect of the random size of scattering particles, their random arrival times, and finite passage times across the observation volume. This random component illustrates the ambiguity present in the measurement of the mean flow velocity by an LDV system and is usually termed *ambiguity noise*. The relative effects of this ambiguity on the estimation of the flow velocity can be obtained from the statistics of $d\phi(t)/dt$, such as its mean value, correlation, or power spectrum. These will be considered in detail in Section 3.3.

Power Spectra of Doppler Signal

As the process $\{x(t)\}$ is stationary, it is possible to determine its power spectral density function from the autocorrelation function

$$R_x(\tau) = E[x(t)x(t + \tau)]$$
$$= \tfrac{1}{2}A^2 R_w(\tau)\cos 2\pi f_0 \tau \tag{3.1.22}$$

which yields the two-sided power spectrum as

$$\Phi_x(f) = \int_{-\infty}^{\infty} R_x(\tau)\,e^{-j2\pi f \tau}\,d\tau, \qquad -\infty < f < \infty$$
$$= \tfrac{1}{4}A^2[\Phi_w(f - f_0) + \Phi_w(f + f_0)] \tag{3.1.23}$$

where $\{\Phi_w(f)\}$ is the two-sided power spectral density function of the weighting function $\{W(t)\}$. Equivalently, for real frequencies only, the one-sided power spectrum of $\{x(t)\}$ is related to the two-sided power spectrum of $\{W(t)\}$ as

$$\Phi_x(f) = \tfrac{1}{2}A^2\Phi_w(f - f_0), \qquad 0 < f < \infty \tag{3.1.24}$$

The Doppler signal $\{x(t)\}$ has a power spectrum which is symmetric about the mean Doppler frequency f_0. Symmetry conditions for the spectrum follow from the fact that $\{W(t)\}$ is an even function of time for any velocimeter setup.

Expressions are derived in Section 3.2 for the power spectra of Doppler signals arising in various optical configurations of the LDV. Although variations in the optical geometries lead to Doppler signals with different power spectra, in general, for uniform flow studies, the signals possess spectra which are narrow-band and centered on the Doppler frequency f_0, with a finite bandwidth (or spectral width). This bandwidth is usually small compared to f_0, and thus it represents another view of the finite passage time of scattering centers across the observation volume. Alternatively, the effect of ambiguity noise is reflected as the introduction of the finite bandwidth to the Doppler signal. Obviously the ambiguity noise can be reduced or the Doppler signal bandwidth can be curtailed by reducing the size of the observation volume, though there are practical limitations.

The center frequency f_0 represents the constant flow velocity. However, if the flow velocity is not uniform, but varies slowly about a mean value, it can be argued that this would lead to an instantaneous variation of the Doppler frequency. As such, for the case of fluid turbulence, the Doppler signal would represent a frequency modulated waveform where the modulating signal would reflect the characteristics of the turbulent component of the flow velocity, while the carrier frequency would be related to the mean flow velocity. The signal $\{x(t)\}$ of equation (3.1.15) or (3.1.17) represents the narrow-band (noise) carrier. Thus, under turbulent flow conditions, the filtered Doppler signal of the LDV would be a narrow-band noise carrier frequency modulated by a low-pass random process. It is this modulation signal that has to be extracted from the Doppler signal for studies on fluid turbulence. The function of the LDV system may be seen as translating fluid turbulence effects into a frequency modulation of the optical frequency about the mean Doppler frequency. Further details in this context are given in Section 3.3, while in Section 3.2 we shall concentrate on techniques for the measurement of the Doppler signal spectra and parameters related to it.

Doppler Signal Power

From the above analysis it is possible to determine the mean square level as the signal power for the filtered Doppler signal $\{x(t)\}$. It is instructive to evaluate its dependence on the various parameters involved, such as the optical geometry, flow conditions, particle concentration, etc. Thus

$$E[x^2(t)] = R_x(0) = \tfrac{1}{2}A^2R_w(0)$$

From equations (2.6.53)–(2.6.55) it may be seen that two typical formats for $\{W(t)\}$ are

(a) $W(t) = \exp\left(-\dfrac{t^2}{2\rho^2}\right)$ Gaussian beam and heterodyne systems

(b) $W(t) = \dfrac{\sin^2 \mu t}{(\mu t)^2}$ rectangular-aperture mask system

For these two cases $R_x(0)$ is $A^2(\pi\rho^2)^{1/2}/2$ and $\pi A^2/3\mu$, respectively.

Including the definition of A^2 as given in equation (3.1.9), and the definitions for ρ and μ proposed in the previous chapter [equation (2.6.55)] we have

(a) $R_x(0) = g_0 \dfrac{U\kappa^2 C_1}{2}\left(\dfrac{\pi}{2}\right)^{1/2}\dfrac{r_0}{U\cos\theta} = \left(\dfrac{\pi}{8}\right)^{1/2} g_0\dfrac{\kappa^2 C_1 r_0}{\cos\theta}$

and similarly

(b) $R_x(0) = g_0\kappa^2 C_1 \dfrac{\lambda L}{3a}$ \hfill (3.1.25)

However, as defined earlier, $g_0 = g(\Delta y\,\Delta z)$, where g is the mean (number) concentration of scattering centers per unit volume of fluid, and Δy, Δz are the dimensions of the observation volume. Using g_0 and the expressions for Δx for the various configurations [equation (2.6.55)], the mean square value of the signal may be expressed as

(a) $R_x(0) = \tfrac{1}{4}(\pi/2)^{1/2}g\kappa^2 C_1(\Delta x\,\Delta y\,\Delta z) = q_1 \cdot g\kappa^2 C_1(\Delta V)$

(b) $R_x(0) = \tfrac{1}{6 8}g\kappa^2 C_1(\Delta x\,\Delta y\,\Delta z) = q_2 \cdot g\kappa^2 C_1(\Delta V)$ \hfill (3.1.26)

where ΔV is the *coherence volume* or the volume of the interference region and q_1 and q_2 are numerical constants. From equation (3.1.26) it is evident that the mean square signal level is totally independent of the fluid velocity and depends only upon the size of the observation volume ΔV, the mean particle concentration (g), the mean scattering cross section of the particles (C_1), and the laser power and photodetector efficiency (κ^2). Thus for any laser velocimeter setup, the signal power is unaffected by the flow conditions, and is only related to the laser power and the mean size and number of particles crossing the observation volume per unit time. Although the present analysis is conducted for the case of uniform flow studies, the results are equally valid for appreciable levels of fluid turbulence.

3.2. Frequency Domain Analysis

In this section we will discuss the simplest method of analyzing signals from LDV systems, namely, the frequency domain method. It will be assumed that the photodetector yields quasicontinuous signals, i.e., even if the concentration of scattering centers is low, each burst will be in the form of a continuous trace rather than a discrete series of photon pulses. The photodetector shot noise will be taken as being of negligible importance. The approach is to measure the spectrum of the photodetector signal directly and normally to display this graphically. Intuitively, one would expect the spectrum to reflect the probability density of the velocity fluctuations in a turbulent or perhaps periodic flow. We will show that to a first approximation this is true. The fundamental advantage of the frequency domain method is its simplicity, i.e., virtually the only apparatus required is a wave analyzer and an XY plotter, both of which are normally standard equipment in a physics or engineering laboratory.

Methods for Measuring the Spectrum

Although techniques for spectral analysis are now quite standard, it is important that the differences between the various approaches are emphasized in relation to the analysis of LDV signals. First of all, the frequencies and quantities of data involved are usually too high for general purpose digital computers, so analogue methods are employed almost exclusively. Supposing the signal from the photodetector is $x(t)$, then an estimate of the power spectral density at frequency $f = \omega/(2\pi)$ is

$$\Phi_x(f) = \frac{1}{B_e T_r} \int_0^{T_r} x^2(t, f, B_e)\, dt \tag{3.2.1}$$

where B_e is the bandwidth of a narrow-band filter centered at frequency f, $x(t, f, B_e)$ is the contribution of $\{x(t)\}$ which passes through the bandpass filter, and T_r is the time over which the record is averaged.

The most efficient type of spectrum analyzer consists of a bank of narrow-band filters connected in parallel, their center frequencies being chosen to cover completely the range of interest. The outputs from these filters are squared and time-averaged and then displayed on the Y trace of an oscilloscope, the X position being proportional to the center frequency of the filter in question. Wave analyzers of this type are commercially available and are capable of computing the power spectrum as defined by equation

(3.2.1) without loss of any information. Unfortunately though, they tend to be very expensive, and instruments of reasonable size and cost invariably have too few channels to provide the resolution required. Also, they lack flexibility in that the range of frequencies covered is frequently very restricted.

On account of the difficulties with filter banks, most analog spectral analysis is carried out using simple wave analyzers of the swept-oscillator type. These are much cheaper than filter banks and also offer more flexibility as regards range and bandwidth, although they suffer one great disadvantage, that they only analyze a single frequency component (as opposed to a complete set of frequencies) at any one instant. From the user's point of view a wave analyzer can be considered essentially a narrow-band filter whose center frequency can be swept (normally at constant rate) across the range of interest. Wave analyzers can be bought as plug-in units for oscilloscopes, in which case the filter output is rectified and displayed on the Y scale after some smoothing. Normally this type of display can only be used for qualitative analysis of signal quality rather than for quantitative measurement of velocity statistics. For quantitative analysis the correct procedure is to compute the true power spectrum by employing a squaring circuit and integrator in conjunction with a wave analyzer, as indicated in the layout of Figure 3.2.1. We will show later on in this section how the power spectrum can be used to measure mean velocities and rms turbulence levels. The accuracy of these measurements is limited mainly by the fact that the wave analyzer only processes a single narrow frequency band at any given instant, so the total sweep generally takes a matter of minutes. The measured power spectrum will then only correspond exactly with the true ensemble-averaged spectrum if the statistical characteristics of the scattering particles (as well as the turbulence) remain stationary. Often in practice it is difficult to ensure that the mean number and size of scattering centers passing the observation volume does not change as the experiment proceeds. For this reason the direct frequency domain methods are normally only used in situations where very high accuracy is unimportant. In fact, for this reason, in the analysis to follow we have used only first-order approximations.

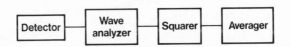

Figure 3.2.1. Layout for measurement of the power spectrum of an LDV signal.

For computing a spectrum, fairly obviously the bandwidth of the wave analyzer should be narrow compared with the Doppler spectrum; otherwise, there will be a significant instrumental broadening. If the bandwidth of the filter is B_e, then, as its risetime will be approximately $1/B_e$, the sweep rate must always be less than B_e^2, otherwise the analyzer filter will not respond fully to abrupt changes in the power spectrum. Usually the averaging time T_r of the integration circuit is considerably greater than $1/B_e$, so the maximum sweep rate is limited to B_e/T_r if true averaging is assumed, or $B_e/(4 \times RC$ time constant) for RC averaging (Bendat and Piersol, 1971).

Doppler Signal Spectrum for Constant Velocity Flow

One of the main characteristics of LDV signals is that, even for constant velocity flow, their spectra have a finite width. If the instrument is to be used for the measurement of turbulence, then it is important that the shape of the constant velocity spectrum be known; otherwise, the extent of the spectrum broadening caused by the turbulence cannot be calculated.

We assume that each particle produces a Doppler pulse

$$x_i(t) = K_i \cdot \kappa \cdot W(t) \cos (\omega_0 t) \tag{3.2.2}$$

the total signal being $x(t) = \sum_i x_i(t - t_i)$. Here $\{t_i\}$ are the random arrival times of the scattering particles at the observation volume. $\{K_i\}$ are constants which characterize the particle sizes, $\{W(t)\}$ is the weighting function, and κ is the weighting constant, dependent upon the over-all sensitivity of the detection system. It is convenient to normalize $x_i(t)$ by setting

$$\int_{-\infty}^{\infty} \kappa W(t)\, dt = 1 \qquad \text{and} \qquad N_p E[K_i^2] = 1$$

where N_p is the expected number of particles crossing the observation volume per second $[N_p = g_0 U$ of equation (3.1.8)]. No useful information is lost by this normalization since, for analogue analysis, the signal amplitude can be adjusted at will by altering the gain of the associated amplifiers. In equation (3.2.2) low-frequency components have not been included as these are generally either filtered out or disregarded.

From Campbell's theorem the autocorrelation of $x(t)$ is

$$R_x(\tau) = N_p^2 \left\{ E[K_i] \int_{-\infty}^{\infty} V(t)\, dt \right\}^2 + N_p E[K_i^2] \int_{-\infty}^{\infty} V(\mu) V(\mu + \tau)\, d\mu \tag{3.2.3}$$

where we have written

$$V(t) = \kappa W(t) \cos (\omega_0 t) \tag{3.2.4}$$

Only the second term on the rhs of equation (3.2.3) is τ-dependent, so the power spectrum of $x(t)$ will be identical to the energy spectrum of $V(t)$ apart from a δ-function peak at the origin, which we will disregard. The shape of the constant velocity Doppler spectrum is thus determined by computing the energy spectrum of $V(t)$.

From equation (3.2.4) the one-sided energy spectrum of $V(t)$ is

$$\Phi_v(\omega) = \tfrac{1}{2}\kappa^2 F[W(t)]^2 * [\delta(\omega - \omega_0)] \tag{3.2.5}$$

where $F[\ ]$ indicates Fourier transformation, and $*$ implies convolution. In writing equation (3.2.5) it has been assumed that the spectrum of $W(t)$ is narrow-band (as compared to ω_0) so that cross-harmonic terms can be disregarded. Note the similarity between equations (3.2.5) and (3.1.24), where, due to the normalizations employed, $A^2 = \kappa^2$.

Referring to equation (2.6.56), we find for the mask system with fringes aligned perpendicular to the flow direction

$$W(t) = \frac{\sin^2 \mu t}{(\mu t)^2} \tag{3.2.6}$$

which gives

$$F[W(t)] = \frac{\pi}{\mu}\Lambda\!\left(\frac{\omega}{2\mu}\right), \qquad -\infty < \omega < \infty \tag{3.2.7}$$

and since $\kappa = \mu/\pi$, from the normalization, we obtain

$$\Phi_v(\omega) = \frac{1}{2}\left(1 - \frac{|\omega - \omega_0|}{2\mu}\right)^2, \qquad |\omega - \omega_0| \le 2\mu$$
$$= 0, \qquad\qquad\qquad\quad |\omega - \omega_0| > 2\mu \tag{3.2.8}$$

For the Gaussian beam system

$$W(t) = e^{-t^2/(2\rho^2)} \tag{3.2.9}$$

which gives

$$\kappa = 1/(\rho\sqrt{2\pi})$$
$$\Phi_v(\omega) = \tfrac{1}{2}\,e^{-\rho^2(\omega - \omega_0)^2}, \qquad 0 \le \omega \le \infty \tag{3.2.10}$$

It is useful to calculate the spectral width of $\Phi_v(\omega)$, which will be denoted by $\Delta\omega$. To define this more precisely, let M_k be the moments of $\Phi_v(\omega)$ defined by

$$M_k = \int_0^\infty \omega^k \Phi_v(\omega)\, d\omega \tag{3.2.11}$$

The mean Doppler frequency is then M_1/M_0 ($=\omega_0$ in this case), and the spectral width is determined from the expression

$$\Delta\omega^2 = \frac{1}{M_0} \int_0^\infty \left(\omega - \frac{M_1}{M_0}\right)^2 \Phi_v(\omega)\,d\omega \qquad (3.2.12)$$

For the mask system the spectral width, from equations (3.2.8) and (3.2.12) is

$$\Delta\omega = 2\mu/\sqrt{10} \qquad (3.2.13)$$

and the spectral width as a ratio of center frequency is

$$\Delta\omega/\omega_0 = a/(b\sqrt{10}) \qquad (3.2.14)$$

For the Gaussian beam system the spectral width as a ratio of the mean frequency is

$$\Delta\omega/\omega_0 = (\omega_0\rho\sqrt{2})^{-1} \qquad (3.2.15)$$

The validity of equations (3.2.8) and (3.2.10) can easily be checked by using an LDV system to measure the velocity of a Perspex disc rotating at constant velocity on a record player turntable. As the concentration of scattering centers is high, the Doppler signal resembles white noise filtered by a bandpass filter of spectral width $\Delta\omega$ and the shape of the power spectrum can be determined by averaging the rectified output from a wave analyzer. This procedure eliminates the need for a squaring amplifier. With the correct scaling (Bendat and Piersol, 1971) the averaged value of the rectified wave analyzer output gives the square root of the power spectral density ($\Phi_v^{1/2}$), sometimes referred to as the frequency spectrum. For the mask system, from equation (3.2.8),

$$\Phi_v^{1/2}(\omega) = \frac{1}{\sqrt{2}}\left(1 - \frac{|\omega - \omega_0|}{2\mu}\right), \qquad |\omega - \omega_0| \le 2\mu$$

$$= 0, \qquad |\omega - \omega_0| > 2\mu \qquad (3.2.16)$$

Figure 3.2.2 shows a comparison between the theoretical frequency spectrum computed from equation (3.2.16) with $b/a = 40$ (i.e., $\mu = \omega_0/80$) and a frequency spectrum measured in the laboratory. The triangular shape of the measured spectrum can be seen quite clearly. The widths of the frequency spectra are greater than the power spectra. For the mask system we have

$$\left(\frac{\Delta\omega}{\omega_0}\right)_{\text{frequency spectrum}} = \frac{1}{\sqrt{6}}\frac{a}{b} \qquad (3.2.17)$$

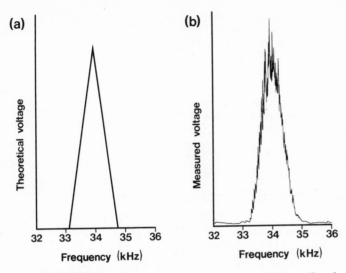

Figure 3.2.2. Frequency spectra for the mask system with $b/a = 40$ and $f_0 = 33.9$ kHz: (a) computed from equation (3.2.16); (b) measured in a rotating-disc experiment.

For the Gaussian beam system we have

$$\left(\frac{\Delta\omega}{\omega_0}\right)_{\text{frequency spectrum}} = \frac{1}{\rho\omega_0} \tag{3.2.18}$$

Rotation of the Optical System

The form of the intensity distribution across the measuring volume is such that equation (3.2.15) applies only when the scattering particles move in the plane of the beams (Figure 2.6.1). However, if the optical system is rotated so that the x axis moves away from the flow direction, then the ratio $\Delta\omega/\omega_0$ becomes larger. This is due to a decrease in ω_0 coupled with an increase in the passage time across the measuring volume. If the rotation is about the z axis such that the flow direction subtends an angle θ_f with the x axis while it remains in the x-y plane, then, from equation (2.6.25), the passage time across the beam between the $1/e$ points will be

$$\Delta t = \frac{2r_0}{U}(\cos^2\theta_f \cos^2\theta + \sin^2\theta_f)^{-1/2} \tag{3.2.19}$$

which reduces to equation (2.6.55) when $\theta_f = 0$. From equation (3.2.15) the relative spectral broadening becomes (as $\omega_0 = (4\pi U/\lambda) \sin \theta \cos \theta_f$)

$$\frac{\Delta\omega}{\omega_0} = \frac{1}{\omega_0 \rho\sqrt{2}} = \frac{U}{\omega_0 r_0}(\cos^2 \theta_f \cos^2 \theta + \sin^2 \theta_f)^{1/2}$$

$$= \frac{\lambda}{4\pi r_0}(\cot^2 \theta + \theta_f^2 \csc^2 \theta)^{1/2} \qquad (3.2.20)$$

As an example, when θ is small, we have

$$\frac{\Delta\omega}{\omega_0} \approx \frac{\lambda \sec \theta_f}{4\pi r_0 \tan \theta} \qquad (3.2.21)$$

and so a rotation of the optical system which increases θ_f from 0° to 45° also increases $\Delta\omega/\omega_0$ by a factor of $\sqrt{2}$. The effective reduction in the resolution of the velocimeter caused by rotating the x axis away from the flow direction can have important practical implications, for example, in the measurement of Reynolds' stresses, to be discussed later in this section.

The effect on the Doppler spectrum of rotating the fringes in the mask system depends on the shape of the apertures in the mask. It is quite obvious that if the fringe pattern shown in Figure 2.2.5a was rotated so that the flow was no longer perpendicular to the fringes, there would be a sharp increase in $\Delta\omega/\omega_0$ since the scattering centers would traverse only a relatively few fringes. The increase would be less marked, however, if the fringe pattern was as pictured in Figure 2.2.5b. To determine the exact shape of the Doppler spectrum consider again a flow velocity U at an angle θ_f to the x axis. Using equation (2.2.7) we see that equation (3.2.6) converts to

$$W(t) = \text{sinc}^2 \left(\frac{\omega_0 a t}{2b}\right) \text{sinc}^2 \left(\frac{\omega_0 c \tan \theta_f t}{2b}\right) \qquad (3.2.22)$$

where the Doppler frequency is now

$$\omega_0 = \frac{2\pi U b \cos \theta_f}{\lambda L} \qquad (3.2.23)$$

From equation (3.2.5) the one-sided power spectrum is

$$\Phi_v(\omega) = 2K_1^2 \left[\Lambda\left(\frac{\omega}{2K_2}\right) * \Lambda\left(\frac{\omega}{2K_3}\right) \right]^2 * \delta(\omega - \omega_0) \qquad (3.2.24)$$

where

$$K_1 = \frac{\kappa \pi b^2}{\omega_0^2 ac \tan \theta_f}, \qquad K_2 = \frac{\omega_0 c \tan \theta_f}{2b}, \qquad K_3 = \frac{\omega_0 a}{2b}$$

The convolution within the square brackets in equation (3.2.24) is not a continuous function but can be evaluated analytically within specified limits, the results being as follows:

For $K_2 < K_3 < 2K_2$

$$\Lambda\left(\frac{\omega}{2K_2}\right) * \Lambda\left(\frac{\omega}{2K_3}\right) = \begin{cases} I_1, & \text{when } 0 < |\omega| \leq 2(K_3 - K_2) \\ \\ I_2, & \text{when } 2(K_3 - K_2) < |\omega| \leq 2K_2 \\ \\ I_3, & \text{when } 2K_2 < |\omega| \leq 2K_3 \\ \\ I_4, & \text{when } 2K_3 < \omega \leq 2(K_2 + K_3) \end{cases} \tag{3.2.25a}$$

For $K_3 \geq 2K_2$

$$\Lambda\left(\frac{\omega}{2K_2}\right) * \Lambda\left(\frac{\omega}{2K_3}\right) = \begin{cases} I_1, & \text{when } 0 < |\omega| \leq 2K_2 \\ \\ I_5, & \text{when } 2K_2 < |\omega| \leq 2(K_3 - K_2) \\ \\ I_3, & \text{when } 2(K_3 - K_2) < |\omega| \leq 2K_3 \\ \\ I_4, & \text{when } 2K_3 < |\omega| \leq 2(K_2 + K_3) \end{cases} \tag{3.2.25b}$$

In the expressions (3.2.25a) and (3.2.25b),

$$I_1 = 2K_2\left(1 - \frac{K_2}{3K_3}\right) - \frac{\omega^2}{2K_3}\left(1 - \frac{\omega}{6K_2}\right)$$

$$I_2 = (K_2 + K_3)\left(1 - \frac{\omega^2}{4K_2K_3}\right) + \frac{\omega(K_2 - K_3)^2}{2K_2K_3} - \frac{1}{K_2K_3}\left(\frac{K_2^3 + K_3^3}{3} - \frac{\omega^3}{8}\right)$$

$$I_3 = (K_2 + K_3) + \frac{\omega^2(K_2 - K_3)}{4K_2K_3} - \frac{\omega}{2K_2K_3}(K_2^2 + 2K_2K_3 - K_3^2)$$

$$\qquad + \frac{1}{3K_2K_3}\left(K_2^3 - K_3^3 + \frac{\omega^3}{8}\right)$$

$$I_4 = (K_2 + K_3)\left(1 + \frac{\omega^2}{4K_2K_3}\right) - \frac{\omega(K_2 + K_3)^2}{2K_2K_3} + \frac{1}{3K_2K_3}\left(K_2^3 + K_3^3 - \frac{\omega^3}{8}\right)$$

$$I_5 = 2K_2\left(1 - \frac{\omega}{2K_3}\right)$$

When $K_3 \leq K_2$, then equations (3.2.25a) apply except that K_2 and K_3 are interchanged.

The validity of equation (3.2.24) has been checked in a rather simple manner that avoided the complexities of equation (3.2.25) (Greated, 1971c). From equation (3.2.24), the frequency spectrum is

$$\Phi_v^{1/2}(\omega) = \sqrt{2} K_1 \left[\Lambda\left(\frac{\omega}{2K_2}\right) * \Lambda\left(\frac{\omega}{2K_3}\right) \right] * \delta(\omega - \omega_0) \qquad (3.2.26)$$

From the moment theorem [equation (1.2.84)], the variance of $\Phi_v^{1/2}(\omega)$ is proportional to the sum of the variances of $\Lambda(\omega/2K_2)$ and $\Lambda(\omega/2K_3)$, which gives

$$\left(\frac{\Delta\omega}{\omega_0}\right)_{\text{frequency spectrum}} = \left(\frac{c^2 \tan^2 \theta_f + a^2}{6b^2}\right)^{1/2} \qquad (3.2.27)$$

In a rotating disc experiment $\Delta\omega/\omega_0$ was measured from the frequency spectrum for varying alignments of the fringe pattern relative to the direction of motion and also for different combinations of the mask parameters a, b, and c. The results of these experiments are shown in Figure 3.2.3, where comparison is made with the theoretical curves given by equation (3.2.27). When the c/a ratio is large (i.e., the mask apertures are two narrow slits), the fringe pattern is narrow in the fringe direction, as indicated in Figure 2.2.5a, and the ratio $\Delta\omega/\omega_0$ increases sharply with increasing θ_f. As the c/a

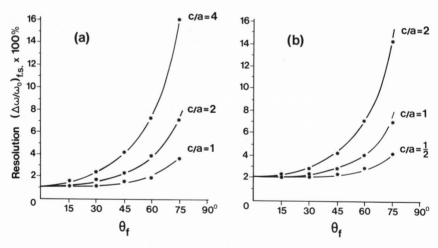

Figure 3.2.3. Comparison of theoretically predicted values of $(\Delta\omega/\omega_0)$ (frequency spectrum) with resolutions from a rotating-disc experiment for (a) $b/a = 40$; (b) $b/a = 20$. The stars are experimental points, and the solid curves are from equation (3.2.27).

ratio decreases, the rate of increase in $\Delta\omega/\omega_0$ with changing θ_f becomes less abrupt, which confirms the conclusions drawn from our intuitive reasoning.

The above analysis shows that with a mask containing two narrow slits, very high spatial resolution can be obtained in the direction of the fringes. The advantages of this, however, are offset by the broad spectral peak produced when the fringes are rotated relative to the flow direction. Choice of the most suitable fringe pattern shape depends on the particular experimental requirements. For example, when one is measuring close to a wall in laminar flow it can be an advantage to have c/a large, whereas in a turbulent flow the c/a ratio would generally be set equal to unity (square apertures) or less.

Spectrum in a Turbulent Flow

In a turbulent flow the center frequency ω_0 is continuously modulated by the velocity fluctuations. This gives rise to a broader Doppler spectrum than would be obtained with a constant flow velocity. By measuring the width of this spectrum it is possible, as we will see, to obtain information on the magnitude of the velocity fluctuations. For the reasons stated earlier in this section our analysis will be confined to first-order approximations. It will be assumed that the ensemble-averaged spectrum is obtained by averaging the energy spectra produced by the individual scattering particles passing through the measuring region. This approach will be elaborated on in Section 3.3.

If the instantaneous flow velocity along the x axis is

$$U(t) = U_0 + u(t)$$

then from equation (3.2.5) the ensemble-averaged power spectrum is

$$E[\Phi_v(\omega, \omega_0)] = \frac{\kappa^2}{2} \int_{-\infty}^{\infty} p(\omega_0) \cdot \{F[W(t)]^2 * \delta(\omega - \omega_0)\} \, d\omega_0 \qquad (3.2.28)$$

where $p(\omega_0)$ is the probability density of $\omega_0(t)$, which is now time-dependent and proportional to the instantaneous flow velocity. If D is the velocity-to-frequency conversion constant, then $\omega_0(t) = DU(t)$. Although $W(t)$ is now, strictly speaking, a function of $\omega_0(t)$, we write

$$W(t) = W(t, U_0) \approx W(t, U(t))$$

which is a good approximation provided that the bandwidth of $W(t)$ is narrow compared with ω_0 or, alternatively, that the rms turbulence level is low.

Equation (3.2.28) can equivalently be written as

$$E[\Phi_v(\omega, \omega_0)] = \tfrac{1}{2}\kappa^2 p(DU(t)) * F[W(t)]^2 \qquad (3.2.29)$$

i.e., the spectrum of the Doppler signal in a turbulent flow is a convoluted form of the velocity probability density function (correctly scaled using the velocity-to-frequency conversion constant). Thus if the bandwidth of $W(t)$ is narrow compared with ω_0, corresponding to a large number of fringes in the real fringe systems, then the Doppler spectrum is directly proportional to $p(DU(t))$.

It is common practice in laser anemometry to measure rms turbulence levels by observing the width of the Doppler spectrum. Applying the moment theorem [equation (1.2.84)] to (3.2.29) gives

$$\sigma_\Phi^2 = (D\sigma_u)^2 + (\Delta\omega)^2 \qquad (3.2.30)$$

where σ_Φ is the standard deviation of the power spectrum function, σ_u is the rms value of the velocity fluctuation, and $\Delta\omega$ is the standard deviation of the function $F[W(t)]^2$, i.e., the spectral width of the power spectrum with constant flow velocity.

To measure the rms turbulence level, the spectral width of the power spectrum estimate should first be determined. Frequently, a sufficiently good approximation can be obtained by assuming the spectrum to be Gaussian in shape, whence the width at half the height is equal to 2.35 standard deviations of the Gaussian function. A correction is then applied for the ambiguity broadening by using equation (3.2.30), $\Delta\omega$ being calculated from the expressions determined earlier in this section. Figure 3.2.4 shows a typical power spectrum recorded in a turbulent flow. The ordinates were obtained by measuring the output from a wave analyzer with a true rms voltmeter and then squaring the readings.

Interference of Low-Frequency Components

With a real fringe instrument, if either the turbulence level is very high or the number of fringes is small, a situation can arise in which the spectrum of the low frequencies overlaps the Doppler spectrum. This is depicted in Figure 3.2.5. If this arises, it is impossible to filter out the unwanted low frequencies without distorting the shape of the Doppler spectrum (unless, of course, some type of tracking filter is used).

In Section 2.2 it was shown that by using polarized beams it is possible to obtain two Doppler signals of the same amplitude but 180° out of phase.

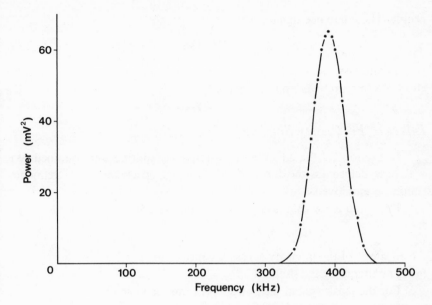

Figure 3.2.4. Typical power spectrum of the Doppler signal measured in a turbulent flow.

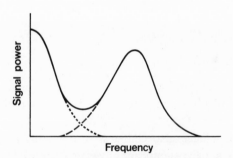

Figure 3.2.5. Effect of low-frequency interference in a highly turbulent flow: (– –) Doppler spectrum; (- - -) low-frequency spectrum; (———) total spectrum.

Suppose that the two signals for a single particle are

$$x_1(t) = W(t)[1 + \cos(\omega_0 t)] \tag{3.2.31}$$

$$x_2(t) = W(t)[1 + \cos(\omega_0 t + \pi)] \tag{3.2.32}$$

where $W(t)$ is low-pass, corresponding to the envelope of the intensity profile. The difference signal is then

$$x_1(t) - x_2(t) = 2W(t) \sin(\omega_0 t + \tfrac{1}{2}\pi) \tag{3.2.33}$$

i.e., is bandpass, the low-frequency term having been suppressed. Thus the effect of spectrum overlap is eliminated.

Effect of Frequency Shifting

In Section 2.2 the advantages of frequency shifting were outlined. We will now determine the form of the Doppler spectrum when frequency shifting is employed.

If the frequency shift is ω_s, then equation (3.2.5) converts to

$$\Phi_v(\omega) = \tfrac{1}{2}\kappa^2 F[W(t)]^2 * \delta(\omega - \omega_0 - \omega_s) \tag{3.2.34}$$

the envelope of the intensity across the measuring volume, and hence $W(t)$, being unaltered by the shift.

For the mask system the power spectrum then becomes

$$\Phi_v(\omega) = \frac{1}{2}\left(1 - \frac{|\omega - \omega_0 - \omega_s|}{2\mu}\right)^2, \qquad |\omega - \omega_0| \le 2\mu$$

$$= 0, \qquad\qquad\qquad\qquad\quad |\omega - \omega_0| > 2\mu \tag{3.2.35}$$

and for the Gaussian beam system

$$\Phi_v(\omega) = \tfrac{1}{2} \exp\left[-\rho^2(\omega - \omega_0 - \omega_s)^2\right], \qquad 0 \le \omega \le \infty \tag{3.2.36}$$

Note that in both cases the spectral width remains unaltered by the shift, while for an upward shift in frequency, $\Delta\omega/\omega_0$ is reduced by a factor $\omega_0/(\omega_0 + \omega_s)$. However, for a turbulent flow the relative broadening $D\sigma_u/\omega_0$ caused by the turbulence also changes by the same factor so frequency shifting does not yield any significant advantage towards separating the two broadening effects.

Frequency shifting is particularly useful if highly turbulent flows are to be measured, since an upward shift is accompanied by a separation of the Doppler and low-frequency components.

Measurement of Temporal Flow Characteristics

Frequency domain analysis of laser Doppler signals is primarily used for the measurement of rms turbulence levels and probability density estimates of the velocity fluctuations. However, it is also possible, by using

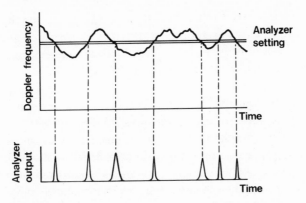

Figure 3.2.6. Form of the wave analyzer output in a turbulent flow.

a wave analyzer, to measure temporal characteristics of both periodic and turbulent flows.

Figure 3.2.6 indicates the form of the wave analyzer output (before squaring and averaging) in a turbulent flow, where the analyzer has been set at the mean Doppler frequency. It is a series of pulses, each pulse arising when the Doppler frequency passes through the passband of the analyzer. The height and time duration of each pulse will in general be different and dependent upon the bandwidth of the wave analyzer. The mean pulse rate, which can be measured with a simple pulse counter, is equal to the zero crossing rate of the velocity fluctuation, which we will refer to as N_z. Assuming Gaussian statistics for the velocity fluctuations, the zero crossing rate is related to the second derivative of the normalized correlation function $\rho_E(\tau)$ for the velocity fluctuations by (Papoulis, 1965)

$$N_z = (1/\pi)[-\rho_E''(0)]^{1/2} \tag{3.2.37}$$

In terms of the number of zeros per second, the turbulence micro time scale from equation (1.3.18) is then

$$\mathcal{T} = \frac{\sqrt{2}}{\pi N_z} \approx \frac{0.45}{N_z} \tag{3.2.38}$$

Methods have also been proposed for extending this idea to the measurement of integral time scales (Durrani and Greated, 1973a). The approach involves amplitude-limiting the rectified wave analyzer output and then time-averaging the resulting train of square wave pulses. This results in a dc level on which is superimposed a random ripple whose magnitude is dependent upon the relative values of the mean pulse rate and the averaging time constant. The rms magnitude of the ripple is measured and it can be shown that this is directly related to the turbulence integral scale.

An important application of laser anemometry is in the measurement of velocities under water waves in the laboratory. If the waves are periodic, frequency domain methods are particularly easy to apply and can be used to give complete velocity traces at various spatial positions. We will suppose that the waves propagate in a laboratory flume (i.e., two-dimensional flow) and have a surface elevation which is approximately sinusoidal. The horizontal component of fluid velocity, measured at some fixed spatial position under the wave, will then be approximately sinusoidal (Figure 3.2.7a) and in phase with the record of surface elevation. The output signal from a laser Doppler anemometer aligned in the flow then has a center frequency ω_0 which varies in proportion to the modulus of the velocity, as indicated in Figure 3.2.7b. The fact that the sign of the velocity is lost is unimportant in this application since observation of the surface elevation shows immediately whether the velocity is positive or negative. To record the velocities, the wave analyzer is set at a fixed frequency ω_f (Figure 3.2.7b) so that the output consists of a series of pulses (Figure 3.2.7c), each pulse occurring when the velocity passes the value ω_f/D, D being the velocity-to-frequency conversion constant. To reconstruct the complete velocity trace, the experiment is

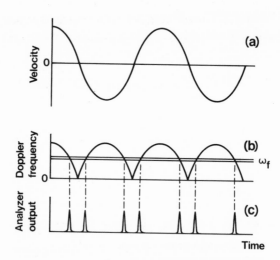

Figure 3.2.7. Wave analyzer operation when measuring under periodic water waves: (a) water velocity; (b) instantaneous frequency; (c) wave analyzer output.

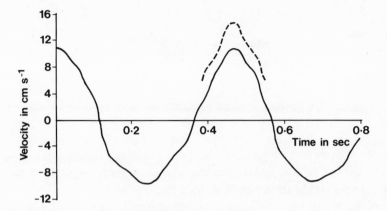

Figure 3.2.8. Typical traces of the horizontal component of velocity measured under a water wave by the frequency domain method. The solid line is the trace just below still-water depth, the dashed line is that at still-water depth.

repeated for a number of different values of ω_f. To obtain the correct phase relationship between the different series of pulses it is convenient to display them on an oscilloscope and trigger the time base from a pointer gauge located above the measuring point. The gauge can form part of a make-and-break circuit which produces the trigger pulse every time a wave crest passes and causes the water surface to touch the gauge. Figure 3.2.8 shows velocity traces at two different depths, reconstructéd from pulse records obtained in the manner just described. The upper trace represents the velocity record measured at still water depth and is discontinuous because the probe volume is only in the water part of the time. More detailed results are given by Lee, Greated, and Durrani (1974).

Measurement of Reynolds' Stresses

We will now consider the problem of measuring the cross product $E[u_1u_2]$ in a statistically stationary turbulent flow, u_1 being the velocity fluctuation in the mean flow direction and u_2 the fluctuation transverse to the flow. This quantity is important because the stress term $\rho_0E[u_1u_2]$ is a dominant parameter in most shear flow calculations (see Section 1.3). The most obvious approach is to measure the $u_1(t)$ and $u_2(t)$ fluctuations instantaneously and then determine the time average of the product $u_1(t)u_2(t)$; however this requires a two-component optical system and two-frequency tracking units to record the instantaneous signal frequencies. A much

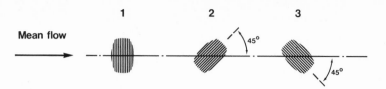

Figure 3.2.9. Orientation of the fringes for the measurement of Reynolds'
stresses.

simpler approach is to use a single optical unit and record three separate power spectra of the signal with the fringes aligned, respectively, at 90°, +45°, and −45° to the mean flow direction.

Referring to Figure 3.2.9, we find the instantaneous Doppler frequency when the fringes are aligned at right angles to the mean flow direction, i.e., in position 1, will be

$$\omega_0^{(1)}(t) = D[U_0 + u_1(t)] \tag{3.2.39}$$

When the fringes are rotated at +45° or −45° to the mean flow direction, i.e., into positions 2 and 3, then both the u_1 and u_2 velocity fluctuations contribute to the instantaneous Doppler frequency. Hence in position 2, we have

$$\omega_0^{(2)}(t) = \frac{D}{\sqrt{2}}[U_0 + u_1(t) - u_2(t)] \tag{3.2.40}$$

Similarly in position 3, we have

$$\omega_0^{(3)}(t) = \frac{D}{\sqrt{2}}[U_0 + u_1(t) + u_2(t)] \tag{3.2.41}$$

From equations (3.2.39), (3.2.40), and (3.2.41), respectively, we obtain

$$\{\omega_0^{(1)}(t) - E[\omega_0^{(1)}(t)]\}^2 = D^2 u_1^2(t) \tag{3.2.42}$$

$$\{\omega_0^{(2)}(t) - E[\omega_0^{(2)}(t)]\}^2 = \tfrac{1}{2}D^2[u_1^2(t) + u_2^2(t) - 2u_1(t)u_2(t)] \tag{3.2.43}$$

$$\{\omega_0^{(3)}(t) - E[\omega_0^{(3)}(t)]\}^2 = \tfrac{1}{2}D^2[u_1^2(t) + u_2^2(t) + 2u_1(t)u_2(t)] \tag{3.2.44}$$

Taking averages in equations (3.2.42)–(3.2.44) and then rearranging gives

$$E[u_1^2(t)] = (1/D^2)\, \text{var}\,[\omega_0^{(1)}(t)] \tag{3.2.45}$$

$$E[u_2^2(t)] = (1/D^2)\{\text{var}\,[\omega_0^{(2)}(t)] + \text{var}\,[\omega_0^{(3)}(t)] - \text{var}\,[\omega_0^{(1)}(t)]\} \tag{3.2.46}$$

$$E[u_1(t)u_2(t)] = (1/2D^2)\{\text{var}\,[\omega_0^{(3)}(t)] - \text{var}\,[\omega_0^{(2)}(t)]\} \tag{3.2.47}$$

After correction for ambiguity broadening, the widths of the three power spectra give var $[\omega_0^{(1)}(t)]$, var $[\omega_0^{(2)}(t)]$, and var $[\omega_0^{(3)}(t)]$ directly. The above three equations then indicate how those spectral widths are used to estimate the rms velocity fluctuations in the mean flow and transverse directions and also the cross product $E[u_1(t)u_2(t)]$. The center frequencies of the spectra will be related by

$$E[\omega_0^{(1)}(t)] = \sqrt{2}E[\omega_0^{(2)}(t)] = \sqrt{2}E[\omega_0^{(3)}(t)] \qquad (3.2.48)$$

Typically the method just described is used when measuring just above a boundary wall in a flow channel. In this situation the Reynolds' stress is negative and the power spectrum of the signal will be broader with the fringes in position 2 than when the fringes are aligned in position 3. Typical spectra recorded adjacent to a wall are shown by Greated (1970).

When correcting for spectrum broadening caused by the finite passage time across the beam, due account should be taken of the fringe rotation, as detailed earlier on in this section.

3.3. Time Domain Analysis

Doppler signal analysis by techniques of the previous section facilitate measurement of the mean flow velocity and the mean square levels of turbulence as observed by an LDV. Here we shall analyze the effect of temporal variations in flow velocity on the LDV signal. We propose to show that the instantaneous frequency of the signal faithfully follows velocity variations at the observation point. We shall develop relationships between the statistics of the flow velocity and the Doppler signal frequency and show how these relationships allow estimation of the temporal characteristics of the flow by processing techniques which involve detecting and analyzing the instantaneous signal frequency. Prior to that it is necessary to investigate in greater detail the effect of turbulent velocity variations on the Doppler signal correlation.

Correlation Function for Doppler Signals

In Section 2.6 an expression was developed for the instantaneous Doppler photocurrent in terms of the instantaneous position $\{x_p(t)\}$ of scattering centers present in the flow [cf. equations (2.6.62) and (2.6.63)]

$$i(t) = \kappa \sum_{p=-\infty}^{\infty} K_p W(\beta x_p(t)) \cos D x_p(t) \tag{3.3.1}$$

where $W(\beta x_p(t))$ represents the spatial weighting function expressed in terms of the position of particles. In the above equation the low-frequency term is not included, since in usual signal processing the Doppler signal output from the photodetector is always passed through a high-pass filter.

Let $\{x(t)\}$ be the voltage related to the Doppler photocurrent $\{i(t)\}$, and to avoid confusion we shall refer to the position of any pth particle at any time t as $\xi_p(t)$, i.e.,

$$x(t) = \kappa \sum_{p=-\infty}^{\infty} K_p W(\beta \xi_p(t)) \cos D \xi_p(t) \tag{3.3.2}$$

In Section 2.6 we specified the dimensions of the observation volume in terms of the region where the light intensity reduces to an arbitrarily small value. However, in theory, the light interference pattern extends indefinitely in all directions. Thus, to include the effect of a multiplicity of particles present both at the beam intersection at any instant and in the flow away from the beam intersection, we consider the dimensions of the observation volume to extend indefinitely along the flow axis (say x axis) and to restrict the volume cross section to $\Delta y \, \Delta z$ in the plane perpendicular to the flow axis. $\Delta y \, \Delta z$ represents the volume cross section as defined by equations (2.6.26), (2.6.31), or (2.6.38). Light scattered by particles outside this region would be negligible and would thus make a negligible contribution to the Doppler photocurrent.

If g is the mean (number/unit volume) concentration of scattering particles present in the fluid, then for the volume defined above, $g_0 = g \, \Delta y \, \Delta z$ is the mean number of particles present per unit length along the flow axis. As such, at any time instant, the probability of exactly M particles lying within a length X in the volume (i.e., in volume $X \, \Delta y \, \Delta z$) would be Poissonian and be given by

$$P(M, X) = \frac{(g_0 X)^M}{M!} e^{-g_0 X} \tag{3.3.3}$$

Further, if we consider any pth particle to be present within a spatial length X of the observation volume (along the flow axis) at any time, then its position within this interval is an independent random variable, and as such,

prob {pth particle lies in interval $\xi_p, \xi_p + d\xi_p$,

i.e., in volume element $d\xi_p \, \Delta y \, \Delta z$, at time t} $= (1/X) \, d\xi_p(t)$

In general, the position of any particle is totally independent of the position of any other particle at the same time instant.

If we consider the number of scattering particles present at any time t within the observation volume of size $X(\Delta y \, \Delta z)$ to be M, then the signal or photocurrent contributed by these particles is

$$x_M(t) = \kappa \sum_{p=1}^{M} K_p W(\beta \xi_p(t)) \cos D\xi_p(t) \tag{3.3.4}$$

such that from equation (3.3.2) we have

$$x(t) = \lim_{\substack{X \to \infty \\ M \to \infty}} x_M(t) \tag{3.3.5}$$

From equation (3.3.4) we have the conditional mean

$$E[x_M(t)|M] = \kappa C_0 \sum_{p=1}^{M} \int_{-X/2}^{X/2} W(\beta \xi_p(t)) \cos D\xi_p(t) \frac{d\xi_p(t)}{X}$$

$$= \kappa C_0 \frac{M}{X} \int_{-X/2}^{X/2} W(\beta y) \cos Dy \, dy \tag{3.3.6}$$

where $C_0 = E[K_p]$, as defined in equation (3.1.9). However

$$E[x_M(t)] = E[E[x_M(t)|M]]$$

$$= \sum_{M=0}^{\infty} E[x_M(t)|M]P(M, X)$$

where $P(M, X)$ is given in equation (3.3.3). Hence

$$E[x_M(t)] = \kappa C_0 g_0 \int_{-X/2}^{X/2} W(\beta y) \cos Dy \, dy$$

which leads, via equation (3.3.5), to the mean value of the Doppler signal:

$$E[x(t)] = \kappa C_0 g_0 \int_{-\infty}^{\infty} W(\beta y) \cos Dy \, dy \tag{3.3.7}$$

Note the similarity with equation (3.1.10). Here it must be remembered that the weighting function is defined in terms of spatial variables rather than time variables [vide equations (2.6.62) and (2.6.63)].

To determine the correlation function for $x(t)$ we define ξ_p as the position of the pth particle at any time t and ζ_p as the position of the same particle at time $t + \tau$ along the flow axis. Hence, we have, say,

$$\zeta_p = \xi_p + \int_t^{t+\tau} V_p(s)\,ds = \xi_p + \eta_p(\tau) \tag{3.3.8}$$

where $\{V_p(t)\}$ is the instantaneous velocity of the pth particle. For a homogeneous isotropic turbulent flow with mean velocity U_0, where the particles in the fluid move with the velocity of the fluid, we have, say,

$$E[\eta_p(\tau)] = U_0\tau, \qquad \text{var}\,[\eta_p(\tau)] = \int_0^\tau \int_0^\tau R_L(s_1 - s_2)\,ds_1\,ds_2$$

$$= \Omega(\tau) \tag{3.3.9}$$

where $R_L(s)$ is the Lagrangian autocorrelation of the fluid fluctuations. As such, the first-order statistics (mean, variance, and probability density function) of $\eta_p(\tau)$ are the same for all particles.

Thus we have

$$E[x_M(t)x_M(t + \tau)|M] = \kappa^2 E\left[\sum_{p,q=1}^{M} K_p K_q W(\beta\xi_p)W(\beta\zeta_p)\cos D\xi_p \cos D\zeta_q\right]$$

$$= \kappa^2 C_0^2 E\left[\sum_{\substack{p,q=1\\p \neq q}}^{M} W(\beta\xi_p)W(\beta\zeta_p)\cos D\xi_p \cos D\zeta_q\right]$$

$$+ \kappa^2 C_1 E\left[\sum_{p=1}^{M} W(\beta\xi_p)W(\beta\zeta_p)\cos D\xi_p \cos D\zeta_p\right] \tag{3.3.10}$$

where $C_1 = E[K_p^2]$ of equation (3.1.9).

It is worth stating that the position of a particle at any time depends only on its own position at a previous instant and its instantaneous velocity, and is independent of the position of any other particle at any time. As such, in the first term of equation (3.3.10), $\{\xi_p\}$ and $\{\zeta_q\}$ are independent random variables with identical distributions. Thus, after an analysis similar to the above, this term reduces to

$$\kappa^2 C_0^2 \left(\frac{M^2 - M}{X^2}\right)\left[\int_{-X/2}^{X/2} W(\beta y)\cos Dy\,dy\right]^2 \tag{3.3.11}$$

while the second term is equal to

$$\kappa^2 C_1 \sum_{p=1}^{M} \int_{-X/2}^{X/2} \int_{-X/2}^{X/2} W(\beta \xi_p) W(\beta \zeta_p)$$

$$\times \cos D\xi_p \cos D\zeta_p p(\zeta_p, \xi_p; t + \tau, t) \, d\zeta_p \, d\xi_p \quad (3.3.12)$$

where

$p(\zeta_p, \xi_p; t + \tau, t) \, d\zeta_p \, d\xi_p$ = prob {pth particle lies in the observation volume within the spatial interval $\zeta_p, \zeta_p + d\zeta_p$ at time $t + \tau$; and it lies in interval $\xi_p, \xi_p + d\xi_p$ at time t}

(These spatial intervals correspond to volume elements $d\xi_p \, \Delta y \, \Delta z$ and $d\zeta_p \, \Delta y \, \Delta z$, respectively, along the flow axis.) However,

$$p(\zeta_p, \xi_p; t + \tau, t) \, d\zeta_p \, d\xi_p = p(\zeta_p, t + \tau | \xi_p, t) p(\xi_p, t) \, d\zeta_p \, d\xi_p$$

$$= p_\eta(\zeta_p - \xi_p; \tau) \, d\zeta_p \frac{d\xi_p}{X} \quad (3.3.13)$$

where $p_\eta(\ )$ is the probability density function of the variable η_p of equation (3.3.8). However, since the first-order distribution function of $\{\eta_p\}$ is identical for all particles present in the flow, equation (3.3.12) reduces to

$$\kappa^2 C_1 \left(\frac{M}{X}\right) \int_{-X/2}^{X/2} \int_{-X/2}^{X/2} W(\beta y_1) W(\beta y_2)$$

$$\times \cos Dy_1 \cos Dy_2 p_\eta(y_1 - y_2; \tau) \, dy_1 \, dy_2 \quad (3.3.14)$$

Combining equations (3.3.11) and (3.3.14) and taking the limits of equation (3.3.5) after averaging over M, we obtain

$$E[x(t)x(t + \tau)] = \left[\kappa C_0 g_0 \int_{-\infty}^{\infty} W(\beta y) \cos Dy \, dy \right]^2$$

$$+ \kappa^2 C_1 g_0 \int\!\!\int_{-\infty}^{\infty} W(\beta y_1) W(\beta y_2) \cos Dy_1 \cos Dy_2$$

$$\times p_\eta(y_1 - y_2; \tau) \, dy_1 \, dy_2 \quad (3.3.15)$$

which reduces to

$$\text{cov}\,[x(t)x(t + \tau)] = \frac{\kappa^2 C_1 g_0}{2} \int_{-\infty}^{\infty} p_\eta(y; \tau) R_w(\beta y) \cos Dy \, dy \quad (3.3.16)$$

where

$$R_w(\beta y) = \int_{-\infty}^{\infty} W(\beta y_1)W(\beta(y_1 + y))\, dy_1$$

= autocorrelation function of the spatially defined
weighting function, i.e., a spatial correlation function

(3.3.17)

It is mathematically trivial to show that for constant velocity flows, where $p_\eta(y; \tau) = \delta(y - U_0\tau)$, equations (3.3.7) and (3.3.16) reduce to (3.1.10) and (3.1.11) or (3.1.14).

It can be shown from equation (2.6.64) that for a Gaussian beam optical setup

$$R_w(\beta y) = \left(\frac{\pi}{2\beta^2}\right)^{1/2} e^{-\beta^2 y^2/2}$$

(3.3.18)

$$\beta = (\cos \theta)/r_0 \simeq 1/r_0$$

and for a rectangular mask system

$$R_w(\beta y) = \frac{2\pi}{3\beta}\left[\frac{6}{(2\beta y)^2}\right](1 - \operatorname{sinc} 2\beta y)$$

(3.3.19)

$$\beta = \pi a/\lambda L$$

For homogeneous turbulent flows, the fluid velocity has a Gaussian probability density function, and thus the probability density function for variable η of equation (3.3.8) may be expressed as

$$p_\eta(y; \tau) = [2\pi\Omega(\tau)]^{-1/2} \exp\left[-\frac{(y - U_0\tau)^2}{2\Omega(\tau)}\right]$$

(3.3.20)

which has been obtained by employing the relationships of equation (3.3.9).

For the Gaussian beam system, the autocorrelation function of the Doppler signal may be determined by substituting equations (3.3.18) and (3.3.20) into (3.3.16) to yield

$$\operatorname{cov}[x(t)x(t + \tau)] = \frac{\kappa^2 C_1 g_0}{\{8\beta^2[1 + \beta^2\Omega(\tau)]/\pi\}^{1/2}} \exp\left[-\frac{1}{2}\frac{U_0^2\tau^2\beta^2 + D^2\Omega(\tau)}{1 + \beta^2\Omega(\tau)}\right]$$

$$\times \cos\left[\frac{DU_0\tau}{1 + \beta^2\Omega(\tau)}\right]$$

(3.3.21)

Hence the normalized autocorrelation function for the Doppler signal under conditions of turbulent flow is

$$\frac{\text{cov}\,[x(t)x(t + \tau)]}{\text{var}\,[x(t)]} = [1 + \beta^2\Omega(\tau)]^{-1/2}\exp\left[-\frac{1}{2}\frac{U_0^2\tau^2\beta^2 + D^2\Omega(\tau)}{1 + \beta^2\Omega(\tau)}\right]$$

$$\times \cos\left[\frac{DU_0\tau}{1 + \beta^2\Omega(\tau)}\right] \tag{3.3.22}$$

Thus the autocorrelation function for the Doppler signal in a Gaussian beam case is a damped cosine function, where the damping depends upon the mean flow velocity and the turbulent effects.

The above expression is the most general relationship for the correlation function of the Doppler signal, and it is valid for all possible conditions of flow. Thus in highly turbulent flows considerable diffusion may occur as the scattering particles move across the observation volume, defined in Section 2.6, such that their velocity changes appreciably as they pass across the beam interference region, as may happen when the interfering beams meet at a very small angle to produce a large observation region. The contribution of this diffusion effect is included in the integral $\Omega(\tau)$ of equation (3.3.9) or (3.3.22). If, however, the Lagrangian integral scale of diffusion is large, i.e., the particle velocities do not change significantly as they pass across the observation volume, then

$$\Omega(\tau) \simeq \sigma_u^2\tau^2$$

where $\sigma_u^2 = $ mean square turbulence level, which yields for the Gaussian beam setup

$$\rho_x(\tau) = (1 + \sigma_u^2\tau^2/r_0^2)^{-1/2}\exp\left[-\frac{1}{2}\tau^2\left(\frac{U_0^2/r_0^2 + D^2\sigma_u^2}{1 + \sigma_u^2\tau^2/r_0^2}\right)\right]$$

$$\times \cos\left(\frac{DU_0\tau}{1 + \sigma_u^2\tau^2/r_0^2}\right) \tag{3.3.23}$$

It may be seen on comparing equations (3.3.22) and (3.3.23) that the effect of diffusion is to reduce the rate of damping of the signal correlation. This is intuitively correct, and may be proved rigorously by considering a simplified [say, $R_L(\tau) = \sigma_u^2\exp(-\lambda|\tau|)$] model for the Lagrangian correlation function of the fluid (λ being the inverse of the Lagrangian integral scale).

Obviously, under conditions of uniform flow, equation (3.3.23) reduces to

$$\rho_x(\tau) = \exp\left(-\frac{U_0^2\tau^2}{2r_0^2}\right)\cos DU_0\tau \tag{3.3.24}$$

It is difficult to obtain a closed-form expression for the correlation function of the Doppler signal arising in a rectangular mask system. However, by employing equations (3.3.19) and (3.3.20), it may be shown that

$$\text{cov}\,[x(t)x(t+\tau)] = \frac{2\pi\kappa^2 C_1 g_0}{\beta}\sum_{k=0}^{\infty}\frac{(2\beta)^{2k}}{(2k+3)!}L_{2k}$$

where

$$L_{2k} = \frac{\partial^{2k}}{\partial D^{2k}}[e^{-D^2\Omega(\tau)/2}\cos DU_0\tau]$$

$$(3.3.25)$$

which may be evaluated by means of the Leibnitz rule for the higher-order differentials of the product of two functions. This yields

$$L_{2k} = \sum_{s=0}^{k}\binom{2k}{2s}(-1)^{k-s}[\Omega(\tau)]^s(U_0\tau)^{2(k-s)}H_{2s}(D[\Omega(\tau)]^{1/2})\,e^{-D^2\Omega(\tau)/2}\cos DU_0\tau$$

$$-\,[\Omega(\tau)]^{1/2}\sum_{s=0}^{k-1}\binom{2k}{2s+1}(-1)^{k-s}[\Omega(\tau)]^s(U_0\tau)^{2(k-s)-1}$$

$$\times\,H_{2s+1}(D[\Omega(\tau)]^{1/2})\,e^{-D^2\Omega(\tau)/2}\sin DU_0\tau$$

where $H_k(x)$ is a Hermite polynomial in x of order k, i.e.,

$$H_k(x) = (-1)^k\,e^{x^2/2}\frac{\partial^k}{\partial x^k}e^{-x^2/2}$$

The above results for the signal correlation, though cumbersome, are exact. Considerable simplification is possible, if we recall that the correlation of the weighting function $\{R_w(\beta y)\}$ does not change significantly with variations in η. Thus equation (3.3.16) may be closely approximated by

$$\text{cov}\,[x(t)x(t+\tau)]$$

$$\approx\frac{\kappa^2 C_1 g_0}{2}R_w(\beta U_0\tau)\int_{-\infty}^{\infty}\frac{\exp\{-(y-U_0\tau)^2/[2\Omega(\tau)]\}}{[2\pi\Omega(\tau)]^{1/2}}\cos Dy\,dy \qquad (3.3.26)$$

where equation (3.3.20) has been used for $p_\eta(y;\tau)$. This leads to

$$\text{cov}\,[x(t)x(t+\tau)] \approx \tfrac{1}{2}\kappa^2 C_1 g_0 R_w(\beta U_0\tau)\,e^{-D^2\Omega(\tau)/2}\cos DU_0\tau \qquad (3.3.27)$$

Because of the (dimensional) scaling involved in defining $\{W(\beta x)\}$, $R_w(\beta U_0\tau)$ is related to the (time) autocorrelation function $R_w(\tau)$ of Section 3.1 [equation (3.1.13) or obtained from equation (2.6.56)] through the flow velocity term, i.e.,

$$R_w(\beta U_0\tau)/R_w(\tau) = U_0$$

Substituting equations (3.3.18) and (3.3.19) into (3.3.27), we easily see that the expression for the Doppler signal power for the turbulence case is identical to that for uniform flow conditions, as in equations (3.1.25). It depends only on the mean particle concentration, laser power, and size of observation volume.

Simplified expressions for the normalized autocovariance of the Doppler signal, originating in the two LDV configurations considered here, may be conveniently obtained from equation (3.3.27) as

$$\rho_x(\tau) \simeq \exp\left[-\frac{U_0^2\tau^2}{r_0^2} - \frac{D^2\Omega(\tau)}{2}\right]\cos DU_0\tau \qquad \text{Gaussian beam system}$$

$$\rho_x(\tau) \simeq \frac{6}{(2\beta U_0\tau)^2}(1 - \text{sinc } 2\beta U_0\tau)\, e^{-D^2\Omega(\tau)/2}\cos DU_0\tau, \qquad \text{rectangular mask system}$$

Instantaneous Frequency of the Doppler Signal

Expressions were developed in Section 3.1 for the instantaneous frequency of the Doppler signal originating in the LDV under conditions of uniform flow. It was shown that the signal frequency was related to the flow velocity and included an additive term reflecting ambiguity noise. Here we extend the analysis to cover the effect of fluid velocity variations, such as fluid turbulence, on the instantaneous signal frequency. This enables us to develop expressions for the fluid velocity "observed" by the LDV and to relate it to various parameters of the flow. It is worth reiterating that it is the signal frequency that contains Doppler information on the instantaneous flow velocity past the observation volume.

The model for the Doppler current or voltage is as developed in Section 2.6 or as in equations (3.3.1) and (3.3.2). The following analysis could be conducted to include the contributions of the low-frequency component of the signal arising, for instance, in a real fringe system. However, it will be assumed that this component is filtered out prior to signal processing. The commonly assumed definition of the instantaneous frequency of the signal is the time derivative of its instantaneous phase angle. This definition was employed in Section 3.1 to determine the instantaneous Doppler signal frequency [equation (3.1.21)]. The instantaneous phase of the random Doppler signal of equations (3.3.1) and (3.3.2) is not immediately obvious. Thus, to determine the instantaneous frequency of the signal and to show how it relates to the flow velocity under conditions of nonuniform flow, we employ an analytic signal representation for the Doppler signal:

$$z(t) = x(t) + j\hat{x}(t) \qquad (3.3.28)$$

where

$$x(t) = \kappa \sum_p K_p W(\beta \xi_p(t)) \cos D\xi_p(t) \qquad (3.3.29)$$

$$\hat{x}(t) = \kappa \sum_p K_p W(\beta \xi_p(t)) \sin D\xi_p(t) \qquad (3.3.30)$$

Obviously the Doppler signal is the real part of $z(t)$. Then

$$z(t) = R(t)\, e^{j\theta(t)} \qquad (3.3.31)$$

with

$$\theta(t) = \tan^{-1} \hat{x}(t)/x(t), \qquad R^2(t) = x^2(t) + \hat{x}^2(t) \qquad (3.3.32)$$

This yields the instantaneous frequency of the analytic signal as

$$\omega_i(t) = \frac{d\theta(t)}{dt} = \frac{x(t)\dot{\hat{x}}(t) - \dot{x}(t)\hat{x}(t)}{x^2(t) + \hat{x}^2(t)} \,\text{rad/sec} \qquad (3.3.33)$$

Since the instantaneous frequency of the analytic signal $\{z(t)\}$ is the same as that of $\{x(t)\}$, we have from equations (3.3.29) and (3.3.30)

$$\omega_i(t) = D \frac{\sum\sum_{p,q} K_p K_q V_p(t) W(\beta \xi_p) W(\beta \xi_q) \cos D(\xi_p - \xi_q)}{\sum\sum_{p,q} K_p K_q W(\beta \xi_p) W(\beta \xi_q) \cos D(\xi_p - \xi_q)}$$

$$+ \beta \frac{\sum\sum_{p,q} K_p K_q V_p(t) W'(\beta \xi_p) W(\beta \xi_q) \sin D(\xi_p - \xi_q)}{\sum\sum_{p,q} K_p K_q W(\beta \xi_p) W(\beta \xi_q) \cos D(\xi_p - \xi_q)} \qquad (3.3.34)$$

where the time variable is implicit in the arguments of $\{\xi_p\}$ or $\{\xi_q\}$; $W'(x) = dW(x)/dx$; and $\{V_p(t)\}$ is the velocity of pth particle at time t, i.e., $V_p(t) = d\xi_p(t)/dt$.

The instantaneous frequency of the Doppler signal is a random variable which varies in time, both with the size and location of scattering particles, as well as with their instantaneous velocities. The Doppler signal $\{x(t)\}$, under nonuniform flow conditions, is therefore a frequency modulated signal where the modulating process is itself random. This modulating process, as indicated by the instantaneous signal frequency, reflects the varying conditions of the flow, as observed by the velocimeter. The (unconditional) mean value of $\omega_i(t)$ will be seen to be exactly equal to DU_0, where U_0 is the uniform mean flow velocity and this indicates that the Doppler signal is randomly frequency modulated about the mean (carrier) frequency.

Results identical to that of equation (3.3.34) for the instantaneous frequency of the Doppler signal are obtained if Van der Pol's definition

(Van der Pol, 1946; Stumpers, 1948) is employed. This definition views the instantaneous frequency as the mean density of zeros, of the signal, averaged over a small time interval:

$$\omega_i(t) = \lim_{h \to 0} \frac{2\pi}{h} \int_{t-h/2}^{t+h/2} \delta(x(\tau))\dot{x}(\tau)U(\dot{x}(\tau)) \, d\tau \qquad (3.3.35)$$

where $U(\ )$ is a unit step function. The integral counts the positive number of zero crossings of $\{x(t)\}$ in the interval $(t - \frac{1}{2}h, \, t + \frac{1}{2}h)$. Equation (3.3.35) may be simplified by using Fourier transforms, since

$$\delta(x(\tau)) = \frac{1}{2\pi} \int_{-\infty}^{\infty} \exp\left[jz_1 x(\tau)\right] dz_1$$

$$\dot{x}(\tau)U(\dot{x}(\tau)) = -\frac{1}{2\pi} \int_{-\infty}^{\infty} \frac{1}{z_2^2} \exp\left[jz_2 \dot{x}(\tau)\right] dz_2$$

Substituting into equation (3.3.35) and taking limits, we obtain an alternative expression for the signal frequency:

$$\omega_i(t) = -\frac{1}{2\pi} \int\int_{-\infty}^{\infty} \frac{1}{z_2^2} \exp\left\{j[z_1 x(t) + z_2 \dot{x}(t)]\right\} dz_1 \, dz_2 \qquad (3.3.36)$$

By inserting values of $\{x(t)\}$ and $\{\dot{x}(t)\}$, the exponential may be expanded into a series of Bessel functions, of which only the zeroth harmonic leads to finite values on integration. Thus we obtain

$$\exp\left[jz_1 x(t) + jz_2 \dot{x}(t)\right] = J_0(\kappa\sqrt{a_1^2 z_1^2 + 2a_3 z_1 z_2 + a_2^2 z_2^2})$$

$$+ \text{ higher-order terms} \qquad (3.3.37)$$

where

$$a_1^2 = \sum_{p,q}\sum K_p K_q W(\beta\xi_p)W(\beta\xi_q) \cos D(\xi_p - \xi_q)$$

$$a_3 = \sum_{p,q}\sum K_p K_q V_p[\beta W'(\beta\xi_p)W(\beta\xi_q) \cos D(\xi_p - \xi_q)$$

$$- DW(\beta\xi_p)W(\beta\xi_q) \sin D(\xi_p - \xi_q)] \qquad (3.3.38)$$

$$a_2^2 = \sum_{p,q}\sum K_p K_q V_p V_q\{[\beta^2 W'(\beta\xi_p)W'(\beta\xi_q) + D^2 W(\beta\xi_p)W(\beta\xi_q)] \cos D(\xi_p - \xi_q)$$

$$+ 2\beta DW'(\beta\xi_p)W(\beta\xi_q) \sin D(\xi_p - \xi_q)\}$$

Applying the geometrical expansion of the Bessel function of equation (3.3.37), we have

$$\exp[jz_1 x(t) + jz_2 \dot{x}(t)] = J_0(\kappa a_1 z_1)J_0(\kappa a_2 z_2) + 2\sum_{m=1}^{\infty} J_m(\kappa a_1 z_1)J_m(\kappa a_2 z_2)\cos m\theta$$

where $\cos\theta = -a_3/a_1 a_2$.

Inserting the above expansion into equation (3.3.36) and integrating term by term, we obtain

$$\omega_i(t) = \frac{1}{a_1^2}(a_2^2 a_1^2 - a_3^2)^{1/2} \quad \text{rad/sec} \tag{3.3.39}$$

which reduces to equation (3.3.34) after some tedious algebraic manipulations.

Since the two approaches lead to identical results, it is categorically confirmed that $\omega_i(t)$ of equation (3.3.34) is the instantaneous frequency of the Doppler signal, irrespective of the flow conditions.

Statistics of Observed Flow Velocity

Referring to equation (3.3.34), we can easily see that for constant fluid velocity [$V_p(t) = U_0$ for all p and t], the instantaneous signal frequency reduces to equation (3.1.21), i.e.,

$$\omega_i(t) = DU_0 - \frac{a\dot{b} - \dot{a}b}{a^2 + b^2} \quad \text{rad/sec} \tag{3.3.40}$$

where a and b are the orthogonal components of the Doppler signal as defined in equation (3.1.18), or, alternatively, as

$$a(t) = \kappa \sum_p K_p W(\beta U_0(t - t_p)) \cos DU_0 t_p$$

$$b(t) = \kappa \sum_p K_p W(\beta U_0(t - t_p)) \sin DU_0 t_p$$

Here $\{t_p\}$ represents the (random) time instants at which the particles cross the center of the observation volume.

In general the instantaneous Doppler signal frequency can be expressed as [see equation (3.3.34)]

$$\omega_i(t) = DU_a(t) + \dot{\phi}(t) \quad \text{rad/sec} \tag{3.3.41}$$

where $U_a(t)$ represents the effective velocity "observed" by the velocimeter at any time instant, and $\dot{\phi}(t)$ is the ambiguity noise. Here we propose to analyze the instantaneous observed velocity and develop expressions relating its correlation function to the Eulerian correlations of the flow.

Referring to equation (3.3.33), we see that since $\{x(t), \dot{x}(t), \text{etc.}\}$ depend on both the instantaneous position and velocity of scattering particles present in the flow, the value of $\{\omega_i(t)\}$ will be conditioned on the instantaneous velocity of the particles. A conditional (joint) probability density function $p(\mathbf{X}(t))$ can be developed for the variables,

$$\mathbf{X}^T(t) = (x(t)\hat{x}(t)\dot{x}(t)\dot{\hat{x}}(t)) \tag{3.3.42}$$

From this joint distribution the statistics of $\omega_i(t)$ can be determined. Since the Doppler signal $\{x(t)\}$ is considered as Gaussian with zero mean, the three other variables in $\mathbf{X}$ are also Gaussian, with zero mean. Then we have

$$p(\mathbf{X}(t)) = \frac{1}{(2\pi)^2|\mathbf{\Gamma}(t)|^{1/2}} \exp\left[-\tfrac{1}{2}\mathbf{X}^T\mathbf{\Gamma}^{-1}(t)\mathbf{X}\right] \tag{3.3.43}$$

where the covariance matrix $\mathbf{\Gamma}(t)$ is given by

$$\mathbf{\Gamma}(t) = \text{cov}\left[\mathbf{X}(t)\mathbf{X}^T(t)\right] = \begin{bmatrix} b_0 & 0 & 0 & b_1(t) \\ 0 & b_0 & -b_1(t) & 0 \\ 0 & -b_1(t) & b_2(t) & 0 \\ b_1(t) & 0 & 0 & b_2(t) \end{bmatrix} \tag{3.3.44}$$

Here, using the statistics of $x(t)$ derived earlier, we get

$$b_0 = \text{var}\,[x(t)] = \text{var}\,[\hat{x}(t)] = \frac{g_0 C_1}{2}\kappa^2 \int_{-\infty}^{\infty} W^2(\beta\xi)\,d\xi$$

$$= \frac{g_0 C_1}{2}\kappa^2 R_w(0) \tag{3.3.45}$$

[note that this is identical to equations (3.1.25) and (3.1.26)] and

$$b_1(t) = \text{cov}\,[x(t)\dot{\hat{x}}(t)] = -\text{cov}\,[\dot{x}(t)\hat{x}(t)]$$

$$= \text{cov}\left[\kappa^2 \sum_{p,q} K_p K_q V_p(t)\{\beta W'(\beta\xi_p)W(\beta\xi_q)\sin D\xi_p \cos D\xi_q \right.$$

$$\left. + DW(\beta\xi_p)W(\beta\xi_q)\cos D\xi_p \cos D\xi_q\}\right]$$

However, noting that $V_p(t)$, the velocity of any pth particle at any location ξ_p at time t, is equal to the fluid velocity $U(\xi, t)$ at the same location and time, we can reduce the above expression to the conditional covariance

$$b_1(t) = \text{cov}\,[x(t)\dot{\hat{x}}(t)|U(\xi, t) \text{ for all } \xi]$$

$$= \frac{\kappa^2 g_0 C_1}{2} D \int_{-\infty}^{\infty} U(\xi, t) W^2(\beta\xi)\,d\xi \qquad (3.3.46)$$

where higher-order harmonic terms are neglected. Similarly,

$$b_2(t) = \text{var}\,[\dot{x}(t)|U(\xi, t)\,\forall\xi] = \text{var}\,[\dot{\hat{x}}(t)|U(\xi, t)\,\forall\xi]$$

$$= \frac{\kappa^2 g_0^2 C_1}{2} \int_{-\infty}^{\infty} U^2(\xi, t)[\beta^2 W'^2(\beta\xi) + D^2 W^2(\beta\xi)]\,d\xi \qquad (3.3.47)$$

Then the mean value of the instantaneous Doppler frequency, conditioned on the statistics of the flow velocity, is obtained from (for a detailed analysis see Durrani and Greated, 1973)

$$E[\omega_i(t)|U(\xi, t)\,\forall\xi] = \iiiint\limits_{-\infty}^{\infty} \left(\frac{x\dot{\hat{x}} - \dot{x}\hat{x}}{x^2 + \hat{x}^2}\right) p(\mathbf{X})\,dx\,d\hat{x}\,d\dot{x}\,d\dot{\hat{x}}$$

$$= (b_1(t))/b_0 \qquad (3.3.48)$$

Thus the mean observed velocity is given by

$$E[U_a(t)|U(\xi, t)\,\forall\xi] = \int_{-\infty}^{\infty} U(\xi, t)\frac{W^2(\beta\xi)}{R_w(0)}\,d\xi \qquad (3.3.49)$$

A comparison with equation (3.3.41) suggests that $E[\dot{\phi}(t)] = 0$.

It was necessary to employ a conditional distribution for $\{x(t)\}$, since $\{x(t)\}$ is a frequency modulated process. Unconditional distributions would not yield the effect of the modulation, but rather the overall average values, just as the frequency spectrum of a randomly modulated FM process does not indicate the instantaneous variation of the frequency content of the signal, but only the overall envelope of the frequency deviations.

For zero turbulence the mean value of the observed velocity reduces to U_0, the uniform flow velocity. Otherwise, the observed velocity would always be a spatially averaged value of the flow velocity in the vicinity of the observation volume. The exact record of the (Eulerian) fluid velocity at a point would only be obtained when $W(\beta\xi) \to \delta(\xi)$.

Further, for a uniform mean flow velocity U_0, $E[U_a(t)] = U_0$, i.e., the unconditional mean value of the observed velocity is always equal to mean flow velocity.

While equation (3.3.49) shows the exact form of the spatial averaging effect arising in the LDV, a similar, though less cumbersome relationship may be developed by noting that in equation (3.3.34) $\{\xi_p(t) - \xi_q(t)\}$ represents the distance between any two particles in the vicinity of the observation volume at any time. The expression for the observed velocity may be simplified, because, for scattering particles in the flow which generate Doppler signals of appreciable strength, $\{\xi_p(t) - \xi_q(t)\}$ would be exceedingly small. Thus the effective velocity observed by the velocimeter at any time would be proportional to the first term in equation (3.3.34), i.e.,

$$U_a(t) = \frac{\sum_p K_p V_p(t) W(\beta\xi_p(t))}{\sum_p K_p W(\beta\xi_p(t))} \tag{3.3.50}$$

which suggests the observed velocity to be a weighted average of the instantaneous velocity of all the particles present in the observation volume, the weighting being proportional to the instantaneous position of the particle. George and Lumley (1973) and Kreid (1974) have also suggested that the velocimeter measures a weighted average velocity similar to equation (3.3.50). The conditional mean of this expression can be easily determined from the statistics of $\{x(t)\}$ and shown to be identical to that of equation (3.3.49).

The second-order statistics of the instantaneous signal frequency are given by

$$E[\omega_i(t)\omega_i(t + \tau)] = D^2 E[U_a(t)U_a(t + \tau)] + R_{\dot{\phi}}(\tau)$$
$$+ DE[U_a(t)\dot{\phi}(t + \tau) + U_a(t + \tau)\dot{\phi}(t)]$$

where $R_{\dot{\phi}}(\tau)$ is the autocorrelation of ambiguity. It will be shown later in this section that $R_{\dot{\phi}}(\tau)$ decays rapidly at the same rate as $R_w(\beta U_0\tau)$, further, that the cross correlation between ambiguity noise and the observed flow velocity is negligible. Thus, for an appreciable lag interval, the correlation function of $\omega_i(t)$ yields the correlation function of the observed flow velocity.

$$R_{\omega_i}(\tau) = D^2 R_{ua}(\tau) + R_{\dot{\phi}}(\tau)$$
$$= D^2 R_{ua}(\tau), \quad \text{for large lag values}$$

The autocorrelation function $R_{ua}(\tau)$ may be determined either from the eightfold probability density function $p[\mathbf{X}(t), \mathbf{X}(t + \tau)]$ or from the joint distribution associated with $U_a(t)$, $U_a(t + \tau)$ of equation (3.3.50). In either case identical results are obtained. First, the correlation of $U_a(t)$ may be determined conditioned on the statistics of the flow, and the observed velocity correlation obtained from the conditional moments. Thus

$$E[U_a(t)U_a(t + \tau)] = E[E[U_a(t)U_a(t + \tau)|U(\xi, t)U(\zeta, t + \tau) \, \forall \xi, \zeta]]$$

$$= E\left[E\left[\frac{g_1(t)g_2(t + \tau)}{q_1(t)q_2(t + \tau)}\right]\right] \tag{3.3.51}$$

where the definitions of g and q are obvious from equation (3.3.50). The conditional moments of g and q may be easily determined from their joint probability distribution, which is considered as Gaussian with zero mean. It may be shown that for appreciable values of lag τ, we have for the conditional moment

$$E\left[\frac{g_1(t)g_2(t + \tau)}{q_1(t)q_2(t + \tau)}\right] = \frac{\hat{b}_1(t)\hat{b}_1(t + \tau)}{\hat{b}_0^2} \tag{3.3.52}$$

where $\hat{b}_1(t) = 2b_1(t)/\kappa^2 D$ and $\hat{b}_0 = 2b_0/\kappa^2$ of equations (3.3.44)–(3.3.46). It is worth reiterating that this value of the conditional moment is obtained for lag values in which the ambiguity correlation or equivalently $R_w(\beta U_0 \tau)$ has decayed to negligible values and particle diffusion effects across the observation volume are considered as negligible.

Hence the correlation function of the observed velocity is given by

$$E[U_a(t)U_a(t + \tau)]$$

$$= E\left[\frac{1}{R_w^2(0)} \int\int_{-\infty}^{\infty} U(\xi, t)U(\zeta, t + \tau)W^2(\beta\xi)W^2(\beta\zeta) \, d\xi \, d\zeta\right] \tag{3.3.53}$$

For homogeneous turbulent flow conditions, with $U(\xi, t)$ having a uniform mean velocity U_0 and a turbulence component $u(\xi, t)$ such that $U(\xi, t) = U_0 + u(\xi, t)$, we may define the following statistics:

$$E[u(\xi, t)] = 0, \qquad \text{for all } \xi \text{ and } t$$

and

$$E[u(\xi_1, t)u(\xi_2, t + \tau)] = R_u(\xi_2 - \xi_1 ; \tau) \tag{3.3.54}$$

where $R_u(\xi_2 - \xi_1 ; \tau)$ represents the space–time velocity correlation at two points placed a distance $\xi_2 - \xi_1$ apart in the direction of the mean flow, for a lag value of τ. Thus

$$R_u(0; \tau) = \text{Eulerian (time) correlation of fluid velocity at a point}$$
$$[= \sigma_u^2 \rho_E(\tau)]$$

$$R_u(\xi_2 - \xi_1 ; 0) = \text{two-point (space) correlation of fluid velocity}$$

$$R_u(0; 0) = \text{mean square level of turbulence } (= \sigma_u^2)$$

Substituting the above definition of $U(\xi, t)$ into equation (3.3.50) or (3.3.49), we have

$$U_a(t) = U_0 + u_a(t)$$

or

$$E[U_a(t)|U(\xi, t) \,\forall\, \xi] = U_0 + \int_{-\infty}^{\infty} u(\xi, t)\frac{W^2(\beta\xi)}{R_w(0)}\, d\xi \qquad (3.3.55)$$

where the time-varying component $\{u_a(t)\}$ reflects the turbulence variations of the fluid velocity. Employing equations (3.3.53) and (3.3.54), we obtain

$$E[U_a(t)] = U_0, \qquad E[u_a(t)] = 0 \qquad (3.3.56)$$

and

$$\text{cov}\,[U_a(t)U_a(t + \tau)]$$
$$= \int_{-\infty}^{\infty} dz\, R_u(z; \tau)\left[\frac{1}{R_w^2(0)}\int_{-\infty}^{\infty} W^2(\beta\xi)W^2(\beta(z + \xi))\, d\xi\right] \qquad (3.3.57)$$

Defining

$$G(\beta z) = \frac{1}{R_w^2(0)}\int_{-\infty}^{\infty} W^2(\beta\xi)W^2(\beta(z + \xi))\, d\xi \qquad (3.3.58)$$

we see that the correlation function of the instantaneous Doppler signal frequency is

$$R_{\omega_i}(\tau) = D^2 \int_{-\infty}^{\infty} R_u(z; \tau)G(\beta z)\, dz + R_{\dot\phi}(\tau) \qquad (3.3.59)$$

The above analysis indicates that the mean value of the instantaneous Doppler signal frequency always yields the mean flow velocity and emphasizes the fact that the Doppler signal is randomly frequency modulated about a mean carrier frequency of DU_0.

The effect of the finite size of the observation volume in an LDV is seen as resulting in a spatial averaging of the flow velocities. This suggests an upper limit to the spatial resolution provided by the LDV. Thus (spatial) variations in fluid velocity of the order of the dimensions of the observation volume also contribute to the correlation of the observed flow velocity. Further, the Eulerian (point) velocity correlation is obtained only when $G(\beta z) \to \delta(z)$, or equivalently $W(\beta z) \to \delta(z)$. Then,

$$\text{cov}\,[U_a(t)U_a(t + \tau)] = R_u(0; \tau) \qquad (3.3.60)$$

In practice the dimensions of the observation volume are exceedingly small compared to the length scales of fluid turbulence. Therefore the correlation function of the instantaneous frequency of the Doppler signal consists of the Eulerian velocity correlation and the correlation of ambiguity noise. Expressions will be developed later for the ambiguity correlation. It will be shown that the ambiguity noise spectrum is broad-band compared to the Eulerian turbulence spectrum, such that the power spectrum of $\{\omega_i(t)\}$ consists of the Eulerian turbulence spectrum riding on top of (i.e., added onto) the ambiguity spectrum.

Corresponding to the space–time correlation function of the turbulent field, we have the frequency–wave-number spectrum:

$$\Phi_u(k;\Omega) = \int\!\!\!\int_{-\infty}^{\infty} R_u(z;\tau)\,e^{-jkz-j\Omega\tau}\,dz\,d\tau$$

Then from equations (3.3.56) and (3.3.57) the power spectrum of the velocity observed by the LDV is

$$\Phi_{ua}(\Omega) = \int_{-\infty}^{\infty} \text{cov}\,[U_a(t)U_a(t+\tau)]\,e^{-j\Omega\tau}\,d\tau \;+\; U_0^2\delta(\Omega)$$

$$= \frac{1}{2\pi}\int_{-\infty}^{\infty} \Phi_u(k;\Omega)\Phi_G(k)\,dk \;+\; U_0^2\delta(\Omega) \tag{3.3.61}$$

where $\Phi_G(k)$ is the wave number spectrum corresponding to the higher-order spatial correlation $\{G_w(\beta z)\}$ of the weighting function, i.e.,

$$\Phi_G(k) = \int_{-\infty}^{\infty} G(\beta z)\,e^{-jkz}\,dz = \left[\int_{-\infty}^{\infty} W^2(\beta z)\,e^{-jkz}\,dz\right]^2 \Big/ R_w^2(0)$$

Ignoring the delta function at $\Omega = 0$, which represents the contribution of the mean flow velocity U_0 to the power spectrum of the observed velocity, we would obtain, ideally for $G(\beta z) \to \delta(z)$, the exact Eulerian velocity spectrum

$$\Phi_{ua}(\Omega) = \Phi_E(\Omega) = \frac{1}{2\pi}\int_{-\infty}^{\infty} \Phi_u(k;\Omega)\,dk \tag{3.3.62}$$

The smoothing effect introduced on the wave number spectrum of the flow field due to finite dimensions of the observation volume is apparent from equation (3.3.61). Thus for the Gaussian beam system, we have from equation (3.3.18)

$$\Phi_G(k) = e^{-k^2/4\beta^2} \tag{3.3.63}$$

and for the mask system, from equation (3.3.19) or equivalently from (3.2.25a)

$$
\Phi_a(k) = \left[\frac{1}{2\pi}\Lambda\left(\frac{k}{2\beta}\right) * \Lambda\left(\frac{k}{2\beta}\right)\right]^2 \frac{1}{R_w^2(0)}
$$

$$
= \begin{cases}
\left[1 - \frac{3}{2}\left(\frac{k}{2\beta}\right)^2 + \frac{3}{4}\left|\frac{k}{2\beta}\right|^3\right]^2, & 0 \leq |k| \leq 2\beta \\[3mm]
\left[2 - 3\left|\frac{k}{2\beta}\right| + \frac{3}{2}\left(\frac{k}{2\beta}\right)^2\left(1 - \frac{1}{6}\left|\frac{k}{2\beta}\right|\right)\right]^2 & 2\beta \leq |k| \leq 4\beta \\[3mm]
0, & \text{otherwise}
\end{cases}
\tag{3.3.64}
$$

In either case, the velocity–wave-number spectrum components upto 2β would be unaffected. Typically 2β is of the order of $200\ \mathrm{cm}^{-1}$ for the dimensions of the observation volume considered in the examples given in Section 2.6. In most circumstances this would be well beyond the ranges of turbulence of interest. Thus, in practice, the difference between the observed velocity spectrum $\Phi_{ua}(\Omega)$ and the Eulerian velocity spectrum is negligibly small. This deviation may be expressed as

$$
\Phi_E(\Omega) - \Phi_{ua}(\Omega) = \frac{1}{2\pi}\int_{-\infty}^{\infty} \Phi_u(k;\Omega)[1 - \Phi_G(k)]\,dk
$$

$$
= \frac{1}{2\pi}[-\Phi_G''(0)]\left[\frac{1}{2}\int_{-\infty}^{\infty} k^2\Phi_u(k;\Omega)\,dk\right]
\tag{3.3.65}
$$

where the latter is obtained by a Taylor's expansion of $\{\Phi_G(k)\}$ about $k = 0$. The approximation is very close since $\{\Phi_G(k)\}$ is broad-band compared to $\{\Phi_u(k,\Omega)\}$. The mean square deviation of the "observed" velocity from that of any point $\{\xi\}$ within the observation volume may be evaluated as

$$
\frac{E[u(\xi,t) - u_a(t)]^2}{E[u^2(\xi;t)]} = -\Phi_G''(0)\left\{\frac{\frac{1}{2}\displaystyle\iint_{-\infty}^{\infty} k^2\Phi(k;\Omega)\,dk\,d\Omega}{\displaystyle\iint_{-\infty}^{\infty} \Phi(k,\Omega)\,dk\,d\Omega}\right\}
\tag{3.3.66}
$$

The term within the braces is the well-known normalized dissipation factor (Hinze, 1959) for the fluid turbulence. This shows that the root mean square deviation of observed velocity is proportional to $1/\beta$, which indicates that the deviation increases linearly with the dimensions of the observation volume. It also suggests a lower bound to the spatial velocity variations that can be resolved by the LDV.

The analysis developed here shows conclusively that the Eulerian statistics of the flow velocity can be obtained from the instantaneous frequency of the Doppler signal. Hardware systems for obtaining the instantaneous signal frequency, such as frequency demodulators, zero-crossing detectors, and phase-locked loops shall be discussed in Chapter 6.

Ambiguity Noise Analysis

We have shown that the instantaneous frequency of the LDV signal for turbulent flow conditions consists of a term proportional to the instantaneous flow velocity at the observation point and an additive ambiguity noise component. To obtain reliable estimates of the flow velocity parameters such as its autocorrelation or (Eulerian) power spectrum from the signal frequency, it is necessary to correct for ambiguity noise. For instance, the power spectrum of the signal frequency is given by

$$\Phi_{\omega_i}(\Omega) = D^2\Phi_{ua}(\Omega) + \Phi_{\dot{\phi}}(\Omega) \tag{3.3.67}$$

A straightforward subtraction of the ambiguity noise spectrum from $\Phi_{\omega_i}(\Omega)$ will yield the turbulence spectrum.

It is exceedingly cumbersome to determine exactly the statistics of ambiguity noise under conditions of random frequency modulation of the Doppler signal as in the case of turbulent flows. We propose a practical simplification to obtain meaningful results.

The statistics of ambiguity noise can be easily determined for the Doppler signal arising under uniform flow conditions. To a close approximation, the ambiguity noise statistics, such as its power spectrum, remain unaffected by the presence of low levels of turbulence and depend only upon the mean flow velocity. It is only when turbulence levels are very high, typically over 15%, that the ambiguity noise spectrum departs significantly from that for uniform flow. For most practical situations, the Eulerian turbulence spectrum may be obtained by subtracting from the (measured) spectra of the Doppler signal frequency the ambiguity noise spectrum corresponding to uniform flow conditions.

For this case, the filtered Doppler signal represents a narrow-band stationary Gaussian process as given by equation (3.1.17), where the ambiguity noise is expressed in terms of orthogonal components of the signal as [equation (3.1.21)]

$$\dot{\phi}(t) = \frac{a(t)\dot{b}(t) - \dot{a}(t)b(t)}{a^2(t) + b^2(t)} \tag{3.3.68}$$

We have already shown that the mean value of $\dot{\phi}$ is zero under all conditions of flow. To determine its correlation we should evaluate

$$R_{\dot{\phi}}(\tau) = E[\dot{\phi}(t)\dot{\phi}(t + \tau)] = E\frac{(a_1\dot{b}_1 - \dot{a}_1 b_1)(a_2\dot{b}_2 - \dot{a}_2 b_2)}{(a_1^2 + b_1^2)(a_2^2 + b_2^2)} \quad (3.3.69)$$

where subscripts 1 and 2 refer to time instants t and $t + \tau$. The quantity $R_{\dot{\phi}}(\tau)$ may be determined from the joint probability distribution of $(a_1, a_2, b_1, b_2, \dot{a}_1, \dot{b}_1, \dot{a}_2, \dot{b}_2)$. Since all the terms are normally distributed, this requires an eightfold Gaussian distribution. $R_{\dot{\phi}}(\tau)$ as a function of Gaussian random variables has been evaluated by Rice (1948) in connection with noise detection in FM receivers, and extended for the LDV case by Durrani and Greated (1973b; 1974a). We quote the results:

$$R_{\dot{\phi}}(\tau) = \frac{1}{2}\left[\frac{\rho_w(\tau)\ddot{\rho}_w(\tau) - \dot{\rho}_w^2(\tau)}{\rho_w^2(\tau)}\right] \ln\left[1 - \rho_w^2(\tau)\right] \quad (\text{rad/sec})^2 \quad (3.3.70)$$

where

$$\rho_w(\tau) = \frac{R_w(\tau)}{R_w(0)} = \frac{E[a_1 a_2]}{E[a_1^2]} = \frac{E[b_1 b_2]}{E[b_1^2]}$$

$\rho_w(\tau)$ is the normalized autocorrelation function of the weighting function $W(t)$ [see equation (3.1.20)].

Equivalently, $R_{\dot{\phi}}(\tau)$ may be expressed in terms of the spatial correlation function $R_w(\beta z)$ discussed in the previous section. Thus

$$R_{\dot{\phi}}(\tau) = \frac{\beta^2 U_0^2}{2}\left\{\left[\frac{d^2}{d(\beta z)^2}\ln\rho_w(\beta z)\right]\ln\left[1 - \rho_w^2(\beta z)\right]\right\}_{z = U_0\tau} \quad (3.3.71)$$

where U_0 is the mean flow velocity and $\rho_w(\beta z)$ is the normalized (spatial) correlation function of the weighting function $\{W(\beta z)\}$. Note that $R_{\dot{\phi}}(\tau)$ tends logarithmically to infinity as $\tau \to 0$, which suggests infinite power for ambiguity noise. In practice, finite bandwidths and ranges of amplifiers associated with the frequency discriminator would limit this to finite values.

The logarithmic singularity also precludes a closed-form solution for $\Phi_{\dot{\phi}}(\Omega)$. However, a series expansion leads to the one-sided power spectrum of ambiguity noise:

$$\Phi_{\dot{\phi}}(f) = 4\int_0^\infty \frac{R_{\dot{\phi}}(\tau)}{(4\pi^2)}\cos 2\pi f\tau\, d\tau \quad (\text{Hz}^2/\text{Hz})$$

$$= -\frac{1}{2\pi^2}\sum_{k=1}^\infty \frac{1}{k}\int_0^\infty \left[\frac{d^2}{d\tau^2}\ln\rho_w(\tau)\right]\rho_w^{2k}(\tau)\cos 2\pi f\tau\, d\tau \quad \text{Hz},$$

$$0 \le f \le \infty \quad (3.3.72)$$

In general, a frequency to voltage conversion device is employed to determine the instantaneous Doppler signal frequency. If Q is the frequency (Hz) to voltage transformation constant of the instrument, then $Q^2\Phi_{\dot\phi}(f)$ is the conventional power spectral density function given in terms of V^2/Hz.

Ambiguity Spectra

We shall consider two typical velocimeter configurations.

A. Gaussian Beam System

The normalized autocorrelation of the weighting function is given by equation (3.3.18) as

$$\rho_w(\tau) = \exp\left(-\frac{\beta^2 U_0^2 \tau^2}{2}\right) = \exp\left(-\frac{\tau^2}{4\rho^2}\right)$$

where ρ is as defined in Section 2.6.6. This leads to

$$R_\phi(\tau) = \tfrac{1}{2}(\beta U_0)^2 \ln\left(1 - e^{-(\beta U_0 \tau)^2}\right) \quad (\text{rad/sec})^2$$

Substituting this into equation (3.3.72), we obtain the ambiguity noise spectrum as

$$\Phi_{\dot\phi}(f) = \frac{\beta U_0}{4\pi^{3/2}} \sum_{m=1}^{\infty} \frac{1}{m^{3/2}} \exp\left[-\frac{1}{m}\left(\frac{\pi f}{\beta U_0}\right)^2\right] \quad \text{Hz} \qquad (3.3.73)$$

It is important to note that $\beta U_0 = 1/\rho\sqrt{2}\ (= 2\pi\,\Delta f$, say) is the bandwidth (rad/sec) of the Doppler signal under uniform flow conditions [equation (3.2.15)]. Defining the normalizing factor $K_1 = 1/\rho\sqrt{2\pi}$ as in equation (3.2.10), we have the ambiguity spectrum as

$$\Phi_{\dot\phi}(f) = \frac{K_1}{4\pi} \sum_{m=1}^{\infty} \frac{1}{m^{3/2}} \exp\left[-\frac{\pi}{m}\left(\frac{f}{K_1}\right)^2\right] \quad \text{Hz}$$

$$= \frac{\Delta f}{2\sqrt{\pi}} \sum_{m=1}^{\infty} \frac{1}{m^{3/2}} \exp\left[-\frac{1}{4m}\left(\frac{f}{\Delta f}\right)^2\right] \quad \text{Hz} \qquad (3.3.74)$$

For $f < K_1$, the effect of the exponential term is small, and the ambiguity spectrum is largely flat. Using the Euler summation formula, we have

$$\Phi_{\dot\phi}(f) = \frac{K_1}{4\pi}\left\{\sum_{m=1}^{M-1} \frac{1}{m^{3/2}} \exp\left[-\frac{\pi}{m}\left(\frac{f}{K_1}\right)^2\right] + \frac{K_1}{f}\left[\text{erf}\left(\frac{\pi f^2}{MK_1^2}\right)\right]^{1/2}\right\} \qquad (3.3.75)$$

With the choice $M = \pi f^2/K_1^2$ and for $f \to \infty$, the above expression tends asymptotically to

$$\Phi_{\dot\phi}(f) \simeq \frac{K_1^2}{4\pi f} \simeq \frac{(\Delta f)^2}{f}, \qquad f \gg (\Delta f)$$

However, $f = \Delta f$ is a frequency well beyond the highest turbulence frequency of interest, so the ambiguity spectrum may be considered flat for most experimental purposes. The velocimeter frequency-to-voltage converter output is always low-pass-filtered. If f_b Hz is the bandwidth of this filter, then the observed ambiguity noise power is given in $(volt)^2$ as

$$\begin{aligned}
N_0 &= Q^2 \Phi_{\dot\phi}(0) f_b \quad V^2 \\
&= 0.2079 \, K_1 Q^2 f_b = 0.1173 \, \beta U_0 Q^2 f_b \\
&= 0.7369 \, Q^2 (\Delta f) f_b \tag{3.3.76}
\end{aligned}$$

since the series in equation (3.3.74), for $f = 0$, sums to 2.61237.

B. Mask System

The normalized autocorrelation of the weighting function is given in equation (3.3.19) as

$$\rho_w(\tau) = \frac{6}{(2\beta U_0 \tau)^2}(1 - \text{sinc } 2\beta U_0 \tau)$$

The ambiguity noise spectrum for this case has been computed numerically, since, inspite of the series expansion of equation (3.3.72), an algebraic solution is not possible. Details of the normalized spectrum are given in Durrani and Greated (1973b). The spectrum is flat with a bandwidth far in excess of any frequencies of interest for turbulence studies. The zero-frequency ordinate which specifies the spectrum completely in the regions of interest is given by

$$\Phi_{\dot\phi}(0) = 2.43099 \, K_2/4\pi \qquad \text{Hz} \tag{3.3.77}$$

where $K_2 = \mu/\pi = \beta U_0/\pi \; (= \Delta f/\sqrt{10})$, as in equations (2.6.55) or (3.2.14) and (3.3.19). Thus this gives an ambiguity noise power over the output filter bandwidth f_b as

$$\begin{aligned}
N_0 &= 0.1935 \, K_2 Q^2 f_b \\
&= 0.0616 \, \beta U_0 f_b Q^2 \quad V^2 \tag{3.3.78} \\
&= 0.612 \, Q^2 (\Delta f) f_b
\end{aligned}$$

Signal-to-Noise Ratios

The ambiguity noise spectra are flat and roll off at the rate of f^{-1} for substantially large values of f. It has been determined (Durrani and Greated 1973b) that for the two common LDV setups, the ambiguity noise has a 3-dB bandwidth of approximately Δf Hz, where Δf is the Doppler signal bandwidth.

On the basis of the flatness of the ambiguity noise spectrum over the relevant frequency range, "signal"-to-noise ratios can be developed for the LDV systems. In a record of the instantaneous frequency of the Doppler signal, the signal of interest is the component proportional to the instantaneous turbulent fluid velocity; therefore, the signal output from the frequency demodulator is $DU_a(Q/2\pi)$ V, where U_a is the observed flow velocity. If the mean velocity level is removed, this leads to the signal power as

$$S_0 = \frac{Q^2 D^2}{4\pi^2} \operatorname{var}(U_a(t)) = \frac{Q^2 D^2}{4\pi^2} \sigma_u^2 \quad \text{V}^2 \tag{3.3.79}$$

where σ_u^2 is the mean square level of turbulence. Here it is assumed that the low-pass filter on the output of the FM demodulator passes the signal proportional to the observed velocity without any attenuation. This yields the following signal-to-noise ratios for the two LDV systems expressed in terms of the parameters of the optical setup, by using equations (2.6.63) and (2.6.64), (3.3.76), and (3.3.78),

$$\eta_{01} = S_0/N_0 = 0.216 \frac{D^2 \sigma_u^2}{\beta U_0 f_b}$$

$$= \frac{34.1}{f_b} \left(\frac{r_0}{\lambda^2} \right) \left(\frac{\sigma_u^2}{U_0} \right) \tan\theta \sin\theta, \qquad \text{Gaussian beam} \tag{3.3.80}$$

$$\eta_{02} = S_0/N_0 = 0.411 \frac{D^2 \sigma_u^2}{\beta U_0 f_b} = \frac{5.17}{f_b} \left(\frac{b^2}{\lambda a L} \right) \left(\frac{\sigma_u^2}{U_0} \right), \qquad \text{Mask system} \tag{3.3.81}$$

Similarly, corresponding to the uniform mean flow velocity U_0, the mean level of the instantaneous frequency $\omega_i(t)$ is $DU_0(Q/2\pi)$ V, which gives the output dc power (D_0) as $(QDU_0/2\pi)^2 = (Qf_0)^2$, where f_0 Hz is the mean Doppler frequency of the signal $\{x(t)\}$. Thus a noise-to-"carrier" ratio, or percentage ambiguity noise, may be defined as

$$(N_0/D_0)^{1/2} = [N_0/(Qf_0)^2]^{1/2} = \{[\Phi_\phi(0) f_b]^{1/2}/f_0\} 100\% \tag{3.3.82}$$

For the Gaussian beam system this is

$$(N_0/D_0)^{1/2} = 28.8 \, (f_b/\rho f_0^2)^{1/2} \% \tag{3.3.83}$$

and for the mask system it is

$$(N_0/D_0)^{1/2} = 43.98\,(a/b)^{1/2}(f_b/f_0)^{1/2}\,\% \qquad (3.3.84)$$

From the above relationships the percentage ambiguity can be computed for any specified flow conditions. If P_0 is the mean square power of the frequency to voltage converter output after removal of the dc level, then the mean square value of the turbulence fluctuations can be computed by using equation (3.3.79). Since $P_0 = S_0 + N_0$,

$$\frac{\sigma_u^2}{U_0^2} = \frac{P_0}{Q^2 f_0^2} - \Phi_\phi(0)\frac{f_b}{f_0^2} \qquad (3.3.85)$$

Figure 3.3.1 illustrates a measured power spectrum of the instantaneous fluid velocity measured by a Gaussian beam LDV system for turbulent flow

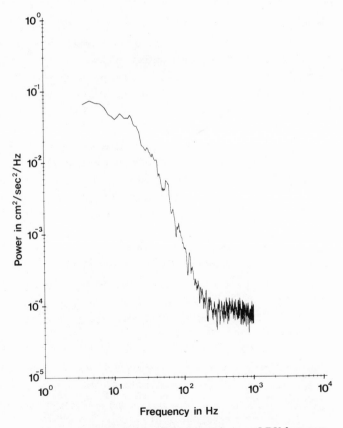

Figure 3.3.1. Power spectrum of the output from an LDV frequency-tracking system recorded behind a grid in a water tunnel. At the high-frequency end the spectrum falls to the constant ambiguity level.

conditions. The Doppler signal was bandpass filtered and then passed through a frequency-to-voltage converter which had an output filter with a bandwidth (≈ 1 kHz) considerably larger than the bandwidth of the (Eulerian) turbulence spectrum. The low-pass characteristics of the turbulence spectrum are immediately obvious. Note that the spectrum decays to constant values around 100 Hz. In this region the turbulence spectrum has decayed to negligible values, and $\Phi_{\omega_i}(f)$ is being dominated by the (flat) ambiguity noise spectrum. This is in accordance with the spectrum model of equation (3.3.67). The measured values of ambiguity noise power satisfy equation (3.3.76) exactly.

Noise Effects

The preceding analysis has been conducted for the Doppler signal, arising in the LDV, which is uncorrupted by any noise effects. In practical situations, noise arises from various sources in the over-all LDV setup; it contaminates all measurements and limits signal processing.

Noise contributions on the Doppler signal appear from three distinct sources: (1) optical noise sources, (2) photodetection effects, and (3) electronic system noise sources.

Optical noise sources may be characterized as diffractive and refractive beam perturbations, coherence degradation, light dispersion from lenses and medium, and laser hum. Imperfections in the optical system such as angular misalignment could also introduce bias to the Doppler signal. These account for noise introduced in the generation and transmission of the laser beams in the velocimeter setup.

Conversion of the Doppler shifted optical signal by a photodetector introduces two noise components—thermal (or Johnson) noise and quantum (or shot) noise. The amplifiers and effective load resistors of the detection system cause thermal noise, while dark currents contribute to internally generated noise. External quantum noise arises from the total radiation incident on the detector, and is thus contributed in part by the Doppler light signal and in part by the background environment. (Noise characteristics of commercially available photodetectors are well documented by Anderson and McMurtry, 1966, and Melchoir *et al.* 1970. Further relevant details are given in Section 1.4.)

Other electronic noise effects arise in the circuitry associated with the signal processing hardware.

The effect of the different noise sources can be lumped together, and can be represented as a single additive noise component on the Doppler signal $\{x(t)\}$. This noise is white and Gaussian due to the independent nature of the noise sources. In practice, it is band-limited by the bandwidth of the detection system following the photodetector.

We shall discuss the effect of this noise on the instantaneous frequency of the Doppler signal arising in the Gaussian beam system under uniform flow conditions. While it is not possible to determine completely the statistics of the instantaneous frequency of the signal corrupted by noise for turbulent flows, it is known that for turbulence levels of practical interest these do not depart significantly from that for uniform flow studies. The performance of any practical frequency detection system used with the LDV will depend upon and be limited by the characteristics of the signal frequency.

Prior to any frequency detection, the photodetected signal is always bandpass-filtered to remove low-frequency components and frequencies that do not contain Doppler information. For steady flows, the filtered Doppler signal uncorrupted by additive noise can be represented as a narrow-band process [see equation (3.1.17)]

$$x(t) = a(t) \cos 2\pi f_0 t + b(t) \sin 2\pi f_0 t$$

In practice the photodetected signal is degraded by noise effects, and thus has the form

$$y(t) = x(t) + n(t) \tag{3.3.86}$$

where $n(t)$ is the additive noise uncorrelated with the signal $x(t)$. Although the noise is white and Gaussian at the photodetector output, after bandpass filtering it reflects the frequency characteristics of the bandpass filter. It is rare for the center frequency of the bandpass filter f_1 ($=\omega_1/2\pi$ Hz) to be coincident with the mean Doppler frequency f_0 ($=\omega_0/2\pi$) and so $n(t)$ will generally have the form

$$n(t) = n_1(t) \cos \omega_1 t + n_2(t) \sin \omega_1 t \tag{3.3.87}$$

where $n_1(t)$, $n_2(t)$ are the orthogonal noise components. Let the offset frequency be

$$\omega_m = \omega_0 - \omega_1 \tag{3.3.88}$$

Then

$$y(t) = y_1(t) \cos \omega_0 t + y_2(t) \sin \omega_0 t$$
$$= H(t) \cos [\omega_0 t - \phi(t)] \tag{3.3.89}$$

where

$$y_1(t) = a(t) + n_1(t) \cos \omega_m t - n_2(t) \sin \omega_m t$$

$$y_2(t) = b(t) + n_1(t) \sin \omega_m t + n_2(t) \cos \omega_m t$$

$$H^2(t) = y_1^2(t) + y_2^2(t), \qquad \phi(t) = \tan^{-1} y_2(t)/y_1(t) \qquad (3.3.90)$$

Processing $\{y(t)\}$ through an ideal frequency demodulator yields the instantaneous frequency

$$\omega_i(t) = \omega_0 - d\phi(t)/dt \quad \text{rad/sec} \qquad (3.3.91)$$

Statistics of the ambiguity noise $\{d\phi(t)/dt\}$ would be affected by the additive noise $\{n(t)\}$. A finite mean value would lead to a bias on measurements of ω_0, while its correlation function or spectral density function would indicate the level below which turbulence measurements cannot be performed.

For the Gaussian beam system we define the Doppler signal correlation function as in equation (3.3.24):

$$R_x(\tau) = S_i \, e^{-\tau^2/4\rho_i^2} \cos \omega_0 \tau \qquad (3.3.92)$$

where S_i is the signal power and $1/\rho_i\sqrt{2}$ rad/sec is the signal bandwidth. Also, considering the bandpass filter characteristics as Gaussian (the most generally applicable case), we have

$$R_n(\tau) = N_i \, e^{-\tau^2/4\rho_n^2} \cos \omega_1 \tau \qquad (3.3.93)$$

where N_i is the noise power and $1/\rho_n\sqrt{2}$ rad/sec is the bandwidth of the bandpass filter.

The derivation of the statistics of $\dot{\phi}(t)$ is very complicated. For Gaussian distributed Doppler signals and noise, it has been fully developed in Durrani and Greated (1974a). We shall simply quote the results.

We can relate $R_x(\tau)$ and $R_n(\tau)$ by defining the following terms:

$\eta_i = S_i/N_i,$ input signal-to-noise ratio or carrier-to-noise ratio

$G_0 = \rho_i^2/\rho_n^2,$ input bandwidth ratio

$G_1 = G_0 - 1$

$\alpha = 1/4\rho_i^2$

Then

$$E[\dot{\phi}] = \frac{\omega_m}{\eta_i + 1} = \frac{b_0}{b_1} \qquad (3.3.94)$$

and

$$R_{\dot{\phi}}(\tau) = \left(\frac{q^2}{1-q^2}\right)\left(\frac{b_1}{b_0} + \frac{U_1^2}{q^2}\right)^2 + \left(\frac{U_1^2}{q^4} - \frac{U_2}{2q^2}\right)\ln(1-q^2) \quad (3.3.95)$$

where

$$b_0 = S_i + N_i, \qquad b_1 = \omega_m N_i$$
$$q^2 = (g^2 + h^2)/b_0^2, \qquad U_1 = (\dot{g}h - g\dot{h})/b_0^2$$
$$U_2 = (1/b_0^2)(\dot{g}^2 + \dot{h}^2 - g\ddot{g} - h\ddot{h}) \qquad (3.3.96)$$

g and h are the correlations of the components $y_1(t)$ and $y_2(t)$, i.e.,

$$g = E[y_1(t)y_1(t+\tau)] = E[y_2(t)y_2(t+\tau)]$$
$$= N_i e^{-\alpha\tau^2}(\eta_i + e^{-\alpha G_1\tau^2}\cos\omega_m\tau)$$

and

$$h = E[y_1(t)y_2(t+\tau)] = -E[y_1(t+\tau)y_2(t)]$$
$$= N_i e^{-\alpha G_0\tau^2}\sin\omega_m\tau \qquad (3.3.97)$$

$\dot{g} = dg/d\tau$, $\ddot{g} = d^2g/d\tau^2$, and similarly $\dot{h} = dh/d\tau$, $\ddot{h} = d^2h/d\tau^2$.

It may be seen that due to the offset center frequencies ($\omega_m \neq 0$) the ambiguity noise has a finite mean level, and its mean square level tends to infinity.

The following cases are of interest.

Case I. $\eta_i \to \infty$, i.e., the absence of additive noise on the signal:

$$E[\dot{\phi}] = 0, \qquad b_1/b_0 = 0, \qquad q^2 = e^{-2\alpha\tau^2}, \qquad U_1 = 0, \qquad U_2 = 2\alpha e^{-2\alpha\tau^2}$$

These give

$$R_{\dot{\phi}}(\tau) = -\alpha\ln(1 - e^{-2\alpha\tau^2}) \quad (\text{rad/sec})^2$$

which is identical to the ambiguity correlation developed earlier for the Gaussian case.

Case II. $\eta_i \to 0$, i.e., the absence of signal; $y(t) = n(t)$. Then

$$E[\dot{\phi}] = \omega_m, \qquad q^2 = e^{-2\alpha G_0\tau^2}, \qquad U_1 = -\omega_m e^{-2\alpha G_0\tau^2},$$
$$U_2 = 2(\omega_m^2 + \alpha G_0)e^{-2\alpha G_0\tau^2}$$

Hence

$$R_{\dot{\phi}}(\tau) = -\alpha G_0\ln(1 - e^{-2\alpha G_0\tau^2}) \qquad (3.3.98)$$

which is the autocorrelation of the instantaneous frequency of a bandpass-filtered Gaussian noise (Rice, 1948).

Case III. $\omega_m = 0$, i.e., the mean Doppler signal frequency is coincident with the center frequency of the bandpass filter. This yields

$$E[\dot\phi] = 0$$

$$R_\phi(\tau) = -\alpha\left[1 + \frac{G_1 e^{-\alpha G_1 \tau^2}}{\eta_i + e^{-\alpha G_1 \tau^2}} - \frac{2\eta_i \alpha (G_1 \tau)^2 e^{-\alpha G_1 \tau^2}}{(\eta_i + e^{-\alpha G_1 \tau^2})^2}\right]$$

$$\times \ln\left[1 - e^{-2\alpha\tau^2}\left(\frac{\eta_i + e^{-\alpha G_1 \tau^2}}{\eta_i + 1}\right)^2\right] \quad (\text{rad/sec})^2 \quad (3.3.99)$$

The ambiguity noise spectrum can be obtained by expanding in series the logarithmic term and then Fourier transforming the series term by term. If the bandwidth f_b of the low-pass filter following the frequency discriminator is such that

$$\omega_b = 2\pi f_b = H/\rho_i\sqrt{2}$$

then the ambiguity noise power is

$$P_0 = \int_0^{f_b} \Phi_\phi(f)\,df \quad \text{Hz}^2 \tag{3.3.100}$$

with

$$\Phi_\phi(f) = \frac{1}{\pi^2}\int_0^\infty R_\phi(\tau)\cos 2\pi f\tau\,d\tau \quad (\text{Hz}^2/\text{Hz})$$

For the three cases considered earlier, we have calculated the ambiguity noise power as

(I) $$P_0 = \frac{\alpha}{4\pi^2}\sum_{s=1}^{\infty}\frac{1}{s}\operatorname{erf}\left(\frac{H}{2\sqrt{s}}\right) \tag{3.3.101}$$

(II) $$P_0 = \frac{\alpha G_0}{4\pi^2}\sum_{s=1}^{\infty}\frac{1}{s}\operatorname{erf}\left(\frac{H}{2\sqrt{G_0 s}}\right) \tag{3.3.102}$$

(III) $$P_0 = \frac{\alpha}{4\pi^2}\sum_{s=1}^{\infty}\frac{1}{s}\frac{1}{(1 + 1/\eta_i)^{2s}}\left[\operatorname{erf}\left(\frac{H}{2\sqrt{s}}\right) + T_s\right] \tag{3.3.103}$$

where

$$T_s = \frac{1}{2s}\sum_{s=1}^{2s}\binom{2s}{r}\frac{1}{\eta_i^r}\left[(2s + G_1 r)\operatorname{erf}\left(\frac{H}{\sqrt{2(2s + G_1 r)}}\right)\right.$$
$$\left. - \frac{G_1^2 Hr(2s - r)}{(2s - 1)(2s + G_1 r)^{3/2}\sqrt{\pi/2}}e^{-H^2/2(2s + G_1 r)}\right] \tag{3.3.104}$$

Obviously as $\eta_i \to \infty$, equation (3.3.103) reverts to equation (3.3.101). As η_i deteriorates, i.e., as the contribution of external noise on the Doppler signal increases, the level of ambiguity noise increases. This increase may be calculated either from equations (3.3.101) and (3.3.104) or, as the ambiguity noise bandwidth is generally very large, using the approach proposed earlier, from the zeroth ordinate of the ambiguity power spectrum, as $P_0 \simeq \Phi_\phi(0) f_b$. We have calculated P_0 for the third case from the power spectral density function given by

$$\Phi_\phi(f) = \frac{\alpha^{1/2}}{\pi^{3/2}} \sum_{m=1}^{\infty} \frac{1}{(1 + 1/\eta_i)^{2m}} (A_m + B_m) \tag{3.3.105}$$

where

$$A_m = \sum_{s=0}^{2m-1} \frac{1}{\eta_i^s} \binom{2m-1}{s} \frac{\exp\{-v^2/[2(2m + G_1 s)]\}}{(2m - 1)(2m + G_1 s)^{1/2}}$$

$$+ \frac{G_1}{\eta_i} \frac{2m + G_1 s - 1 + G_1(2m - s - 1)v^2/\{2m[2m + G_1(s + 1)]\}}{(2m - 1)[2m + G_1(s + 1)]^{3/2}}$$

$$\times \exp\left(-\frac{v^2}{2[2m + G_1(s + 1)]}\right)$$

and

$$B_m = \frac{1}{\eta_i^{2m-1}} \left\{ \exp \frac{-v^2}{2[2m(G_1 + 1) - G_1]} \right\} [2m(G_1 + 1) - G_1]^{-1/2}$$

$$+ \frac{1}{2mn\eta_i^{2m}} \left(\frac{G_1 + 1}{2m}\right)^{1/2} \exp\left[\frac{-v^2}{4m(G_1 + 1)}\right]$$

where $v^2 = 2\pi^2 f^2/\alpha = (f/\Delta f)^2$, Δf being the Doppler signal bandwidth for zero additive noise. For computational purposes equation (3.3.105) may be summed up to N terms, and the remainder determined by the Euler summation formula. This remainder term is equal to

$$\frac{\alpha^{1/2}}{v\pi^{3/2}} \operatorname{erf}\left(\frac{v^2}{4N - 2}\right)^{1/2} + \frac{G_1}{(\eta_i + 1)^2}\left[(\eta_i - 1)\operatorname{erf}(c_1)\right.$$

$$\left. + \frac{4\eta_i c_1}{\sqrt{\pi}} \exp(-c_1^2)\right] \tag{3.3.106}$$

where $c_1 = v/[2(2N + G_1 - 1)]^{1/2}$. As $\eta_i \to \infty$, equation (3.3.105) reduces to

$$\Phi_\phi(f) = \frac{1}{2\pi}\left(\frac{\alpha}{2\pi}\right)^{1/2} \sum_{m=1}^{\infty} \frac{1}{m^{3/2}} \exp\left(\frac{-\pi^2 f^2}{2m\alpha}\right)$$

which is identical to equation (3.3.74).

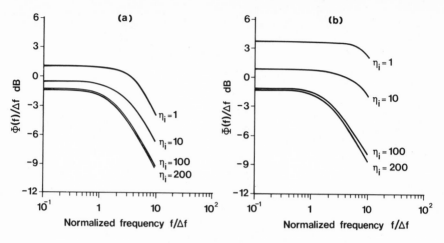

Figure 3.3.2. Ambiguity noise spectra for Doppler signal plus noise in a Gaussian beam system with (a) $G_1 = 5$; (b) $G_1 = 20$.

Figures 3.3.2a and b illustrate the power spectrum of the ambiguity noise for several values of the input signal-to-noise ratios η_i, and two representative values of the input bandwidth ratio G_1. These spectra were computed by summing equation (3.3.105) over 25 terms and then adding on the remainder of (3.3.106). The logarithmic plots, $(10 \log_{10} [\Phi_{\dot\phi}(f)/\Delta f]$ dB, indicate an upper bound of 10 dB/decade for the falloff of the spectra. For higher values of η_i, and independently of G_1, the spectra tend asymptotically to the ambiguity spectrum predicted by equation (3.3.74). For small values of η_i, the ambiguity noise is largely contributed by the additive noise, and the output (ambiguity) noise spectral density increases abruptly around $\eta_i = 1$, suggesting a threshold effect. Note that in all cases the ambiguity spectrum is flat over frequencies up to $f = \Delta f$ Hz. Thus the earlier considerations of wideband ambiguity noise are verified.

Using equations (3.3.76) and (3.3.105), we can calculate the percentage increase in ambiguity noise power due to the presence of additive noise on the Doppler signal for various values of η_i and G_1. This percentage increase is given by

$$\hat\eta_0 = \left\{ \frac{[\Phi_{\dot\phi}(0)f_b]_{\eta_i = \text{finite}}}{[\Phi_{\dot\phi}(0)f_b]_{\eta_i \to \infty}} - 1 \right\} \times 100\%$$

Values of $\hat\eta_0 \%$ for representative values of η_i and G_1 are listed in Table V.

Table V. Values of $\eta_0\%$ for Representative Values of η_i and G_i

η_i	G_1				
	5	10	15	20	25
10	23.25	40.81	56.81	71.94	86.20
100	2.79	4.62	6.26	7.79	9.09
200	1.56	2.48	3.30	4.06	4.55

The ambiguity noise level is sensitive not only to the input signal-to-noise ratio but also the bandwidth ratio G_0 (or G_1). Thus, while a large IF bandwidth of the processing system (or the bandpass filter) would allow analysis of large velocity fluctuations of the medium, it would also result in a corresponding increase in the output ambiguity noise.

Chapter 4

THE PHOTON
CORRELATION METHOD

4.1. Principles of Photon Counting

While in the previous chapter we considered the statistics of continuous
LDV signals generated by the passage of scattering centers through the
measuring volume, it was noted in Chapter 1 that it is actually more correct
to think of the output from the photodetection device as a series of discrete
pulses, each pulse corresponding to the ejection of an electron from the
detector surface. When the pulse rate is high, i.e., the observed intensity is
large, then, since the detection system always has a finite bandwidth, the
series of pulses is effectively smoothed to form a continuous signal (the case
so far considered). Even for high intensities, though, it is important to note
that the quantum nature of the detection process always gives rise to shot
noise superimposed on the continuous signal.

In this chapter we consider the case where intensities, and hence electron
emission rates, are low enough for the individual pulses at the detector output
to be counted and analyzed. One can imagine in this situation that the shot
noise has completely dominated the signal. The intensity level at which this
type of analysis becomes possible is relative in the sense that one can always
count individual emissions provided that the response time of the detection
and analyzing systems is sufficiently rapid. In practice it is not normally

feasible to reduce response times much below about 10 nsec. Photon correlation methods are most powerful in situations where scattering is small, particularly, for example, in unseeded wind tunnel flows (Abbis *et al.*, 1972; Meneelly *et al.*, 1972) or other gas flow situations. At low particle concentrations the intensity can be considered as quasicontinuous, i.e., the intensity varies continuously during the periods of time when particles are present within the measuring volume. However, during these periods the photodetector output is a series of discrete pulses.

The measuring time required for estimating some given velocity statistics is generally greater with the photon correlation method than for analogue analysis of the detector signal, but this disadvantage is offset by the greatly increased sensitivity. In order to implement the method in practice one needs to pay careful attention to the characteristics of the detector and normally only high-quality photomultipliers will be satisfactory. One of the characteristics of photomultipliers is that, due to the statistical nature of the multiplication process, the output pulses, corresponding to each electron ejection from the cathode surface, do not all. have the same height. This problem is normally overcome by incorporating a discriminator within the photomultiplier housing. It will be assumed throughout this chapter that a discriminator is used and adjusted so that equal-height pulses are obtained from the photomultiplier–discriminator unit.

Probability Distribution of Counts

To understand the principle of the photon correlation method, consider first the probability distribution of counts $P(N, t)$ that arises when an LDV system is used to measure the velocity of a rotating disc [$P(N, t)$ is the probability of a photon count of N in a time interval of duration t sec]. Figure 4.1.1 shows a laboratory setup for this measurement that uses a real fringe backscatter system and where the disc rotates at constant angular speed on a record player turntable. The configuration shown makes use of a mask to form the fringe pattern, but a beam splitter can be used equally well. It is important to note here that the fringe pattern formed on the edge of the disc is in effect imaged through the pinhole onto the detector surface. This is in contrast to the type of experiment used to study the statistics of light sources and where the detector observes the scattered field over less than a coherence area (Mandel and Wolf, 1965; Tartaglia and Chen, 1973).

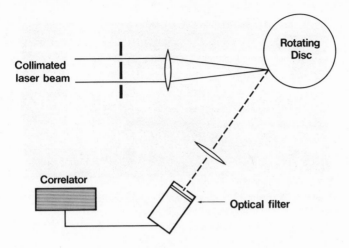

Figure 4.1.1. Laboratory setup for measuring the speed of a rotating disc.

Figure 4.1.2 shows a probability distribution recorded from a disc experiment for the case when the disc is stationary. If the disc moves slightly, the most probable number of counts in the observation time will generally change, since the orientation of the scattering centers forming the surface has changed. Thus the peak of the probability distribution moves either to the right or to the left. When the disc rotates at constant speed, the distribution of Figure 4.1.2 is thus continuously modulated and gives rise to a broad probability distribution. Figure 4.1.3, which was recorded when the disc was rotating, shows this broadening effect.

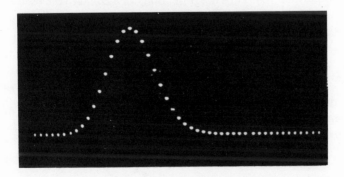

Figure 4.1.2. Probability distribution for backscattered light from a stationary disc. Sample time = 2 μsec.

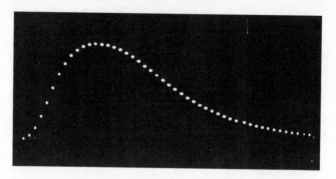

Figure 4.1.3. Probability distribution for backscattered light from a
rotating disc. Sample time = 2 μsec.

Constant Velocity Count Correlation

To formulate the problem mathematically we need to consider the case
in which a random arrangement of scattering centers are moving through a
measuring volume across which the spatial variation of intensity is known
as in the case of the continuous LDV signal studied in Chapter 3. Let $I(t)$
be the instantaneous variation of field intensity observed by the detector as
a single scattering center moves across the measuring volume with constant
velocity; $I(t)$ is a continuous function which is in fact proportional to the
LDV signal studied earlier, the constant of proportionality being dependent
upon the efficiency of the detector. For photon correlation analysis we need
to take into account the discrete nature of the detection process and in
Chapter 1 we noted that the probability of a count being recorded is proportional to the intensity. Thus the probability of a count in the time interval
$(t, t + \Delta t)$ is $\alpha I(t) \Delta t$, where α is the overall quantum efficiency of the detector
and is a constant for any particular optical system. The probability of a
count N in a time $t + \Delta t$ is then seen to be

$$P(N, t + \Delta t) = P(N - 1, t)\alpha I(t) \Delta t + P(N, t)[1 - \alpha I(t) \Delta t] \quad (4.1.1)$$

This is a difference equation which is known to have a solution (Bénard,
1972; Troup, 1972) [see Section 1.2, equation (1.2.51)]

$$P(N, t) = \frac{1}{N!} \left[\alpha \int_0^t I(\tau)\, d\tau \right]^N \exp\left[-\alpha \int_0^t I(\tau)\, d\tau \right] \quad (4.1.2)$$

Equation (4.1.2) represents a nonhomogeneous Poisson process whose
instantaneous rate depends upon the field intensity $\{I(t)\}$. When $\{I(t)\}$ is

time-independent, equation (4.1.2) reverts to the common Poisson distribution.

It is fairly obvious that in order to use records of photon counts observed in an apparatus like the one just described for measuring velocity, we must introduce some time parameters into our analysis. The simplest method of doing this is to form count correlations, and of course simplicity of computational procedure is important in this type of system since the speeds involved are very high. To perform a count correlation the number of counts occurring in consecutive nonoverlapping time intervals T are observed as indicated in Figure 4.1.4. If $N(kT, \overline{k + 1T})$ is the number of counts in the time interval $(kT, \overline{k + 1T})$ (three in the illustration of Figure 4.1.4), then the

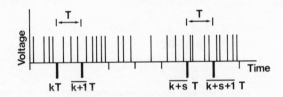

Figure 4.1.4. Typical series of photon pulses with the notation for the sampling procedure indicated.

unnormalized count autocorrelation $R_a(sT)$ is defined by

$$\tilde{R}_a(sT) = E[N(kT, \overline{k + 1T})N(\overline{k + sT}, \overline{k + s + 1T})], \quad k, s = 1, 2, \ldots \quad (4.1.3)$$

In practice, electronic instruments used for photon correlation experiments often use some form of clipping procedure which gives rise to an approximation to $R_a(sT)$ as defined in equation (4.1.3). The approximations introduced by such procedures will be discussed in Chapter 6 and in the theory to follow we will only concern ourselves with the form of the true count correlation as defined by equation (4.1.3).

In order to compute $\tilde{R}_a(sT)$ in a practical situation one usually has to assume that the process is statistically stationary, whence ensemble averages can be replaced by time averages. The digital correlator then accumulates values

$$r_a(sT) = \sum_{k=1}^{M} N(kT, \overline{k + 1T})N(\overline{k + sT}, \overline{k + s + 1T}) \quad (4.1.4)$$

each value of s corresponding to a different channel on the correlator; M is the number of products accumulated. The unnormalized count correlation is $\tilde{R}_a(sT) = r_a(sT)/M$. Notice that r_a gradually grows with time while $\tilde{R}_a$ converges toward a limiting value.

From equation (4.1.2) it is seen that the probability of having N counts over the kth interval of duration T is

$$P_k(N, t) = \frac{1}{N!}\left[\alpha \int_{kT}^{\overline{k+1}T} I(\tau)\, d\tau\right]^N \exp\left[-\alpha \int_{kT}^{\overline{k+1}T} I(\tau)\, d\tau\right] \qquad (4.1.5)$$

We now define

$$m(kT) = \int_{kT}^{\overline{k+1}T} I(\tau)\, d\tau \qquad (4.1.6)$$

Thus the count correlation function, conditioned on the intensity scattered by the passage of a single particle across the observation volume, is

$$E[N(kT, \overline{k+1}T)\, N(\overline{k+s}T, \overline{k+s+1}T)|m(kT)\, m(\overline{k+s}T)]$$

$$= \alpha^2 \int_{kT}^{\overline{k+1}T} \int_{\overline{k+s}T}^{\overline{k+s+1}T} I(\tau)I(v)\, d\tau\, dv + \alpha m(kT)\delta(sT) \qquad (4.1.7)$$

In the above equation the conditional moment is used because, since we are considering only the passage of a single particle, the mean intensity variation is known, i.e., $m(kT)$ and $m(\overline{k+s}T)$ are known. For the case of scattering centers arriving randomly in the observation volume, the expectation of the lhs of equation (4.1.7) is required. Thus

$$\tilde{R}_a(sT) = E[E[N(kT, \overline{k+1}T)\, N(\overline{k+s}T, \overline{k+s+1}T)|m(kT)m(\overline{k+s}T)]]$$

$$= \alpha^2 \int_{kT}^{\overline{k+1}T} \int_{\overline{k+s}T}^{\overline{k+s+1}T} E[I(\tau)I(v)]\, d\tau\, dv + \alpha\delta(sT) \int_{kT}^{\overline{k+1}T} E[I(\tau)]\, d\tau \qquad (4.1.8)$$

For small values of the counting interval T and for a stationary probability distribution for $I(t)$ this reverts to

$$E[N(kT, \overline{k+1}T)\, N(\overline{k+s}T, \overline{k+s+1}T)]$$

$$= \alpha^2 T^2 R_I(sT) + \alpha T m_0 \delta(sT) \qquad (4.1.9)$$

where

$$R_I(sT) = E[I(\tau)I(\tau + sT)]$$

for all τ and

$$m_0 = E[I(\tau)]$$

Equation (4.1.9) shows that the count correlation is proportional to the integrated intensity correlation (integrated over the detector surface) function of the radiation scattered by particles crossing the observation volume. Thus, since the spatial variation of intensity is known across the measuring volume, the count correlation gives a direct measure of the velocity of the scattering centers.

In order to apply equation (4.1.9), the intensity correlation $R_I(sT)$ must be calculated for a particular optical configuration and seeding condition. We will restrict the analysis in this chapter to real fringe LDV configurations. Generalization to include heterodyne systems would complicate the formulas because in correlation analysis there is no signal prefiltering, i.e., all the frequency components are retained. In practical application of the photon correlation method, real fringe geometries are used almost exclusively, the scattered light being collected at an angle to the optical axis in the forward-scattering mode. The reason for this is that the sensitivity of the detection process necessitates that background light levels be reduced to an absolute minimum.

For both mask and Gaussian beam optics the intensity variation observed by the detector for a single particle passing across the measuring volume can be written as

$$\psi_i(t) = K_i \psi(t) \qquad (4.1.10)$$

where

$$\psi(t) = AW(t)(1 + \cos \omega_0 t) \qquad (4.1.11)$$

The coefficient K_i depends upon the size of the scattering particle, and the constant A is related to the constant κ in Section 2.6 by the expression $A\eta = \kappa$. As in Section 3.2 and equation (2.6.56), we have considered the weighting to be a function of time and written it as $W(t)$.

The energy spectrum of the pulse is

$$\Phi_{\psi_i}(\omega) = K_i^2 A^2 \{F[W(t)]\}^2 * \{\delta(\omega) + \tfrac{1}{4}\delta(\omega + \omega_0) + \tfrac{1}{4}\delta(\omega - \omega_0)\} \qquad (4.1.12)$$

where F stands for Fourier transform. In deriving equation (4.1.12) we have disregarded double harmonic terms in ω_0 as these are negligible in all practical situations.

The pulse correlation function is then

$$\begin{aligned} R_{\psi_i}(\tau) &= \int_{-\infty}^{\infty} \psi_i(t)\psi_i(t + \tau)\, d\tau = F^{-1}[\Phi_{\psi_i}(\omega)] \\ &= \tfrac{1}{2}K_i^2 A^2 F^{-1}[\{F[W(t)]\}^2](2 + \cos \omega_0 \tau) \\ &= \tfrac{1}{2}K_i^2 A^2 R_w(\tau)(2 + \cos \omega_0 \tau) \end{aligned} \qquad (4.1.13)$$

where

$$R_w(\tau) = \int_{-\infty}^{\infty} W(t)W(t + \tau)\,d\tau$$

For a continuous stream of particles we define

$$E[K_i] = C_0, \qquad E[K_i]^2 = C_1$$

as in Section 3.1. Then, according to equation (1.2.63), if there are N_p particles per second on average, the intensity correlation function will be

$$R_I(\tau) = E[I(t)I(t + \tau)] = \tfrac{1}{2}N_pC_1A^2R_w(\tau)(2 + \cos\omega_0\tau)$$
$$+ N_p^2\left[C_0\int_{-\infty}^{\infty}\psi(t)\,dt\right]^2 \qquad (4.1.14)$$

The mean intensity is

$$m_0 = N_pC_0\int_{\infty}^{\infty}\psi(\tau)\,d\tau$$

and, from equation (4.1.9), the count correlation will be

$$R_a(sT) = \alpha^2T^2[\tfrac{1}{2}N_pC_1A^2R_w(sT)(2 + \cos\omega_0 sT) + m_0^2]$$
$$+ \alpha Tm_0\delta(sT) \qquad (4.1.15)$$

The pedestal level $m_0^2\alpha^2T^2$ and the delta function term are not used for the measurement of flow parameters, and for practical purposes are generally ignored. Thus in the analysis to follow we will only concern ourselves with the form of the time-lag-dependent part of the count autocorrelation function. This will be normalized to unity value at the origin (zero value for infinite time lag) and referred to as $R_a(sT)$. Thus applying equation (2.6.56) for constant flow velocity, the normalized count correlation functions are, for the Gaussian beam system

$$R_a(sT) = \frac{1}{3}\exp\left[\frac{-(sT)^2}{4\rho^2}\right](2 + \cos\omega_0 sT) \qquad (4.1.16)$$

and for the mask system

$$R_a(sT) = \frac{2(1 - \text{sinc}\,2\mu sT)}{(2\mu sT)^2}(2 + \cos\omega_0 sT) \qquad (4.1.17)$$

Alternatively, in line with the notation employed in Section 3.1, the instantaneous intensity can be written as (Durrani and Greated, 1974b)

$$I(t) = \int_{-\infty}^{\infty} \psi(t - \tau) \, d\tilde{N}(\tau) \qquad (4.1.18)$$

where $\kappa d\tilde{N}(\tau) = dN(\tau)$ as defined in equation (3.1.5).

Here $\{d\tilde{N}(t)\}$ represents the number of scattering centers present within the observation volume in the time interval $(t, t + dt)$. Now, $d\tilde{N}(t)$ is a stochastic process and can be characterized by the following parameters:

$$E[d\tilde{N}(t)] = C_0 N_p \, dt, \qquad \text{var}\,[d\tilde{N}(t)] = C_1 N_p \, dt$$

$$\text{cov}\,[d\tilde{N}(\tau) \, d\tilde{N}(t)] = 0, \qquad \text{for } t \neq \tau \qquad (4.1.19)$$

Using equation (4.1.14), we see that the statistics of the scattered intensity distribution are

$$R_I(sT) = C_1 N_p \int_{-\infty}^{\infty} \psi(\tau)\psi(\tau + sT) \, d\tau + N_p^2 \left[C_0 \int_{-\infty}^{\infty} \psi(\tau) \, d\tau \right]^2 \qquad (4.1.20)$$

$$m_0 = N_p C_0 \int_{-\infty}^{\infty} \psi(\tau) \, d\tau \qquad (4.1.21)$$

Hence, equation (4.1.15) follows.

If the weighting constant A is normalized such that

$$\int_{-\infty}^{\infty} W(t) \, dt = 1/A$$

then as $\{W(t)\}$ is low-pass compared to the Doppler frequency ω_0, this yields $m_0 \simeq N_p C_0$.

Equations (4.1.16) and (4.1.17) indicate that for the two LDV systems the count correlations are periodic and decay with $R_w(sT)$. For the sake of illustration, the correlation function for a mask system has been plotted (Figure 4.1.5) with $\mu = \omega_0/20$, i.e., effectively 20 fringes in the measuring volume. Notice that it has a periodic component in which the number of cycles reflects the number of fringes in the measuring volume. The crests and troughs have been marked for comparison with a correlation measured experimentally (Figure 4.1.6) by using the rotating disc system just described. For this test the sampling time was adjusted so that points on the correlation display coincided as nearly as possible with the crests and troughs.

It is important to note that the above relationships [equations (4.1.16) and (4.1.17)] are valid only under conditions of constant velocity. Turbulent variations in fluid flows lead to a time-varying ω_0, and thus to concomitant

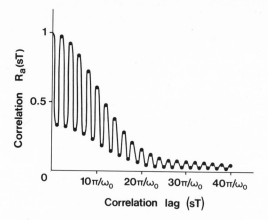

Figure 4.1.5. Normalized count correlation function for a mask LDV
system with $\mu = \omega_0/20$.

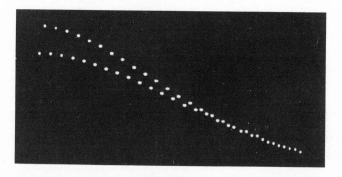

Figure 4.1.6. Count correlation function for backscattered light from
a rotating disc. Mask LDV system with $\mu = \omega_0/20$. Sample time
13 μsec.

frequency-modulation effects on the counting distribution $P(N, t)$. The effect
of these turbulent modulations will be considered in the next section.

4.2. Low-Turbulence Flows

In this section the effect of turbulent velocity fluctuations on the form
of the count correlation function will be considered.

Assume initially that the Lagrangian integral time scale is large compared with the passage time across the measuring region, i.e., each particle

maintains a constant velocity as it traverses the region, although of course the velocities of the individual particles will in general be different. It is then easy to visualize that the correlation $R_a(sT)$ can be constructed from a number of quasisteady velocity values, the final time-averaged correlation being formed by averaging with respect to the velocity variable. Justification for this procedure was given in Section 3.3 [equation (3.3.16)], although now it must be remembered that the low-frequency components of the Doppler signal are not filtered out. Thus

$$R_a(sT) = E[R_a(sT, U)] = \int_{-\infty}^{\infty} p(U)R_a(sT, U)\,dU \qquad (4.2.1)$$

where $p(U)$ is the probability density function for the velocity.

Consider first the Gaussian beam system. Since the instantaneous frequency is $\omega_0 = DU$, equation (4.1.16) can be written as

$$R_a(sT, U) = \frac{1}{3}\exp\left[\frac{-(sT)^2}{4\rho^2}\right](2 + \cos DUsT) \qquad (4.2.2)$$

where D is the velocity-to-frequency conversion constant.

Strictly speaking, the passage time ρ in equation (4.2.2) is a function of the instantaneous velocity since the size of the measuring volume is fixed. However, restricting the analysis to low turbulence levels we may take ρ to a good approximation as constant and equal to the distance across the measuring volume divided by the mean velocity. This approximation is also valid at high turbulence levels when a large number of fringes is employed in the optical system. The effect of very high turbulence levels will be considered in Section 4.6.

Thus for a Gaussian velocity fluctuation with

$$p(U) = \frac{1}{(2\pi\sigma_u^2)^{1/2}}\exp\left[-\frac{(U - U_0)^2}{2\sigma_u^2}\right], \qquad -\infty < U < \infty \qquad (4.2.3)$$

equations (4.2.1)–(4.2.3) may be combined to give

$$E[R_a(sT, U)] = \frac{1}{3(2\pi\sigma_u^2)^{1/2}}\exp\left[\frac{-(sT)^2}{4\rho^2}\right]$$

$$\times \int_{-\infty}^{\infty}\exp\left[-\frac{(U - U_0)^2}{2\sigma_u^2}\right](2 + \cos DUsT)\,dU \qquad (4.2.4)$$

Performing the integration, we see that the form of the normalized count correlation in a turbulent flow, with Gaussian beam optics is

$$R_a(sT) = \frac{1}{3}\exp\left[\frac{-(sT)^2}{4\rho^2}\right]\left\{2 + \exp\left[-\frac{(D\sigma_u)^2(sT)^2}{2}\right]\cos DU_0sT\right\} \quad (4.2.5)$$

The only difference between the above expression and the corresponding equation for constant velocity flow [equation (4.1.16)] is the exponential damping term. The damping effect of the turbulence can be seen in the experimentally measured correlations shown in Figures 4.2.1 and 4.2.2. Both of these were recorded in a wind tunnel without added seeding particles, using a forward-scattering real fringe system and 2 mW of laser power. Figure 4.2.1 shows the correlation behind a very fine grid of wires where the turbulence level was low. In this case virtually all of the damping is due to

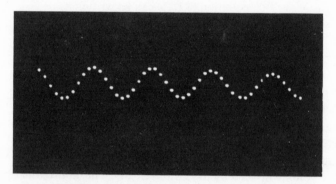

Figure 4.2.1. Count correlation function measured behind a fine grid in a wind tunnel, i.e., low turbulence level. Sample time = 1 μsec.

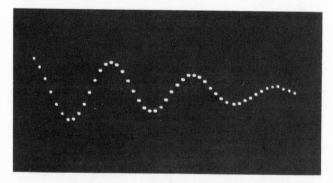

Figure 4.2.2. Count correlation function measured behind a coarse grid in a wind tunnel, i.e., high turbulence level. Sample time 1 μsec.

the fringe geometry, the damping due to the second exponential term in equation (4.2.5) being very small. Figure 4.2.2, on the other hand, shows the correlation behind a coarse grid of bars where the turbulence level was higher. Note the higher damping rate in this case.

For mask system optics the expression for the count correlation corresponding to equation (4.2.5) is

$$R_a(sT) = \frac{2(1 - \text{sinc } 2\mu sT)}{(2\mu sT)^2}\left\{2 + \exp\left[-\frac{(D\sigma_u)^2(sT)^2}{2}\right]\cos DU_0 sT\right\} \quad (4.2.6)$$

Before considering further experimental situations, we will briefly discuss the importance of the above analysis in estimating flow parameters.

4.3. Estimation of Flow Parameters

Once the count correlation for a turbulent flow is obtained, the most obvious approach to estimate mean flow velocity and rms turbulent intensity is to perform a Fourier transformation to convert the correlation to a frequency spectrum. Then the spectral width gives the rms turbulent intensity, after correction for ambiguity, as in the direct frequency analysis of LDV signals discussed in the previous chapter. This approach will be discussed in some detail in Section 4.8. Although very powerful, it can only be used where computing facilities are available, and generally speaking an on-line link between the correlator and the computer is essential. Another approach is to make a least squares fit to equations (4.2.5) and (4.2.6), but again this entails lengthy computations. For the moment we will only be concerned with simpler methods which have been devised in order to avoid the necessity for any extensive calculations.

The mean velocity measurement is a fairly simple matter since one needs only to measure the time interval between successive crests and troughs to obtain the mean Doppler frequency. Generally speaking, the time lag corresponding to a crest or trough will not fall at an exact multiple of the sample time T, so one must interpolate between the values. If as in Figure 4.3.1 three consecutive points on the count correlation at time lags $\overline{k - 1}T, kT$, and $\overline{k + 1}T$ are $r_{a,k-1}, r_{a,k}$, and $r_{a,k+1}$, respectively, then it can easily be verified that a Lagrangian interpolation gives for the parabola passing through these points

$$r_a(v) = \frac{1}{2T^2}[(v^2 - vT)r_{a,k-1} + (2T^2 - 2v^2)r_{a,k} + (v^2 + vT)r_{a,k+1}] \quad (4.3.1)$$

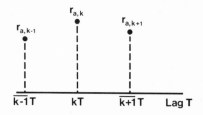

Figure 4.3.1. Notation for Lagrangian interpolation.

(where $v = \tau - kT$, and τ is the correlation lag), and that $\partial r_a/\partial \tau$ is zero when

$$v = \frac{T(r_{a,k-1} - r_{a,k+1})}{2r_{a,k-1} - 4r_{a,k} + 2r_{a,k+1}} \qquad (4.3.2)$$

The heights of maxima and minima are obtained by substituting values obtained from equation (4.3.2) back into (4.3.1) and can be used for estimating rms turbulence levels. The positions of the crests and troughs can of course alternatively be measured by graphical interpolation.

For the computation of rms turbulence levels we will assume now that the Lagrangian integral time scale of the turbulence is long compared to the passage time across the measuring volume, so that equations (4.2.5) and (4.2.6) apply. Otherwise, corrections have to be applied in the manner to be described in the next section. The damping rate of the periodic component in the count correlation is related to the turbulence level, and measurement of this parameter can easily be accomplished by noting the rate at which the relative heights of successive crests and troughs decrease. Birch *et al.* (1973) suggest that this can be done by first drawing in the line which corresponds to the low frequency of the LDV signal as indicated in Figure 4.3.2 (full line). The heights of the first trough and the first crest are then measured relative to this line, i.e., h_1 and h_2 in Figure 4.3.2. From equations (4.2.5) and (4.2.6), assuming the damping term due to the finite member of fringes to be negligible, we easily see that in terms of h_1 and h_2 the relative turbulent intensity is given by

$$\frac{\sigma_u}{U_0} = \frac{1}{\pi}\left[\frac{2}{3}\ln\left(\frac{h_1}{h_2}\right)\right]^{1/2} \qquad (4.3.3)$$

where U_0 is the mean flow velocity.

Although this is convenient in that it gives an explicit expression for the turbulence level in terms of parameters which can be directly measured from the count correlation, it tends to be too inaccurate for all but the roughest

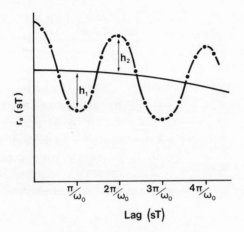

Figure 4.3.2. Notation for computing damping rate of the correlation function.

estimates, especially when the number of fringes is small. A more accurate method is to measure the damping ratio

$$D_r = \frac{r_a(4\pi/\omega_0) - r_a(3\pi/\omega_0)}{r_a(2\pi/\omega_0) - r_a(\pi/\omega_0)} \qquad (4.3.4)$$

Figure 4.3.3 shows how this ratio varies with the changes in turbulent

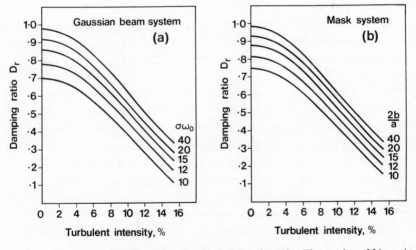

Figure 4.3.3. Variation of damping ratio with turbulent intensity. The number of fringes is effectively (a) $\sigma\omega_0$; (b) $2b/a$.

intensity (a) for the Gaussian beam and (b) for the mask LDV systems. Each curve corresponds effectively to a given number of fringes in the measuring volume, the values having been computed by substituting various values of $D\sigma_u$ into equations (4.2.5) and (4.2.6). For any measured D_r value the corresponding relative turbulent intensity can be read off these graphs for the particular optical geometry in use. Notice that for small values of relative turbulent intensity the damping of the periodic component is almost entirely due to the effect of having a finite number of fringes in the measuring volume, and D_r varies slowly with increasing intensity. In this region it becomes difficult to obtain accurate estimates of the turbulent fluctuations, but measurement becomes easier as the turbulence level increases.

Effect of Background Noise

It has been noted in previous chapters that one of the greatest practical difficulties in performing a laser anemometer measurement is that of obtaining a signal free, as far as possible, from background noise. In practical measuring situations there will always be some background noise contaminating the signal, and in the photon correlation method this will usually come primarily from background light picked up by the photomultiplier. Much of this can be eliminated in laboratory experimental facilities by operating in a dark room, and obviously an optical filter in front of the photomultiplier is essential in this connection. In wind tunnels and other similar rigs, flare from the side walls will usually be the major source of noise but with some care, by using suitable combinations of spatial filters in the form of masks and pinholes, it is not normally difficult to keep this down to acceptable levels.

In the frequency domain method of LDV signal analysis, background noise, being for all practical purposes white and uncorrelated with the signal itself, shows up as a constant increase in level on the spectrum. The various forms of noise that arise are discussed in Section 1.4. In the photon correlation method, as the counts will be Poisson-distributed, background noise shows up as an overall increase in the predicted level together with a delta-function peak at the origin. One disadvantage with the digital photon counting methods is that there is no simple means of filtering off low-frequency noise which can arise if light from moving scattering centers outside the measuring volume falls onto the detector surface. This will cause the overall level of the correlation to drop more rapidly than predicted by theory.

Measurement Accuracy

Estimation of the accuracy of measurements recorded with the photon correlation method is an area which has so far not been fully investigated although there have been fairly extensive studies made of the accuracy obtainable in some simpler experimental situations than laser anemometry (Degiorgio and Lastovka, 1971 ; Saleh, 1973). Two possible approaches come to mind. One is to derive direct variance estimates for $\tilde{R}_a$ and the flow parameters measured from it as functions of measuring time. The other approach is to calculate lower bounds for these variances using the Cramer–Rao inequality (Helstrom, 1968; Kendall and Stuart, 1961), the aim here being to establish relationships giving the maximum possible accuracy obtainable with the system. For a more detailed explanation of how these methods are applied, the reader is referred to the papers by Durrani and Greated (1973c), Costas (1950), and Davenport *et al.* (1952). Here we will only attempt to consider the simplest possible situation.

It is important to realize that for a given sample time and seeding condition the accumulated count correlation at the origin grows at a rate which is independent of the velocity. As the counts arrive in a random manner (only their expected rate of arrival is governed by the integrated intensity), then obviously one has to average over a reasonable time period to obtain a steady and accurate correlation curve. If the correlation function is accumulated over only a very short period of time, then it will be completely dominated by the shot-noise process. For the case of a very low count rate each product in equation (4.1.4) will be either zero or unity, and the products themselves will be Poisson-distributed. Since the variance of a Poisson process is the same as the mean value, it is easily seen that

$$\text{var}\,[r_a(sT)] = r_a(sT) \tag{4.3.5}$$

whence

$$\text{var}\,[\tilde{R}_a(sT)] = \tilde{R}_a(sT)/M \tag{4.3.6}$$

i.e., the variance is inversely proportional to the number of products accumulated. Equation (4.3.6) can give a useful indicator of the number of products required but it does not directly enable one to estimate the accuracy of a velocity measurement. Also, it must be remembered that background noise can make a considerable contribution to the correlation.

In practical systems clipping procedures are often introduced in order to reduce the amount of computation involved. These will be described in some detail in Chapter 6. Here it is worth noting that clipping introduces additional errors, the general conclusion being that, for Gaussian intensity statistics, single clipping results in an undistorted correlation with increased variance, whereas double clipping results in a distortion of the correlation shape.

4.4. Effect of Particle Diffusion

Photon correlation methods are frequently used for velocity measurements in wind tunnels, and it is common practice to use an optical arrangement similar to that depicted in Figure 2.2.6, with a very small angle between the two beams forming the fringe pattern. In this situation the size of the measuring volume may be such that the mean passage time cannot be considered as being negligibly small compared with the Lagrangian time scale. Account should then be taken of the effect caused by the velocities of particles changing as they pass across the measuring region.

The optical intensity variation associated with the passage of a single scattering center is then

$$\psi_i(t) = AK_iW(t)\{1 + \cos[\omega_0 t + q(t)]\} \qquad (4.4.1)$$
$$= K_i\psi(t)$$

where

$$q(t) = \int v(t)\,dt$$

represents the effect on the instantaneous frequency of Doppler shifted radiation introduced by the instantaneous variation of the particle velocity. Thus $\{v(t)\}$ is proportional to the instantaneous deviation of the particle velocity from the mean velocity since in equation (4.4.1) the instantaneous frequency of $\psi_i(t)$ is equal to $\omega_0 + v(t)$. Similar modulation effects relevant to other types of measurements are considered by Bendjaballah and Perrot (1971), Fleury and Boon (1973), Picinbono (1971), and Rousseau (1971).

Consistent with the analysis of Section 4.2, $W(t)$ in equation (4.4.1) will be considered a function of the mean flow velocity rather than the instantaneous velocity. We will also assume that the statistics of the turbulent velocity fluctuations, i.e., the statistics of $\{v(t)\}$ are Gaussian, knowing this to be a good approximation to nearly all practical situations. It follows from equation (4.4.1) that $\{q(t)\}$ is also a Gaussian process.

The intensity correlation in this case is seen to be

$$R_I(sT) = C_1 N_p \int_{-\infty}^{\infty} E[\psi(\tau)\psi(\tau + sT)]\, d\tau$$

$$+ N_p^2 \left\{ C_0 \int_{-\infty}^{\infty} E[\psi(\tau)]\, d\tau \right\}^2 \tag{4.4.2}$$

This expression is analogous to equation (4.1.14) for the constant velocity case. Substituting equation (4.4.1) into (4.4.2) leads to

$$E[\psi(t)\psi(t + sT)] = A^2 W(t)W(t + sT)(1 + E[\cos\{\omega_0 t + q(t)\}]$$

$$+ E[\cos\{\omega_0(t + sT) + q(t + sT)\}])$$

$$+ \tfrac{1}{2}E[\cos\{2\omega_0 t + \omega_0 sT + q(t) + q(t + sT)\}]$$

$$+ \tfrac{1}{2}E[\cos\{\omega_0 sT + q(t + sT) - q(t)\}] \tag{4.4.3}$$

In the above expression, as $\{W(t)\}$ is low-pass compared to ω_0, the terms containing $\omega_0 t$ average to zero in the integration of equation (4.4.2). Hence the only terms of interest here are

$$E[\psi(t)\psi(t + sT)]$$

$$= A^2 W(t)W(t + sT)$$

$$\times (1 + \tfrac{1}{2}\operatorname{Re}\{\exp j[\omega_0 sT + q(t + sT) - q(t)]\}) \tag{4.4.4}$$

From the statistics of $v(t)$ it may be shown that

$$E[e^{jq(t+sT)-jq(t)}] = \exp\left[-(D\sigma_u)^2 \int_0^{sT} (sT - v)\rho_v(v)\, dv\right] \tag{4.4.5}$$

where $\rho_v(v)$ is the normalized autocorrelation function of $\{v(t)\}$, σ_u^2 is the mean square turbulent velocity fluctuation, and D is the scaling constant relating $\{v(t)\}$ to the instantaneous flow velocity, i.e., $(E[v^2])^{1/2} = D\sigma_u$ since the rms velocity fluctuation is assumed to be the same in both Eulerian and Lagrangian frames of reference. Substitution of equations (4.4.4) and (4.4.5) into equation (4.4.2) then yields the expression for the intensity correlation function as

$$R_I(sT) = A^2 R_W(sT)N_p C_1\{1 + \tfrac{1}{2}\cos\omega_0 sT \exp[-(D\sigma_u)^2\Omega(sT)]\} + m_0^2 \tag{4.4.6}$$

where

$$\Omega(sT) = \int_0^{sT} (sT - \tau)\rho_L(\tau)\, d\tau$$

and $\rho_L(\tau)$ is the normalized Lagrangian autocorrelation function for the flow. Although $v(t)$ is measured in radians per second and the velocity fluctuations in meters per second, the normalized autocorrelation functions will be identical, i.e.,

$$\rho_v(\tau) = \rho_L(\tau) \qquad (4.4.7)$$

Finally, applying equation (2.6.56), we see the expressions for the count correlations are for the Gaussian beam system

$$R_a(sT) = \frac{1}{3}\exp\left[\frac{-(sT)^2}{4\rho^2}\right]\{2 + (\cos \omega_0 sT)\exp\left[-(D\sigma_u)^2\Omega(sT)\right]\} \qquad (4.4.8)$$

and for the mask system

$$R_a(sT) = \frac{2[1 - \text{sinc}(2\mu sT)]}{(2\mu sT)^2}\{2 + (\cos \omega_0 sT)\exp\left[-(D\sigma_u)^2\Omega(sT)\right]\} \qquad (4.4.9)$$

Equations (4.4.8) and (4.4.9) give the forms of the count autocorrelation functions in terms of the Lagrangian correlation function for the velocity fluctuations. In the case when the measuring volume is so small that the passage time across the beam is short compared with the Lagrangian integral time scale of the turbulence, then for the values of sT under consideration $\rho_L(sT)$ will be approximately unity whence $\Omega(sT)$ becomes equal to $(sT)^2/2$. Equations (4.4.8) and (4.4.9) then reduce to (4.2.5) and (4.2.6).

In most practical situations the exact shape of the velocity correlation will not be known, but it will often be possible to estimate the Lagrangian integral time scale of the turbulence. The effect of varying this integral time scale on the count correlation can be formulated by assuming a model for the turbulence. We will take

$$\rho_L(\tau) = \exp(-\Lambda|\tau|) \qquad (4.4.10)$$

since this is the most convenient to deal with and gives a good approximation, especially when the flow field is approximately isotropic. The use of a more sophisticated model is unnecessary since small changes in the velocity correlation shape will have a negligible influence on the count correlation. In equation (4.4.10) Λ is the Lagrangian integral time scale for the turbulence.

Substituting for $\rho_L(\tau)$ from equation (4.4.10) into (4.4.5) and noting relationship (4.4.7) gives

$$E[e^{jq(t+sT)-jq(t)}] = \exp\left\{-\frac{(D\sigma_u)^2}{\Lambda}\left[sT - \frac{1}{\Lambda}(1 - e^{-\Lambda sT})\right]\right\} \qquad (4.4.11)$$

from which the expressions for the normalized count autocorrelations come to be for the Gaussian beam system

$$R_a(sT) = \frac{1}{3}\exp\left[\frac{-(sT)^2}{4\rho^2}\right]$$

$$\times \left\{2 + (\cos \omega_0 sT)\exp\left[\frac{-(D\sigma_u)^2}{\Lambda}\left(sT - \frac{1 - e^{-\Lambda sT}}{\Lambda}\right)\right]\right\} \qquad (4.4.12)$$

and for the mask system

$$R_a(sT) = \frac{2[1 - \operatorname{sinc}(2\mu sT)]}{(2\mu sT)^2}$$

$$\times \left\{2 + (\cos \omega_0 sT)\exp\left[-\frac{(D\sigma_u)^2}{\Lambda}\left(sT - \frac{1 - e^{-\Lambda sT}}{\Lambda}\right)\right]\right\} \qquad (4.4.13)$$

It can easily be seen that equations (4.4.12) and (4.4.13) revert back to (4.2.5) and (4.2.6) when the turbulent fluctuations are such that the Lagrangian integral time scale is long compared to the passage time across the measuring volume, i.e., when $\Lambda sT \ll 1$. To make this check use a three-term expansion for the last exponential on the right-hand sides.

4.5. *Effect of Frequency Shifting*

Optical frequency shifting techniques are as powerful when applied with photon correlation analysis as they are when used for shifting the frequencies of continuous analogue Doppler signals. As an illustration, Figure 4.5.1a shows a count correlation recorded in the separated flow behind a step where the turbulence level is so high that the velocity fluctuations about the mean value give rise to negative velocities. At a glance one can see that the record is almost useless for the purpose of determining any flow parameters as the periodic component has completely disappeared. Figure 4.5.1b, on the other hand, shows a correlation recorded in exactly the same flow situation, but this time with the optical frequencies shifted, using a pair of Bragg cells. This now resembles a correlation recorded in a low-turbulence situation, and a damping rate can be easily measured.

With minor modification the theoretical expressions already derived for the form of $R_a(sT)$ can be used when there is a frequency shift of ω_s. If one visualizes that the overall size of the measuring volume remains unaltered but that the fringes are now continuously moving across the region,

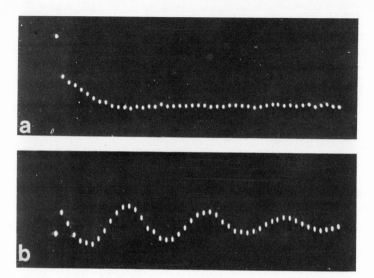

Figure 4.5.1. Count correlation in a reversing flow situation: (a) without optical frequency shift; (b) with optical frequency shift. Both were recorded under the same flow conditions.

then it is easily seen that equation (4.1.11) should be changed to

$$\psi(t) = AW(t)[1 + \cos(\omega_0 + \omega_s)t] \qquad (4.5.1)$$

In this section and in Sections 4.6 and 4.7 we will restrict ourselves to Gaussian beam optics for brevity. The analysis follows through as before, and the resulting expression for the normalized count autocorrelation corresponding to equation (4.2.5), is

$$R_a(sT) = \frac{1}{3} \exp\left[\frac{-(sT)^2}{4\rho^2}\right]$$

$$\times \left\{ 2 + \left[\exp\left(-\frac{(D\sigma_u)^2(sT)^2}{2}\right) \right] \cos(DU_0 + \omega_s sT) \right\} \qquad (4.5.2)$$

By employing equations (4.5.2) and (4.3.4) it is simple to compute a set of graphs corresponding to Figure 4.3.3 for various values of ω_s. These can be used for calculating values of the turbulent intensities from measured damping ratios, in the same manner as was described in Section 4.3.

4.6. *Highly Turbulent Flows*

The expressions for the count correlation derived in Section 4.2 are strictly valid only when the turbulence levels are low or alternatively when there are a very large number of fringes within the measuring volume, making the ambiguity broadening of the spectrum very small. What we did effectively was to consider the passage time across the beam as constant instead of being inversely proportional to the velocity. For very high-turbulence flows, when frequency shifting is not used, it is important to consider $W(t)$ as a function of velocity as well as time.

Defining the distance across the beam as $r_x = r_0/(2^{1/2} \cos \theta)$, then from equation (2.6.53), we have

$$W(t) = \exp \left(\frac{-t^2 U^2}{2r_x^2} \right) \tag{4.6.1}$$

for the Gaussian beam system, and so equation (4.2.5) is converted to

$$R_a(sT, U) = \frac{1}{3} \left[\exp \left(\frac{-(sT)^2 U^2}{4r_x^2} \right) \right] (2 + \cos DUsT) \tag{4.6.2}$$

Also

$$R_a(sT) = E[R_a(sT, U)] = \int_{-\infty}^{\infty} p(U) R_a(sT, U) \, dU \tag{4.6.3}$$

where $p(U)$ is given by equation (4.2.3) and $R_a(aT, U)$ by equation (4.6.2). The integration is performed as follows. Writing

$$G_1 = \int_{-\infty}^{\infty} \frac{1}{(2\pi\sigma_u^2)^{1/2}} \exp \left[-\frac{(U - U_0)^2}{2\sigma_u^2} \right] \exp \left[\frac{-(sT)^2 U^2}{4r_x^2} \right] \cos (DUsT) \, dU \tag{4.6.4}$$

and

$$G_2 = \int_{-\infty}^{\infty} \frac{1}{(2\pi\sigma_u^2)^{1/2}} \exp \left[-\frac{(U - U_0)^2}{2\sigma_u^2} \right] \exp \left[\frac{-(sT)^2 U^2}{4r_x^2} \right] dU \tag{4.6.5}$$

then

$$R_a(sT) = \tfrac{1}{3}(G_1 + 2G_2) \tag{4.6.6}$$

After some manipulations

$$G_1 = \frac{1}{3C_2^{1/2}} \exp \left[-\frac{U_0^2}{2\sigma_u^2} + \frac{U_0^2 - \sigma_u^4 D^2 (sT)^2}{2\sigma_u^2 C_2} \right] \cos \left(\frac{DU_0 sT}{C_2} \right) \tag{4.6.7}$$

where

$$C_2 = 1 + \frac{\sigma_u^2(sT)^2}{2r_x^2} \tag{4.6.8}$$

The expression for G_2 can be obtained by substituting $D = 0$ in equation (4.6.7). Then from equation (4.6.6),

$$R_a(sT) = \frac{1}{3C_2^{1/2}} \exp\left(-\frac{U_0^2}{2\sigma_u^2} + \frac{U_0^2}{2\sigma_u^2 C_2}\right)$$

$$\times \left\{2 + \exp\left[\frac{-\sigma_u^2 D^2(sT)^2}{2C_2}\right] \cos\left(\frac{DU_0 sT}{C_2}\right)\right\} \tag{4.6.9}$$

Foord *et al.* (1974) quoted without proof a formula identical to the above. Note the similarity with equation (3.3.23).

For low turbulence levels this reduces to equation (4.2.5) because in this case $\sigma_u/U_0 \ll 1$ and hence for the part of the correlation curve of interest, $\sigma_u sT \ll r_x$, $\forall(sT)$. Thus,

$$\frac{U_0^2}{2\sigma_u^2 C_2} - \frac{U_0^2}{2\sigma_u^2} = \frac{-U_0^2(sT)^2}{2[2r_x^2 + \sigma^2(sT)^2]} \simeq \frac{-U_0^2(sT)^2}{4r_x^2} = \frac{-(sT)^2}{4\rho^2} \tag{4.6.10}$$

Equation (4.2.5) is then obtained if C_2 is set equal to unity in the other terms in equation (4.6.9).

4.7. Periodic Flows

The photon correlation method can also be used for measuring the amplitude of velocity fluctuations in periodic flows, e.g., vortex flows behind cylinders. We will apply the same integration technique for computing the shape of the correlation function as we used for turbulent flow. The amplitude fluctuation will be taken as small compared with the mean velocity, or, alternatively, a large number of fringes will be assumed. This allows us to ignore the velocity dependence of the weighting function.

Let the velocity in the mean flow direction be

$$U(t) = U_0 + a_m \sin(\omega_m t + \phi_m) \tag{4.7.1}$$

U_0 being the mean velocity; a_m, ω_m, and ϕ_m are, respectively, the amplitude, frequency, and random phase of the modulation (velocity fluctuation).

The velocity probability density is

$$p(U) = (1/\pi)[a_m^2 - (U - U_0)^2]^{-1/2}, \qquad |U - U_0| < a_m$$
$$= 0, \qquad\qquad\qquad\qquad |U - U_0| \geq a_m \qquad (4.7.2)$$

Applying equation (4.6.3) to this situation gives

$$E[R_a(sT, U)] = \frac{1}{3\pi} \int_{U_0-a_m}^{U_0+a_m} \frac{1}{[a_m^2 - (U - U_0)^2]^{1/2}}$$

$$\times \exp\left[\frac{-(sT)^2 U^2}{4r_x^2}\right](2 + \cos DUsT)\, dU \qquad (4.7.3)$$

where we have taken the Gaussian beam system with

$$W(t) = \exp\left(-\frac{t^2 U^2}{2r_x^2}\right) \qquad (4.7.4)$$

Equation (4.7.3) can alternatively be written as

$$E[R_a(sT, U)] = F_1 + F_2 \qquad (4.7.5)$$

where

$$F_1 = \frac{1}{3\pi} \int_{U_0-a_m}^{U_0+a_m} \frac{2}{[a_m^2 - (U - U_0)^2]^{1/2}} \exp\left[\frac{-(sT)^2 U^2}{4r_x^2}\right] dU$$

$$F_2 = \frac{1}{3\pi} \int_{U_0-a_m}^{U_0+a_m} \frac{1}{[a_m^2 - (U - U_0)^2]^{1/2}} \exp\left[\frac{-(sT)^2 U^2}{4r_x^2}\right] \cos DsTU\, dU$$

Now for relatively small velocity fluctuations $U \simeq U_0$, whence

$$F_1 = \frac{2}{3} \exp\left[\frac{-(sT)^2 U_0^2}{4r_x^2}\right] \qquad (4.7.6)$$

$$F_2 = \frac{1}{3\pi} \exp\left[\frac{-(sT)^2 U_0^2}{4r_x^2}\right] \int_{U_0-a_m}^{U_0+a_m} \frac{1}{[a_m^2 - (U - U_0)^2]^{1/2}} \cos DsTU\, dU$$

$$(4.7.7)$$

$$= \frac{1}{3\pi} \exp\left[\frac{-(sT)^2 U_0^2}{4r_x^2}\right] \int_{-a_m}^{a_m} \frac{1}{(a_m^2 - u^2)^{1/2}} \cos DsT(u + U_0)\, du \qquad (4.7.8)$$

where

$$U - U_0 = u$$

The integral in equation (4.7.8) can easily be evaluated by expanding the cosine term. This gives

$$F_2 = \frac{1}{3}\exp\left[\frac{-(sT)^2 U_0^2}{4r_x^2}\right](\cos DsTU_0)J_0(a_m DsT) \qquad (4.7.9)$$

where J_0 is the zero-order Bessel function. Finally then, the normalized count autocorrelation function is

$$R_a(sT) = \frac{1}{3}\exp\left[\frac{-(sT)^2 U_0^2}{4r_x^2}\right][2 + J_0(a_m DsT)\cos DU_0 sT] \qquad (4.7.10)$$

Notice the similarity in the forms of equations (4.7.10) and (4.2.5). For the turbulent flow the cosine term is damped by an exponential factor, whereas for periodic flow it is replaced by Bessel function damping. This causes a beating effect in the correlation curve. Figure 4.7.1 shows a count correlation recorded in the periodic wake behind a thin rod in a wind tunnel. The beating effect can be seen quite clearly. If this correlation was transformed to the

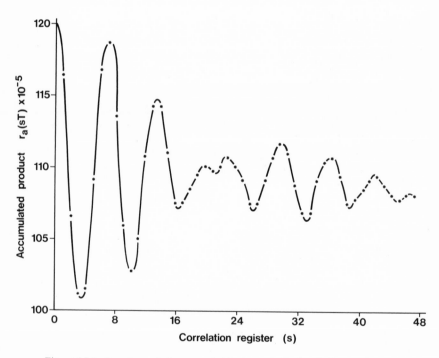

Figure 4.7.1. Count correlation recorded in the periodic flow behind a cylinder.

frequency domain (by the method described in Section 4.8), then the spectrum would exhibit two distinct peaks, i.e., would be a convolved form of the velocity probability density.

The amplitude of the velocity fluctuation as a ratio of the mean velocity can most easily be determined by observing the number of cycles in the cosine wave between zero lag and the first or second minimum of the Bessel function. The first and second minima of $J_0(a_m DsT)$ occur when $a_m DsT = 2.405$ and 5.520, respectively. Suppose that there are n_b complete cycles between zero lag and the first minimum. Then from equation (4.7.10) $DU_0 sT = n_b \cdot 2\pi$ and also $a_m DsT = 2.405$. This gives $a_m/U_0 = 2.405/(2\pi n_b)$. Of course if the damping due to the finite number of fringes [the exponential term in equation (4.7.10)] is too great, then the beating effect may be obscured and either curve fitting or transformation to the frequency domain would then be essential.

4.8. Frequency Transformation of Count Autocorrelations

In the earlier sections of this chapter estimation techniques have been developed and closed-form expressions have been derived for the photon count autocorrelation function obtained for radiation scattered by the passage of particles across the flow volume in an LDV setup. In Section 4.3 simplified techniques were presented for extracting characteristics of the flow from a record of the count autocorrelation. In general, these methods yield estimates of limited accuracy. A more accurate approach which fully utilizes all the available data is to transform the autocorrelation curve into the frequency domain, and to determine the flow parameters directly from the (count) power spectrum.

Consider $\{R_a(sT); s = 0, 1, 2, \ldots, (N - 1)\}$ as an estimate of the count autocorrelation. Then the following *finite Fourier transform* would yield a power spectrum estimate at any frequency f:

$$\Phi(f) = T \sum_{s=1-N}^{N-1} R_a(sT) e^{-j2\pi fsT}, \qquad -\frac{1}{2T} \le f \le \frac{1}{2T} \qquad (4.8.1)$$

where $R_a(-sT) = R_a(sT)$ for an autocorrelation function.

Computationally, $\Phi(f)$ may be determined at discrete (equidistant) frequency intervals $(f = q \Delta f; q = 0, 1, 2, \ldots, (N - 1)]$ by the use of standard *fast Fourier transform* subroutines. To obtain positive-definite spectrum estimates it is usual to multiply $R_a(sT)$ by a lag window (Blackman and Tukey, 1958). The most common, and computationally least expensive, is the Bartlett lag window $\{1 - |s|/N; s = 0, 1, 2, \ldots, (N - 1)\}$. This leads to the spectrum estimate

$$\Phi(f) = T\left[R_a(0) + 2 \sum_{s=1}^{N-1} \left(1 - \frac{|s|}{N}\right) R_a(sT) \cos 2\pi f sT \right] \qquad (4.8.2)$$

It may be easily seen that

$$E[\Phi(f)] = T \int_{-1/2T}^{1/2T} \Phi_T(f_1) \frac{\sin^2 \pi(f - f_1)NT}{N \sin^2 \pi(f - f_1)T} df_1 \qquad (4.8.3)$$

where $\{\Phi_T(f)\}$ is the true spectrum of the process for which $R_a(sT)$ is the autocorrelation estimate.

Equation (4.8.3) indicates that the spectrum estimate $\Phi(f)$ is a smeared or convolved version of the true spectrum; the convolution or smearing effect is represented by the spectral window $\{(\sin^2 \pi NfT)/(N \sin^2 \pi fT)\}$, which is a finite Fourier transform of the Bartlett lag window. This spectral window is usually referred to as *Fejer's kernel* and is (i) evidently positive, (ii) integrates to unity, and (iii) approaches a delta function for large N, and thus leads to an asymptotically unbiased estimate of the spectrum.

However, for the usual case of finite values of N, the frequency resolution offered by the spectral estimator of equation (4.8.2) or (4.8.3) is limited by the bandwidth of the spectral window [be it a Fejer kernel or any other kernel (Durrani and Nightingale, 1972)]. For instance, for a sine wave plus additive (band-limited) Gaussian white noise

$$\Phi_T(f) = A_0\delta(f - f_0) + \sigma_\eta^2$$

Equation (4.8.3) leads to

$$E[\Phi(f)] = A_0 T \frac{\sin^2 \pi(f - f_0)NT}{\sin^2 \pi(f - f_0)T} + \sigma_\eta^2$$

which indicates that the spectral peak of f_0 is smeared out by the major lobe of the spectral window. The spectrum estimator of equation (4.8.1) or (4.8.2) would only yield reliable estimates provided the bandwidth of the narrowest peak in the true spectrum of $\{R_a(sT)\}$ is comparatively larger (twice or more) than the bandwidth of the spectral window, i.e., only when $\{R_a(sT)\}$ represents a broad-band process, or, alternatively when the correlation record is long.

Currently available photon correlators operate at minimum lag values of the order of $(T=)$ 50 nsec, and accumulate simultaneously $(N=)$ 50–100 sampled values of the count correlation function in parallel channels, operating in real time (further details in Section 6.3). Hardware complexity and operating speeds restrict the total number of channels to within this range. This, however, leads to spectrum estimates with very poor frequency resolution if the finite Fourier transform technique is employed. For instance for a 50-channel correlator which accumulates the correlation function at lag intervals of 50 nsec, the above approach would yield independent spectral estimates with a frequency resolution of 400 kHz. In general, spectral peaks for data associated with LDV systems would be narrower than 400 kHz, and thus they would be totally swamped by the spectral window of the estimator.

High-Resolution Spectral Analysis

Two new estimators have been recently proposed for deriving the power spectral density functions from a record of the autocorrelation function of a stochastic process (Lacoss, 1971). They are specially suited to the analysis of count correlations which have been computed over only a limited number of consecutive and equidistant lag values.

One spectral estimator leads to minimum variance unbiased estimates of the spectrum (we will refer to this as the *MLL transformation*), and the other estimator tends to maximize the entropy of the spectrum (*ME transformation*). Details of their derivation are beyond the scope of this text. Suffice it to say that the MLL case involves the design of an optimal (minimum error variance or maximum likelihood) filter, while the ME method requires the design of an N term (one step ahead) prediction error filter based on N sample points (consecutive lag values) of the autocorrelation function.

We define an $(N \times N)$ correlation matrix **R** with elements

$$R_{ij} = R_a(|i - j|T), \qquad \{i, j = 0, 1, 2, \ldots, (N - 1)\}$$

and a vector of complex exponentials

$$\mathscr{E}^T(f) = [1e^{-j2\pi fT} e^{-j4\pi fT} \cdots e^{-j2\pi(N-1)T}]$$

The MLL estimator is given by

$$\Phi_1(f) = TN[\mathscr{E}^T(f)\mathbf{R}^{-1}\mathscr{E}^*(f)]^{-1} \qquad (4.8.4)$$

where * denotes complex conjugate. The ME estimator is expressed as

$$\Phi_2(f) = TN\gamma_0^2[\mathscr{E}^T(f)\boldsymbol{\Gamma}\boldsymbol{\Gamma}^T\mathscr{E}^*(f)]^{-1} \tag{4.8.5}$$

where the vector

$$\boldsymbol{\Gamma}^T = [\gamma_0\gamma_1\cdots\gamma_{N-1}]$$

is the first column or the first row of the matrix $\mathbf{R}^{-1}$.

Using the above definition, we may recast equation (4.8.2) into

$$\Phi(f) = \frac{T}{N}[\mathscr{E}^T(f)\mathbf{R}\mathscr{E}^*(f)] \tag{4.8.6}$$

In general, spectrum estimates derived from equation (4.8.6) have a frequency resolution of $(NT)^{-1}$ Hz. The estimators of equation (4.8.4) and (4.8.5) possess frequency resolution of the order of $(N^{3/2}T)^{-1}$ Hz and $(N^2T)^{-1}$ Hz, respectively. Thus for a 50-channel correlator computing correlation values at lag intervals of 50 nsec, the three estimates given above would yield frequency resolution of the order of 400 kHz, 57 kHz (MLL), and 8 kHz (ME), respectively.

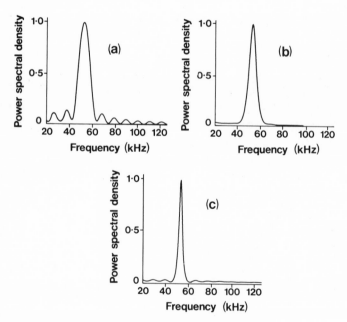

Figure 4.8.1. Transformations of a count correlation recorded in a laminar flow: (a) direct Fourier transformation; (b) maximum log likelihood; (c) maximum entropy.

The high-resolution spectral estimators require inversion of the co-variance matrix, which is a Toeplitz matrix. This may be performed in N^2 operations (Zohar, 1969), and then the spectrum estimates may be formed at discrete frequency intervals by employing fast Fourier transform techniques on elements of the inverse covariance matrix. Obviously the high-resolution spectral estimators involve more computing than the conventional estimators. However, the finer frequency resolution so achieved is more than adequate compensation.

Figures 4.8.1a–c show the spectra obtained from a photon count autocorrelation for a Gaussian beam setup in a laminar flow. For the three cases, the (rms bandwidth)/(center frequency) is 16.3%, 13.1%, and 6.5%, respectively. Calculations of the correct spectral width from theoretical considerations of the optical geometry and the mean flow velocity showed that the maximum entropy spectrum width is almost exact, and indicated that the value determined by the direct transformation method was in error by almost 10%.

Chapter 5

CROSS-CORRELATION TECHNIQUES

Cross-correlation techniques have been applied extensively in the analysis of signals from various types of transducers used for flow measurement purposes. For example Beck *et al.* (1973) describe how flow velocity can be determined by cross-correlating signals arising from two conductivity probes placed a short distance apart in a pipeline. In this case, as with the optical probing systems, it is assumed that the flow carries suspended particles which cause changes in the electrical conductivity signals as they pass the transducers. For industrial application cross-correlation techniques are particularly powerful, mainly because of their simplicity and the ease with which the results can be interpreted. If the two transducers are placed a distance d_0 apart in a flow with velocity U, then the cross correlation formed between the signals from the two transducers has a maximum (peak) at a lag value corresponding to the passage time d_0/U. Hence the flow velocity can be determined immediately by observing the position of the peak. Generally speaking, a distinctive peak can be observed even with very poor signal-to-noise ratios, and the only parameter which needs to be known accurately to determine the velocity is the distance between the two transducers.

Cross-correlation methods are particularly convenient for the analysis of signals from the two-beam type laser anemometers described in Section

2.1. In this chapter we will describe how the cross-correlation function of the signals from the two detectors can be used for the estimation of turbulence parameters as well as mean velocities. In Section 5.1 the signals will be assumed continuous and in Section 5.2 we will show how the expressions are modified if a photon-counting detection system is employed.

5.1. Form of the Correlation Function

Delta Function Beam Profile

We first analyze the case of an idealized optical configuration where the two beams are in the form of infinitely narrow strips placed at a distance d_0 apart in the mean flow direction as indicated in Figure 5.1.1 i.e., the intensity profiles in the mean flow direction are delta functions. It is assumed that the optical system is symmetric and that both detectors have the same sensitivity η. The light scattered by particles present in the flow crossing beam 1 is collected by detector 1 and gives a signal $\eta I_1(\mu)$, where $I_1(\mu)$ is the integral of the light intensity over the surface of the detector. Similarly, the light scattered by particles crossing beam 2 is collected by detector 2 and gives a signal output $\eta I_2(\mu)$.

The cross correlation of the signals from the two detectors at lag $(\mu - v)$ is

$$E[\eta I_1(\mu)\eta I_2(v)] = \eta^2 E[I_1(\mu)I_2(v)] \tag{5.1.1}$$

If $\{t_i\}$ are the random arrival times of scattering centers at beam 1 and τ_k are the random arrival times at beam 2, then the two intensity records can be expressed as

$$I_1(\mu) = \sum_i \beta_i \delta(\mu - t_i) \tag{5.1.2}$$

$$I_2(v) = \sum_k \beta_k \delta(v - \tau_k) \tag{5.1.3}$$

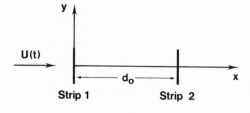

Figure 5.1.1. Two-strip optical geometry for cross-correlation analysis.

where $\{\beta_i\}$ is a random variable dependent upon the size distribution of scattering particles in the flow. This corresponds to the representation given in Section 4.1. Hence

$$E[I_1(\mu)I_2(\nu)] = E\left[\sum_i \sum_k \beta_i\beta_k\delta(\mu - t_i)\delta(\nu - \tau_k)\right] \tag{5.1.4}$$

We now write

$$E[\beta_i] = B_0, \qquad E[\beta_i^2] = B_1 \tag{5.1.5}$$

$$\sum_k E[\delta(\mu - t_k)] = N_p \tag{5.1.6}$$

The two constants B_0 and B_1 then characterize the size distribution of scattering centers in the flow, and N_p represents the mean number of arrivals per second. Equation (5.1.4) can then be expressed in terms of the passage time between the two beams, in the following way. Let $\xi = \nu - \mu$. Then

$$E\left[\sum_k \sum_i \beta_i\beta_k\delta(\mu - t_i)\delta(\nu - \tau_k)\right]$$

$$= \sum_k \sum_i E[\beta_i]E[\beta_k] \cdot \text{prob}\,[i\text{th scattering center arrives at beam 1 at} \\ \text{time instant } \mu \text{ and } k\text{th scattering center} \\ \text{arrives at beam 2 at time instant } \nu]$$

$$+ \sum_k E[\beta_k^2] \cdot \text{prob}\,[k\text{th scattering center arrives at time } \mu \text{ at beam} \\ 1, \textit{and same} \text{ scattering center arrives at beam 2} \\ \text{at time } \mu + \xi]$$

$$= B_0^2 N_p^2 + B_1 \sum_k \text{prob}\,[k\text{th particle takes time } \xi \text{ to traverse distance} \\ \{d_0\} \text{ across two beams} \mid \text{it arrives at beam 1} \\ \text{at time } \mu] \cdot \text{prob}\,[k\text{th particle arrives at} \\ \text{beam 1 at } \mu]$$

$$= B_0^2 N_p^2 + B_1 N_p\{\text{prob}\,[\text{particle passage time across beams} \\ \text{distance } d_0 \text{ is } \xi]\} \tag{5.1.7}$$

Consider now the form of the cross-correlation function in a turbulent flow with instantaneous flow velocity

$$U(t) = U_0 + u(t) \tag{5.1.8}$$

in a direction perpendicular to the two strips of light (Figure 5.1.1). It will be assumed that the velocity of each scattering center does not change in magnitude as it passes between the two beams. This is only valid when the distance d_0 between the two beams is small compared with the Lagrangian integral length scale (Greated, 1975). With this assumption we have

$$d_0 = [U_0 + u(t)]\xi \qquad (5.1.9)$$

Hence

$$\xi = \frac{d_0}{U_0 + u(t)} = \frac{d_0}{U_0}\left[1 + \frac{u(t)}{U_0}\right]^{-1} \qquad (5.1.10)$$

Expanding equation (5.1.10) as a negative binomial series and retaining only the first two terms gives

$$\xi = \frac{d_0}{U_0} - \frac{d_0 u(t)}{U_0^2} + \cdots \qquad (5.1.11)$$

which leads to

$$E[\xi] \approx \frac{d_0}{U_0}, \qquad \text{var}[\xi] \approx \frac{d_0^2}{U_0^2}\frac{\sigma_u^2}{U_0^2} \qquad (5.1.12)$$

As $u(t)$ and ξ are related by equation (5.1.9), the probability density of the passage time can be derived from the relationship (Papoulis, 1965)

$$p(\xi) = p(u)\left|\frac{du}{d\xi}\right| = p(u)\frac{d_0}{\xi^2} \qquad (5.1.13)$$

Equation (5.1.13) enables one to compute $p(u)$ explicitly from the cross-correlation function. In most practical situations $p(u)$ is Gaussian to a close approximation, i.e.,

$$p(u) = \frac{1}{(2\pi\sigma_u^2)^{1/2}}\exp\left[-\frac{u^2}{2\sigma_u^2}\right] \qquad (5.1.14)$$

Substitution into equation (5.1.13) gives

$$p(\xi) = \frac{d_0}{(2\pi\sigma_u^2\xi^4)^{1/2}}\exp\left[-\frac{1}{2\sigma_u^2}\left(\frac{d_0}{\xi} - U_0\right)^2\right] \qquad (5.1.15)$$

From equations (5.1.1) and (5.1.7) the cross-correlation function is given by

$$E[\eta I_1(\mu)\eta I_2(\mu + \xi)] = \eta^2[B_0^2 N_p^2 + B_1 N_p p(\xi)] \qquad (5.1.16)$$

where $p(\xi)$ is given by equation (5.1.15).

Thus the rms width of the cross-correlation peak is proportional to the velocity fluctuation. Strictly speaking, the mean velocity is best estimated by computing moments of the cross-correlation function about the origin. However, for practical purposes the time lag corresponding to the peak value is generally taken as being equal to the expected passage time. From

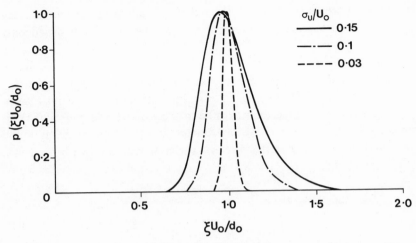

Figure 5.1.2. Values of the probability density of particle passage time from equation (5.1.18), normalized to unity at the peaks.

equation (5.1.12) we have

$$\text{peak} = \frac{d_0}{U_0}, \qquad \frac{\text{rms width}}{\text{peak}} = \frac{\sigma_u}{U_0} \qquad (5.1.17)$$

For the purpose of illustrating the shape of the cross-correlation curve at different turbulence levels, equation (5.1.15) can conveniently be written in terms of nondimensional parameters as follows:

$$p\left(\frac{\xi U_0}{d_0}\right) = \frac{d_0}{U_0} p(\xi) = \frac{d_0^2}{(2\pi)^{1/2}\sigma_u \xi^2 U_0} \exp\left[-\frac{U_0^2}{2\sigma_u^2}\left(\frac{d_0}{\xi U_0} - 1\right)^2\right] \qquad (5.1.18)$$

Figure 5.1.2 shows values of $p(\xi U_0/d_0)$ obtained from equation (5.1.18) plotted for three turbulence levels, $\sigma_u/U_0 = 0.03, 0.1$, and 0.15. The peak values have been normalized to unity for ease of comparison. Note that at high turbulence levels the curves become skewed while the peaks are shifted toward the origin.

Effect of Finite Beam Size

The above analysis has been conducted under the assumption that the passage time across each beam is negligibly small. However, if the width of the beams in the flow direction is not extremely small compared with d_0, then there will be a broadening of the correlation peak caused by the finite passage time across the beams. This will be in addition to the broadening caused by the turbulent fluctuations, analogous to the ambiguity broadening in an LDV system.

The two focal spots or strips of light in the measuring region are generally formed by the focusing of two unapertured laser beams with either spherical lenses (to form two spots) or cylindrical lenses (two strips). When cylindrical lenses are used their axes lie in the y direction (Figure 5.1.1). In either case, with the origin of coordinates at the center of beam 1, the integrated intensities over the detector surfaces associated with a particle at position (x, y) (Figure 5.1.1) will be

$$I_1(x, y) = I_0 \exp\left(-\frac{x^2}{r_0^2} + \frac{y^2}{r_y^2}\right), \qquad \text{beam 1} \qquad (5.1.19)$$

$$I_2(x, y) = I_0 \exp\left[-\frac{(x - d_0)^2}{r_0^2} + \frac{y^2}{r_y^2}\right], \qquad \text{beam 2} \qquad (5.1.20)$$

I_0 being the intensity when the particle is at the origin $(0, 0)$. If the beams are focused by cylindrical lenses, then $r_y = r_u$, the unapertured laser beam radius, and r_0 is the diffraction-limited waist radius given by equation (2.6.4). For beams focused by spherical lenses, $r_y = r_0$.

From equations (5.1.19) and (5.1.20) we can write the intensity associated with the passage of a single scattering center as

$$I_i(\tau) = I_0(y)(\pi r_0^2)^{1/2} W(\tau - t_i), \qquad \text{beam 1} \qquad (5.1.21)$$

$$I_j(\tau) = I_0(y)(\pi r_0^2)^{1/2} W(\tau - \tau_j), \qquad \text{beam 2} \qquad (5.1.22)$$

where

$$W(t) = \frac{1}{(\pi r_0^2)^{1/2}} \exp\left(-\frac{U_0^2 t^2}{r_0^2}\right) \qquad (5.1.23)$$

$I_0(y)$ is now the intensity scattered by a particle at position $(0, y)$. For a low-turbulence flow the value of y will remain approximately constant as the particle traverses the two beams. For a continuous stream of scattering centers it is seen that the integrated intensity over the detector surfaces is

$$I_1(\mu) = \sum_i \int_{-\infty}^{\infty} \beta_i W(\zeta)\delta(\zeta - \mu + t_i)\, d\zeta, \qquad \text{beam 1} \qquad (5.1.24)$$

$$I_2(\nu) = \sum_k \int_{-\infty}^{\infty} \beta_k W(\gamma)\delta(\gamma - \nu + \tau_k)\, d\gamma, \qquad \text{beam 2} \qquad (5.1.25)$$

The above expressions are similar to equations (2.6.62) and (2.6.63) for the LDV systems, where β_i corresponds to κK_p. Equation (5.1.4) is now recast into

$$E[I_1(\mu)I_2(v)]$$

$$= E\left[\sum_k \sum_i \beta_i \beta_k \iint_{-\infty}^{\infty} W(\zeta)W(\gamma)\delta(\zeta - \mu + t_i)\delta(\gamma - v + \tau_k)\,d\zeta\,d\gamma\right] \quad (5.1.26)$$

Since $v = \mu + \xi$, equation (5.1.26) reduces to

$$E[I_1(\mu)I_2(v)]$$

$$= B_0^2 N_p^2\left[\int_{-\infty}^{\infty} W(\zeta)\,d\zeta\right]^2 + B_1 N_p \iint_{-\infty}^{\infty} W(\zeta)W(\gamma)p(\zeta - \gamma + \xi)\,d\zeta\,d\gamma \quad (5.1.27)$$

For a Gaussian velocity fluctuation the probability density $p(\ )$ in equation (5.1.27) is given by (5.1.15).

Equation (5.1.27) can be rewritten in a more convenient form since

$$\iint_{-\infty}^{\infty} W(\zeta)W(\gamma)p(\zeta - \gamma + \xi)\,d\zeta\,d\gamma = \int_{-\infty}^{\infty} p(z)\,dz \int_{-\infty}^{\infty} W(\zeta)W(\zeta + \xi - z)\,d\zeta \quad (5.1.28)$$

and since

$$\int_{-\infty}^{\infty} W(\zeta)W(\zeta + \xi - z)\,d\zeta = R_w(\xi - z) \quad (5.1.29)$$

is the autocorrelation of $\{W(z)\}$. Hence equation (5.1.27) is recast into

$$E[I_1(\mu)I_2(v)]$$

$$= B_0^2 N_p^2\left[\int_{-\infty}^{\infty} W(\zeta)\,d\zeta\right]^2 + B_1 N_p \int_{-\infty}^{\infty} p(z)R_w(\xi - z)\,dz \quad (5.1.30)$$

With $W(t)$ defined by equation (5.1.23), i.e., Gaussian beam profiles, we have

$$\int_{-\infty}^{\infty} W(\tau)\,d\tau = \frac{1}{U_0} \quad (5.1.31)$$

and

$$R_w(\xi - z) = \frac{1}{(2\pi U_0^2 r_0^2)^{1/2}} \exp\left[-\frac{U_0^2}{2r_0^2}(\xi - z)^2\right] \quad (5.1.32)$$

Hence, from equation (5.1.29), the cross-correlation function is

$$E[I_1(\mu)I_2(\nu)]$$

$$= \frac{B_0^2 N_p^2}{U_0^2} + \frac{B_1 N_p}{(2\pi U_0^2 r_0^2)^{1/2}} \int_{-\infty}^{\infty} p(\xi - z) \exp\left(-\frac{U_0^2 z^2}{2r_0^2}\right) dz \qquad (5.1.33)$$

Equation (5.1.33) indicates that the cross correlation consists of a constant pedestal level $(B_0 N_p^2)$ plus a time-lag dependent part. This time-lag dependent part is a convolution of the beam intensity correlation function with the probability density function of the transit time of particles between the two beams. Thus, the finite passage time across the beams causes an additional broadening of the cross-correlation peak, i.e., additional to the broadening caused by the turbulent fluctuations.

For a constant flow velocity U it is seen from equation (5.1.33) that the cross correlation peaks at a time lag d_0/U and has an rms width of r_0/U, whence

$$\frac{\text{rms width}}{\text{peak}} = \frac{r_0}{d_0} \qquad (5.1.34)$$

For *turbulent flow* the relationship between the rms width of the correlation peak and the rms turbulence level is obtained by applying the moment theorem [equation (1.2.84)]. Thus

$$\left(\frac{\text{rms width}}{\text{peak}}\right)^2 = \left(\frac{\sigma_u}{U_0}\right)^2 + \left(\frac{r_0}{d_0}\right)^2 \qquad (5.1.35)$$

Although the beam waist radius r_0 can easily be calculated from equation (2.6.4) if the laser beam radius is known, it is sometimes more convenient to estimate r_0 by autocorrelating the signal from one of the two photo-detectors. If the turbulence level is assumed to be low, then $U(t) \approx U_0$ and so by Campbell's theorem [equation (1.2.63)], the autocorrelation of either $I_1(t)$ or $I_2(t)$ will be equal to $R_w(\tau)$, the autocorrelation of $W(t)$ together with a pedestal level. Thus the rms width of the autocorrelation function (centered about zero frequency) is approximately equal to the rms width of the cross-correlation function for constant velocity flow.

Effect of Background Noise

In most practical situations the signals received from the two photo-detectors are degraded by background noise which can generally be considered as uncorrelated with the signals arising from the passage of the particles. Equations (5.1.2) and (5.1.3) can then be rewritten as

$$I_1(\mu) = \lambda_1(\mu) + \sum_i \beta_i \delta(\mu - t_i) \qquad (5.1.36)$$

$$I_2(\nu) = \lambda_2(\nu) + \sum_k \beta_k \delta(\nu - \tau_k) \qquad (5.1.37)$$

Here $\lambda_1(\mu)$ and $\lambda_2(\nu)$ are the noise components which will be in the form of random fluctuations with nonzero mean. The intensity cross correlation is now

$$\begin{aligned}
E[I_1(\mu)I_2(\nu)] = {} & E[\lambda_1(\mu)\lambda_2(\nu)] + E\left[\lambda_1(\mu)\sum_k \beta_k \delta(\nu - \tau_k)\right] \\
& + E\left[\lambda_2(\nu)\sum_i \beta_i \delta(\mu - t_i)\right] \\
& + E\left[\sum_i \sum_k \beta_i \beta_k \delta(\mu - t_i)\delta(\nu - \tau_k)\right] \qquad (5.1.38)
\end{aligned}$$

The last term in equation (5.1.38) represents the cross correlation in a noise-free system while the other three terms on the rhs are constant pedestal levels which raise the overall height of the correlation function. Therefore, provided that the noise sources are uncorrelated with each other and also with the signals from the scattering particles, their only effect is to raise the pedestal level of the cross-correlation function.

Relationship to Autocorrelation

As an alternative to cross-correlating the signals from two separate detectors it is possible to image the scattered light from both focal spots onto a single detector, as indicated in Figure 2.1.1 and then autocorrelate the resulting signal.

Let the integrated intensity over the surface of the detector be $I_3(\mu)$, where

$$I_3(\mu) = I_1(\mu) + I_2(\mu) \qquad (5.1.39)$$

The autocorrelation of $I_3(\mu)$ is then

$$\begin{aligned}
E[I_3(\mu)I_3(\mu + \tau)] = {} & E[I_1(\mu)I_1(\mu + \tau)] + E[I_2(\mu)I_2(\mu + \tau)] \\
& + E[I_1(\mu)I_2(\mu + \tau)] + E[I_2(\mu)I_1(\mu + \tau)] \qquad (5.1.40)
\end{aligned}$$

The first two terms on the rhs of equation (5.1.40) represent the auto-correlations of signals arising from the two beams separately. The third

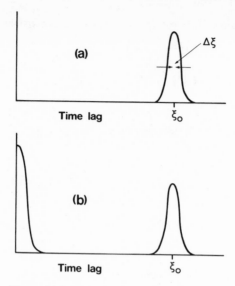

Figure 5.1.3. Form of (a) the cross-correlation function; and (b) the auto-correlation function in a turbulent flow. The pedestal levels have not been included.

term leads only to a constant contribution as the probability of a particle drifting back across beam 1 after it has crossed beam 2 is vanishingly small. The last term on the rhs is the cross correlation of the signals arising from the two beams separately, for which expressions have been derived earlier in this section [equations (5.1.17) and (5.1.30)]. Figure 5.1.3 indicates the form that the auto- and cross-correlation functions take in a turbulent flow. Contributions due to the first three terms on the rhs of equation (5.1.40) tend to introduce noise on the cross-correlation peak which reduces the accuracy with which velocity measurements can be made. For this reason the cross correlation of signals from two separate detectors is generally to be preferred.

Diffusion Effects

In the foregoing analysis it has been assumed that, although the instantaneous velocity of each scattering particle is generally different, the individual particles maintain a constant velocity as they traverse the distance d_0 between the two beams. However, if d_0 is not small compared with the ratio $U_0 \Lambda$, Λ being the Lagrangian integral time scale of the velocity fluctuations, this approximation is not valid and the effect of particle diffusion between the two beams becomes significant.

Suppose that a particle passes across beam 1 at time $t = 0$ and traverses beam 2 at time $t = \xi$. Let the distance traveled in time $\xi_0 = d_0/U_0$ be d and define

$$d - d_0 = \Delta d, \qquad \xi_0 - \xi = \Delta \xi \tag{5.1.41}$$

Then for low turbulence levels $\Delta d \ll d_0$, whence

$$\Delta d \approx U_0(\xi_0 - \xi) = U_0 \Delta \xi \tag{5.1.42}$$

This leads to

$$E\left[\left(\frac{\Delta d}{d_0}\right)^2\right] = U_0^2 E\left[\left(\frac{\Delta \xi}{d_0}\right)^2\right] = E\left[\left(\frac{\Delta \xi}{\xi_0}\right)^2\right] \tag{5.1.43}$$

From equation (5.1.17) it is seen that the square root of the rhs of equation (5.1.43) is equal to the rms width of the cross-correlation function divided by ξ_0. For low turbulence levels ξ_0 is equal to the time lag at the peak of the cross-correlation function (Figure 5.1.3).

By use of the classical theory of turbulent diffusion outlined in Section 1.3, the lhs of equation (5.1.43) can be expressed in terms of the Lagrangian correlation function for the turbulence. Writing the Lagrangian correlation coefficient for the velocity fluctuation in the mean flow direction as $\rho_L(\tau)$, we have, from equation (1.3.25),

$$E\left[\left(\frac{\Delta d}{d_0}\right)^2\right] = \frac{2\sigma_u^2}{U_0^2 \xi_0} \int_0^{\xi_0} \left(1 - \frac{\tau}{\xi_0}\right) \rho_L(\tau) \, d\tau \tag{5.1.44}$$

The general expression relating the rms width of the cross-correlation function to the rms turbulence level is thus

$$\frac{\text{rms width}}{\text{peak}} = \frac{\sigma_u}{U_0}\left[\frac{2}{\xi_0} \int_0^{\xi_0} \left(1 - \frac{\tau}{\xi_0}\right) \rho_L(\tau) \, d\tau\right]^{1/2} \tag{5.1.45}$$

Two limiting forms of equation (5.1.45) are important : (i) short passage times, i.e., $\xi_0 \ll \Lambda$, and (ii) long passage times, i.e., $\xi_0 \gg \Lambda$, where Λ is the Lagrangian integral scale,

$$\Lambda = \int_0^\infty \rho_L(\tau) \, d\tau \tag{5.1.46}$$

For short passage times equation (5.1.45) reduces to (5.1.17), i.e.,

$$\frac{\text{rms width}}{\text{peak}} = \frac{\sigma_u}{U_0} \tag{5.1.47}$$

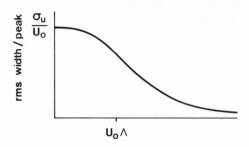

Figure 5.1.4. Variation, with beam separation, of the cross-correlation rms width divided by peak value.

For long times, equation (5.1.45) reduces to

$$\frac{\text{rms width}}{\text{peak}} = \frac{\sigma_u}{U_0}\left(\frac{2\Lambda}{\xi_0}\right)^{1/2} \tag{5.1.48}$$

i.e., the width of the cross-correlation peak has been reduced by a factor determined by the ratio of the Lagrangian integral time scale to the mean passage time between the beams. The manner in which the peak width varies as the beams are set at different separations in a given flow situation is shown in Figure 5.1.4. Notice that at small separations, i.e., small compared with $U_0\Lambda$, the ratio of the rms width to the mean is a constant, while at large separations the ratio dies asymptotically to zero.

It is possible, at least in principle, to apply the foregoing analysis to measure diffusion coefficients in a turbulent flow. The cross-correlation function is first measured with the beams spaced a very short distance apart, i.e., a distance considerably shorter than the expected value of $U_0\Lambda$. The rms width and the position of the cross-correlation peak are then measured, and equation (5.1.47) is applied to compute the rms turbulence level. The beams are then separated to a distance greater than the expected value of $U_0\Lambda$ and the rms width and position of the peak are again measured. With the rms turbulence level known equation (5.1.48) can then be applied to compute the Lagrangian integral scale and hence the longitudinal diffusion coefficient. It is also possible to devise ways of measuring transverse diffusion coefficients by similar techniques.

Measurement Accuracy

We will now derive an expression for the variance of the mean velocity estimated from the cross-correlation function assuming a continuous stream of scattering particles. It is important to know this in order that suitable measuring times can be chosen, consistent with a specified measurement accuracy. If the cross-correlation function for the intensity is

$$R_{12}(\xi) = E[I_1(\mu)I_2(\mu - \xi)] \tag{5.1.49}$$

then the estimated value of $R_{12}(\xi)$ will be

$$\hat{R}_{12}(\xi) = \frac{1}{T_m} \int_0^{T_m} I_1(\mu)I_2(\mu - \xi) \, d\xi \tag{5.1.50}$$

where T_m is the total measuring time.

In our case the signals from both detectors resemble band-limited white noise as they arise from a random distribution of particles passing across the beams. The bandwidth B of the noise will be inversely proportional to the passage time across each beam. For simplicity it will be assumed that ac detectors are employed, i.e., the mean value of the signals are zero. It is then straightforward to show (Bendat and Piersol, 1971) that for sufficiently long measuring times the rms error in $R_{12}(\xi)$ is approximately

$$\varepsilon = \left\{ \frac{\text{var}[\hat{R}_{12}(\xi)]}{R_{12}^2(\xi)} \right\}^{1/2} = \frac{1}{(2BT_m)^{1/2}} \left[1 + \frac{R_1(0)R_2(0)}{R_{12}^2(\xi)} \right]^{1/2} \tag{5.1.51}$$

where $R_1(\xi)$ and $R_2(\xi)$ are the autocorrelation functions for the two signals separately.

In the region of the cross-correlation peak, $R_1(0)R_2(0) \approx R_{12}^2(\xi)$, and the mean square error becomes

$$\varepsilon = (BT_m)^{-1/2} \tag{5.1.52}$$

In order to interpret this as a velocity measurement error we will assume that the mean velocity is obtained by recording the time lag (ξ_p) corresponding to the peak of the cross-correlation function, i.e., the value of ξ where $\partial R_{12}(\xi)/\partial \xi = 0$. Similar results are obtained if the first moment divided by the zeroth moment about the origin is used as the mean velocity estimator.

Considering the case of constant flow velocity U, the cross-correlation function takes the form [from equation (5.1.33)]

$$R_{12}(\xi, \xi_p) = K_c \exp\left[-2B^2(\xi - \xi_p)^2\right] \tag{5.1.53}$$

where we have written $K_c = B_1 N_p/(2\pi U^2 r_0^2)^{1/2}$ and $B = U/(2r_0)$.

Following the simplified approach of Jordan (1973), we will assume that the random variations in $\hat{R}_{12}(\xi)$, caused by the finite sampling time, are not large enough to distort significantly the shape of the cross-correlation peak.

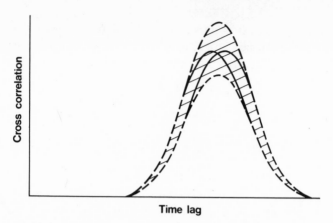

Figure 5.1.5. Confidence band represented by equation (5.1.52). The full lines represent two possible Gaussian curves having the same peak values and which fall predominantly within this band.

Thus, corresponding to the range of $\hat{R}_{12}(\xi)$, there is a range of Gaussian curves having the same shape and peak heights which can be drawn through the plotted $\hat{R}_{12}(\xi)$ points, each of these curves having a different peak lag value. This is illustrated in Figure 5.1.5, where the shaded area represents the confidence band defined by equation (5.1.52) and the solid lines represent two Gaussian curves with different peak lag values which fall predominantly within this band. The extent of the range of possible peak lag values can be found approximately by simply geometrical considerations as follows.

From equation (5.1.53), if the peak lag changes from ξ_p to $\xi_p + \Delta\xi$, then the cross-correlation function will be

$$R_{12}(\xi, \xi_p + \Delta\xi) = K_c \exp\left[-2B^2(\xi - \xi_p - \Delta\xi)^2\right] \qquad (5.1.54)$$

and by expanding the exponential term in equation (5.1.54) it is seen that

$$\frac{R_{12}(\xi, \xi_p + \Delta\xi)}{R_{12}(\xi, \xi_p)} = 1 + 4B^2\Delta\xi(\xi - \xi_p) \qquad (5.1.55)$$

We will set $(\xi - \xi_p) = 1/2B$, considering this as a representative value. Equation (5.1.55) can then be rewritten as

$$R_{12}(\xi, \xi_p + \Delta\xi) - R_{12}(\xi, \xi_p) \approx R_{12}(\xi, \xi_p)2B \cdot \Delta\xi \qquad (5.1.56)$$

Now (considering $\Delta\xi$ as a random variable) it will become clear after a little thought that

$$\{\text{var}\,[R_{12}(\xi, \xi_p + \Delta\xi) - R_{12}(\xi, \xi_p)]\}^{1/2} \approx \{\text{var}\,[\hat{R}_{12}(\xi, \xi_p)]\}^{1/2}$$

$$\approx \frac{R_{12}(\xi, \xi_p)}{(BT_m)^{1/2}} \qquad (5.1.57)$$

Combining equations (5.1.56) and (5.1.57) gives

$$\{\text{var}\,[\Delta\xi]\}^{1/2} = \frac{1}{2B^{3/2}T_m^{1/2}} \qquad (5.1.58)$$

In terms of the beam radius r_0 and the flow velocity U, since $B \approx \frac{1}{2}U/r_0$, the mean square error in the velocity estimate U is approximately

$$\frac{\{\text{var}\,[U]\}^{1/2}}{U} = \frac{\{\text{var}\,[\Delta\xi]\}^{1/2}}{d_0/U} = 1.4r_0^{3/2}U^{-1/2}T_m^{-1/2}d_0^{-1} \qquad (5.1.59)$$

The above expression [equation (5.1.59)] can be used directly to give order-of-magnitude estimates of the measuring time required in a given flow measurement situation. As an example, suppose that $d_0 = 1$ cm, $r_0 = 0.5$ mm, the flow velocity is approximately 1 msec^{-1}, and the velocity measurement is required to 1 % accuracy. Substituting these values into equation (5.1.59) and setting the lhs equal to 0.01 gives the measuring time required as $T_m = 0.025$ sec.

Measurement of Particle Sizes

In certain industrial applications, where fluids are used to transport solid particles, it is important to know particle size distributions as well as velocities of the moving particles. Methods of adapting the cross-correlation technique to give this information have been proposed by Beck *et al.* (1973) and Lading (1973) among others.

Generally it is assumed that the transported particle sizes are much greater than the beam spot sizes. In this situation the length of the pulse associated with the passage of a single particle is proportional to the cross-sectional length of the particle in the flow direction, and hence the signals from the two photodetectors are characterized both by the flow velocity and the particle sizes. Thus by following both detectors with appropriate bandpass filters the contributions arising from the individual particle sizes can effectively be separated. By computing a number of cross-correlation functions, each associated with a different filter center frequency, a complete particle size-versus-velocity distribution can be built up. The details of this procedure are described by Lading (1973).

5.2. *Photon Counting Cross Correlation*

The use of photon counting techniques for signal analysis in a two-beam cross-correlation system results in a particularly sensitive and versatile instrument. To apply the method, two separate detectors are used, both fitted with discriminator units adjusted for single-photon response. Thus two signals are fed to the digital correlator, both in the form of a discrete series of unit height pulses. The optical arrangement shown in Figure 2.1.2 can conveniently be used and has been shown to give good results in practice (Durrani and Greated, 1975; Greated, 1975). An important feature of this scheme is that no laser radiation is allowed to fall directly onto the detector surfaces. Thus, high signal-to-noise ratios can be achieved.

Let $I_1(t_1)$ be the intensity of scattered radiation falling onto photo-detector 1 at time t_1 (i.e., the intensity integrated over the detector surface) due to particles passing across beam 1. Similarly let $I_2(t_2)$ be the intensity falling onto photodetector 2 at time t_2 due to particles passing across beam 2.

In a counting interval $(kT, \overline{k+1}T)$ the conditional probability of registering N counts for channel 1 is given by

$$P[N(kT, \overline{k+1}T)] = \frac{1}{N!} \left[\alpha \int_{kT}^{\overline{k+1}T} I_1(\tau)\, d\tau \right]^N \exp \left[-\alpha \int_{kT}^{\overline{k+1}T} I_1(\tau)\, d\tau \right] \quad (5.2.1)$$

where T is the sample time and α the overall quantum efficiency of the detector. Assuming that photodetector 2 has the same quantum efficiency, i.e., a symmetric system, the conditional probability of registering M counts in the interval $(\overline{k+sT}, \overline{k+s+1}T)$ is

$$P[M(\overline{k+sT}, \overline{k+s+1}T)$$

$$= \frac{1}{M!} \left[\alpha \int_{\overline{k+sT}}^{\overline{k+s+1}T} I_2(\tau)\, d\tau \right]^M \exp \left[-\alpha \int_{\overline{k+sT}}^{\overline{k+s+1}T} I_2(\tau)\, d\tau \right] \quad (5.2.2)$$

where s is the number of the delay register.

Thus the conditional joint moments between the two channels may be expressed as

$$E[N(kT, \overline{k+1}T) \cdot M(\overline{k+sT}, \overline{k+s+1}T)|m_1(sT)m(\overline{k+sT})]$$

$$= \alpha^2 \int_{kT}^{\overline{k+1}T} \int_{\overline{k+sT}}^{\overline{k+s+1}T} I_1(\mu) I_2(\nu)\, d\mu\, d\nu \quad (5.2.3)$$

where

$$m_{1,2}(kT) = \int_{kT}^{\overline{k+1}T} I_{1,2}(\tau)\, d\tau \qquad (5.2.4)$$

The counting cross correlation is then

$$\tilde{R}_c(sT) = E[N(kT, \overline{k+1}T) \cdot M(\overline{k+sT, k+s+1}T)]$$

$$= E[E\{N(kT, \overline{k+1}T) \cdot M(\overline{k+sT, k+s+1}T) | m_1(kT), m_2(\overline{k+sT})\}]$$

$$= \alpha^2 \int_{kT}^{\overline{k+1}T} \int_{\overline{k+sT}}^{\overline{k+s+1}T} E[I_1(\mu)I_2(\nu)]\, d\mu\, d\nu \qquad (5.2.5)$$

For small values of the sample time T it follows from equation (5.2.5) that

$$\tilde{R}_c(sT) = \alpha^2 T^2 E[I_1(kT)I_2(\overline{k+sT})] \qquad (5.2.6)$$

Thus the counting cross-correlation function is directly proportional to the cross correlation of the intensities. Expressions for the intensity cross-correlation function in a turbulent flow were derived in Section 5.1.

The digital correlator generally accumulates the product

$$r_c(sT) = \sum_{k=1}^{K} N(kT, \overline{k+1}T) \cdot M(\overline{k+sT, k+s1}T) \qquad (5.2.7)$$

where K is the number of products accumulated. The nonnormalized count cross-correlation function is then $\tilde{R}_c(sT) = r_c(sT)/M$.

Measured Cross-Correlation Functions

Figure 5.2.1 shows typical counting cross-correlation functions obtained in a laboratory wind tunnel (a) behind a fine wire grid (low turbulence), and (b) behind a coarse grid (high turbulence). The insertion of the coarse grid into the tunnel in this case caused a slight reduction in mean velocity that showed up as a shift in the position of the peak lag value. Otherwise, the working conditions were the same. The optical configuration was as illustrated in Figure 2.1.2, with the scattered light collected at 30° to the illuminating beams. Note that increasing this angle has the effect of improving the spatial resolution in the direction of the optical axis. The light sources were 2-mW HeNe lasers, and the air flow was unseeded. This gives some idea of the high sensitivity of the technique.

In this case the beam separation was 8 mm, which was estimated as being small compared with the product $U_0\Lambda$, so equation (5.1.17) can be

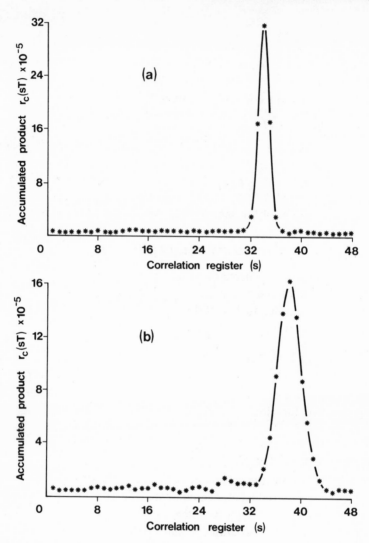

Figure 5.2.1. Count cross-correlation functions obtained in (a) a low-turbulence flow; (b) a high-turbulence flow. Sample time in both cases is $T = 40\,\mu\text{sec}$.

applied to estimate the mean velocities and turbulence levels. Thus, as the peaks occur at lag values of 1.36 and 1.52 msec, respectively, for the high- and low-turbulence flows, the corresponding mean velocities are 5.88 and 5.26 msec^{-1}. The simplest method of measuring rms widths is to assume the peaks to be Gaussian in shape. The standard deviation (equal to the rms width) is then equal to the width of the peak at half of its height divided by 2.35. From the two counting cross-correlation functions shown in Figure 5.2.1 the widths of the peaks at half-height are (a) 86 and (b) 188 μsec, which give turbulence levels of 2.7% and 5.3%, respectively. Corrections for the finite passage time across the beams have been disregarded in this calculation. With the aid of a computer it would be possible to obtain better estimates of both mean velocities and turbulence levels by evaluating the moments, or, alternatively, a curve fitting procedure could be employed. Both of these methods have the advantage that they take full account of all the computed points on the cross correlogram.

One disadvantage of the cross-correlation technique is that only a small fraction of the total number of values computed by the correlator are actually used in evaluating the mean velocity and turbulence level. This is immediately obvious when one examines Figure 5.2.1. By incorporating a suitable time delay into channel 1 (i.e., the upstream channel), however, it is possible to have the bell-shaped correlation peak effectively cover the complete display. This is done by setting the time delay to a value just less than the smallest expected passage time of particles across the two beams. Determination of the exact position of the peak and also the magnitude of the peak rms width then becomes much simpler. Because of the time scales involved a digital delay register is generally required for this purpose.

Since the spacing of the beams in a cross-correlation system is normally at least two orders of magnitude greater than the typical fringe spacing in an LDV system, the correlation delay times involved are very much greater. This makes cross-correlation methods particularly convenient to apply in high-velocity flow situations.

Chapter 6

HARDWARE SYSTEMS FOR LDV SIGNAL PROCESSING

To interpret the photodetector signal in an LDV in terms of the associated flow parameter, an electronic processing unit is required. A number of techniques exist for analyzing the signal, and several systems specially designed for LDV signal analysis are now commercially available. In the main, the choice of a particular technique or electronic system depends upon the flow conditions, or more specifically, on the scattered radiation. Thus, for highly seeded flows, where the Doppler signal is essentially a continuous (frequency modulated) random signal, the techniques employed are the same as, or are variants on, conventional FM detection schemes. While for unseeded flows, where the received signal forms a series of pulses or random bursts (as discussed in Section 3.1), highly sensitive systems are used, such as photon correlators, or frequency-burst processing systems.

6.1. Frequency Detection Systems

In the earlier chapters it has been shown that the Doppler signal arising in the LDV is a frequency-modulated signal where the information on the flow statistics is contained in the modulation. Thus to estimate the flow parameters it is necessary to extract the instantaneous frequency of the Doppler signal.

Several excellent texts cover the topic of conventional FM detection techniques, notably Clarke and Hess (1971) and Taub and Schilling (1971). We shall therefore concentrate on the broad principles of FM detection as they apply to the LDV signal and leave the reader to pursue detailed analyses available in standard texts on communication theory and detection systems.

It must be borne in mind that in almost all analogue processing schemes the signal obtained from the photodetector is filtered to remove the low-frequency content and to eliminate the effects of $1/f$ detector noise and background radiation.

Limiter Discriminator

Figure 6.1.1a gives a block diagram of one of the simplest forms of frequency detectors, sometimes called the pulse-count frequency demodulator. The photodetected Doppler signal is bandpass-filtered. The filter cutoff frequency is chosen to be close to the mean Doppler frequency representing the mean flow velocity, and the filter bandwidth is made sufficiently large to accommodate Doppler signal frequency variations due to fluid turbulence effects. The limiter circuit, usually a Schmitt trigger, removes any amplitude variations of the signal and produces a signal which represents the zero crossings of the bandpass-filtered Doppler signal. The monostable multivibrator generates pulses of fixed duration when triggered at each zero up-crossing (or down-crossing) of the limiter output. The associated low-pass filter (LPF) averages out (or counts) the pulses to yield a signal whose amplitude is inversely proportional to the instantaneous interval between adjacent zero-upcrossings, i.e., directly proportional to the instantaneous frequency of the bandpass-filtered Doppler signal. The attendent sketches of the signal in Figure 6.1.1b illustrate the above discussion. The basic simplicity of system design is one of the reasons for the popularity of the pulse-counting discriminator in LDV applications.

When the instantaneous Doppler signal frequency is high, the pulses $\{v_a(t)\}$ are closely spaced, and the average value of the pulses at the low-pass filter output is high. Conversely when the instantaneous frequency decreases, the interval between pulses $\{v_a(t)\}$ becomes large, and the low-pass filter output falls in amplitude. Thus $V_0(t)$ is proportional to the instantaneous frequency.

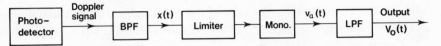

Figure 6.1.1a. Pulse counting frequency demodulator.

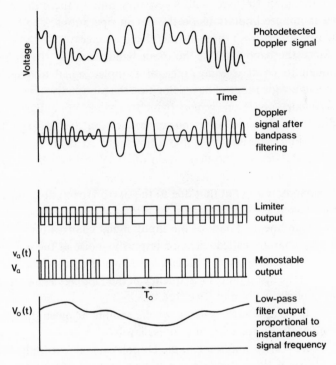

Figure 6.1.1b. Waveforms in pulse counting frequency demodulator.

The frequency-to-voltage conversion constant of the system may be easily determined. If the monostable output sequence is of amplitude V_a and each pulse is of duration T_0, then for a sinusoidal Doppler signal of constant frequency ω, the pulse sequence $\{v_a(t)\}$ would be periodic, with an average value of $\omega T_0 V_a/2\pi$, such that the output signal from the low-pass filter is $V_0(t) = (\omega T_0 V_a/2\pi)H(0)$, where $H(0)$ is the dc gain of the filter. Hence the conversion constant is $(T_0 V_a/\pi)H(0)$. However, it may be seen that if the input signal frequency exceeds (π/T_0) $(V_a > \pi/T_0)$, the monostable would trigger at every alternate zero up-crossing. Hence, for this system the frequency range of detection is limited to $1/2T_0$ Hz. This bound does not take into consideration the recovery time of the monostable. If this is assumed as T_r, then the highest frequency that can be demodulated is $1/2(T_0 + T_r)$ Hz.

Commercial discriminator units designed on the above principle are now readily available, with a choice of center frequencies ranging from 1 Hz to 10 MHz. Since beyond 10 MHz the pulse duration of the monostable should be less than 100 nsec, with a recovery time of the order of 10 nsec, logic speeds impose limitations on the circuit operations. The pulse-count discriminator suffers from three distinct disadvantages:

(a) Since the bandwidth of the input bandpass filter (BPF) has to be large enough to cover a wide range of Doppler signal frequencies corresponding to a wide range of flow velocities, the input noise power accepted by the frequency-detection system (which depends upon the input filter bandwidth for wide-band input noise, see Section 3.3) is large. Further, it has been found experimentally that a threshold exists for such systems at an input "signal"-(carrier)-to-noise ratio of 10 dB, below which the output signal-to-noise ratio falls drastically.

It is worth pointing out that due to the narrow-band noise structure of the Doppler signal, even for uniform flow studies, there are frequent occasions when the instantaneous phase of the input signal changes through 2π rad. This leads to what are called clicks or impulsive noise at the output of the frequency discriminator, since sudden phase inversions produce an impulse (of area 2π) on the instantaneous frequency of the Doppler signal. A rigorous treatment of clicks is given in Rice (1963).

We shall discuss later systems which exhibit a lower threshold and accept comparatively reduced input noise levels.

(b) Whenever the amplitude of the Doppler signal $\{x(t)\}$ falls below the threshold level of the limiter or the trigger level of the monostable, the output signal $V_0(t)$ drops to zero (drop-out effect). Thus, an output signal drop-out occurs whenever the scattered radiation collected by the photodetector does not contain a Doppler component of appreciable strength, for instance, whenever the LDV observation volume is depleted of scattering particles. For this reason the pulse-counting discriminator is ineffective in analyzing flows with low scattering particle concentrations. Several variations have been proposed to overcome the drop-out problem, the most popular being a system in which the output signal $V_0(t)$ is maintained constant when the input signal level falls below threshold (Wilmshurst and Rizzo, 1974).

In practice, a small though finite threshold level is usually set up to stop the monostable from being triggered by the noise on the input signal. This provides a valuable method of signal selection and noise rejection.

For a given threshold level it is possible to determine the mean duration of a drop-out interval if we consider the Doppler signal as narrow-band and normally distributed, as in uniform flow studies [see equation (3.1.17)]. Then according to Rice (1944) the mean number of occasions per unit time the envelope $H(t)$ of the Doppler signal passes downwards (or upwards) across the level H_0 is

$$N = \left[\frac{-R_w''(0)}{2\pi R_w(0)}\right]^{1/2} H_0 \exp\left[-H_0^2/2R_x(0)\right] \qquad (6.1.1)$$

where $R_w''(\tau) = d^2 R_w(\tau)/d\tau^2$, with $R_w(\tau)$ as the autocorrelation of the weighting function, and $R_x(0)$ the mean square level of the Doppler signal. Now the probability that the envelope $H(t)$ is less than H_0 is $1 - \exp\left[-H_0^2/2R_x(0)\right]$. Hence, the average duration of the drop-out interval is given by

$$T_d = \{1 - \exp\left[-H_0^2/2R_x(0)\right]\}/N \quad \text{sec}$$

$$= \left[-\frac{2\pi R_w(0)}{R_w''(0)}\right]^{1/2} \frac{1}{H_0}\left[\exp\frac{H_0^2}{2R_x(0)} - 1\right]$$

$$\doteq \left[-\frac{2\pi R_w(0)}{R_w''(0)}\right]^{1/2} \frac{H_0}{2R_x(0)} \qquad \text{for small } H_0 \qquad (6.1.2)$$

This satisfies the intuitive argument that for a very small threshold level, the drop-out duration is exceedingly small and increases with increase in threshold level. The average time interval between drop-outs may be similarly obtained as

$$\overline{T}_d = \text{Prob}\{H(t) > H_0\}/N$$

$$= \left[-\frac{2\pi R_w(0)}{R_w''(0)}\right]^{1/2} \frac{1}{H_0} \qquad (6.1.3)$$

(c) Even under steady flow conditions, estimation of the mean Doppler frequency by the zero-crossing techniques (used in the pulse counting discriminator) leads to a bias due to the finite bandwidth of the filtered Doppler signal. This may be easily seen by considering two common optical configurations of the LDV.

For a mask system, the autocorrelation function of the filtered Doppler signal is given by [refer to equation (3.3.27)]

$$R_x(\tau) = R_x(0)\left[\frac{6}{(2\mu\tau)^2}(1 - \text{sinc } 2\mu\tau)\cos 2\pi f_0\tau\right]$$

where μ is as described by equation (2.6.55) and f_0 is the mean Doppler frequency. Similarly for the Gaussian beam system we have

$$R_x(\tau) = R_x(0)\exp\left(-\tau^2/4\rho^2\right)\cos 2\pi f_0\tau$$

According to Rice (1944), for narrow-band stationary, normally distributed processes, the mean rate of zero crossings is given by

$$N_z = \frac{1}{\pi}\left[-\frac{R_x''(0)}{R_x(0)}\right]^{1/2} \tag{6.1.4}$$

where $R_x''(\tau) = d^2R_x(\tau)/d\tau^2$.

Using the above expressions, we have

$$N_{z1} = 2(f_0^2 + \mu^2/10\pi^2)^{1/2} \qquad \text{mask system}$$

$$N_{z2} = 2(f_0^2 + 1/8\pi^2\rho^2)^{1/2} \qquad \text{Gaussian beam system}$$

Thus the respective biases are

$$N_{z1}/2 - f_0 \simeq \mu^2/20\pi^2 f_0^2 = a^2/20b^2$$

$$N_{z2}/2 - f_0 \simeq 1/16\pi^2\rho^2 f_0^2 = \lambda^2/32\pi^2 r_0^2\tan^2\theta$$

where the last two expressions have been obtained via equation (2.6.55) and are related to the parameters of the optical setup. Using the definitions of mean square signal bandwidth as given in equations (3.2.11)–(3.2.15), it may be seen that the bias is proportional to the square of the ratio of the rms bandwidth to center frequency (f_0) of the Doppler signal.

The bias may be further increased if any additive noise is present on the signal. An analysis which covers this aspect is given in Durrani *et al.* (1973).

Frequency Tracking Systems

Several systems have been proposed for processing LDV signals to provide a voltage proportional to instantaneous frequency of the signal and to track any variations in this frequency. Most of these systems are based on FM demodulators commonly employed in communication systems, such as the phase-locked loop, the FM demodulator with feedback, or the automatically tracking narrow-band filters (Deighton and Sayle, 1971; Iten and Dandliker, 1972; Wilmshurst *et al.* 1971).

Figure 6.1.2 gives a schematic representation of a frequency tracker. It employs a limiter discriminator with a voltage-controlled oscillator (VCO) in the feedback loop. The VCO generates a sinusoidal signal with a frequency

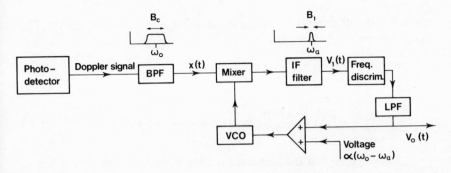

Figure 6.1.2. Frequency tracker.

proportional to voltage applied to its input. $\{x(t)\}$ represents the bandpass-filtered Doppler signal; the bandwidth B_c of the first filter is considerably larger than the IF filter bandwidth B_1. The IF filter is in general tuned around a frequency ω_a different from the center frequency of the Doppler signal ω_0. The bandwidth B_1 is called the acceptance bandwidth of the demodulator. It is usual to employ a single tuned IF filter to avoid instability in the loop.

Consider the instantaneous (filtered) Doppler signal at the input to the frequency tracker to be

$$x(t) = H(t) \cos \left[\omega_0 t + \phi(t) \right] \tag{6.1.5}$$

where $H(t)$ is the signal envelope, ω_0 corresponds to the mean Doppler frequency, and $\phi(t)$, the instantaneous phase, contains the FM information. The VCO output may be written as

$$y(t) = A \cos \left[(\omega_0 - \omega_a)t + K \int V_0(t) \, dt \right] \tag{6.1.6}$$

where $A = \text{const}$ and K is the oscillator control constant.

From the above equations, the IF component of the product $\{x(t)y(t)\}$ applied to the frequency discriminator unit is

$$V_1(t) = \{AH(t)/2\} \cos \left[\omega_a t + \phi(t) - K \int V_0(t) \, dt \right] \tag{6.1.7}$$

However, $V_0(t)$ is the input to the VCO and is proportional to the instantaneous frequency of $V_1(t)$,

$$V_0(t) = C \frac{d}{dt} \left[\phi(t) - K \int V_0(t) \, dt \right]$$

where C is the discriminator frequency-to-voltage conversion constant. This yields

$$V_0(t) = [C/(1 + KC)]\dot{\phi}(t) \qquad (6.1.8)$$

whence

$$V_1(t) = \frac{AH(t)}{2} \cos \left[\omega_a t + \frac{1}{(1 + KC)} \phi(t) \right] \qquad (6.1.9)$$

Thus it is seen that the frequency tracker output voltage $V_0(t)$ is directly proportional to the instantaneous rate of change of phase of the Doppler input signal. This output is reduced by a factor of $(1 + KC)$ as compared with that of the limiter discriminator unit discussed earlier.

The VCO tracks the Doppler signal frequency very closely, and for a small input phase variation $(\delta\omega_0)t$, i.e., Doppler signal frequency shift of $\delta\omega_0$ by equation (6.1.7), the oscillator frequency would change by $(\delta\omega_0)KC/(1 + KC)$. This leads to a sensitivity relationship,

$$\frac{\delta\omega_{VCO}}{\delta\omega_{Doppler}} \approx \frac{KC}{1 + KC}$$

Similarly the frequency variation in $V_1(t)$ for an incremental change $\delta\omega_0$ in the Doppler frequency is given by $\delta\omega_0/(1 + KC)$.

Further, comparing equations (6.1.5) and (6.1.9), we see that within the loop, the feedback has reduced the frequency deviation by a factor of $1/(1 + KC)$. This enables the use of a comparatively narrow-band IF filter (centered on ω_a) to process the same modulation and to accommodate the same range of variation of instantaneous Doppler signal frequency as with the wide-band filter of Figure 6.1.1. Since the acceptance bandwidth B_1 determines the effective noise power input to the frequency discriminator in the loop, we see that a narrow-band filter causes a substantial reduction in this input noise power, and thus leads to greater noise immunity and to an extension of the threshold of detection for the tracker. Obviously this reduction is proportional to the ratio of the IF filter bandwidth used with the tracker to the bandwidth of the IF filter in the frequency discriminator of Figure 6.1.1.

The maximum tracking rates of the system can be shown to be $\sim 0.5(1 + KC)B_1 f_b$ Hz/sec, where f_b Hz is the bandwidth of the low-pass filter following the frequency discriminator. If the input rate of change of frequency exceeds this value, the system tends to lose lock, i.e., lose track of the instantaneous signal frequency, and the output voltage $V_0(t)$ decays to zero. This can occur when highly turbulent flows are investigated where the Doppler signal undergoes exceedingly rapid changes in frequency.

A rigorous derivation for the maximum tracking rate would involve the cumbersome transient analysis of the frequency tracker, which is a nonlinear feedback system. However, the following intuitive argument may be used to arrive at a close approximation. Consider the Doppler signal to be an FM carrier, where the modulating signal is sinusoidal:

$$x(t) = A \cos (2\pi f_0 t + A_m \sin 2\pi f_m t)$$

Then the instantaneous frequency of the signal is

$$f_i(t) = f_0 + f_m A_m \cos 2\pi f_m t$$

The instantaneous frequency deviation of the signal is $f_m A_m \cos 2\pi f_m t$. Then for the frequency tracker to demodulate the signal, $|f_m A_m|$ should be less than the maximum acceptable frequency deviation which is determined by the IF filter bandwidth. Hence $|f_m A_m| \leq 0.5 B_1 (1 + KC)$. Further, for the modulating signal to be detected without distortion, it should lie within the bandwidth of the low-pass filter, i.e., $f_m \leq f_b$.

From above, the instantaneous rate of change of input signal frequency is

$$\frac{df_i}{dt} = -A_m f_m^2 \sin 2\pi f_m t$$

such that

$$\max \left| \frac{df_i}{dt} \right| = A_m f_m^2 \leq 0.5(1 + KC) B_1 f_b$$

The Autodyne Tracking Filter

Figure 6.1.3 shows an autodyne tracking system for frequency demodulating of Doppler signals (Durrani, Greated, and Wilmshurst, 1973). Specific details of hardware design are given in Wilmshurst and Rizzo (1974). The instantaneous signal frequency is detected by separating the Doppler signal into two orthogonal components and then performing an operation similar to that given by equation (3.3.33) on the two components. The two orthogonal components are generated by mixing the Doppler signal with 90° phase shifted outputs of a voltage-controlled oscillator. The input voltage to the oscillator completes the loop and gives an estimate of the signal frequency.

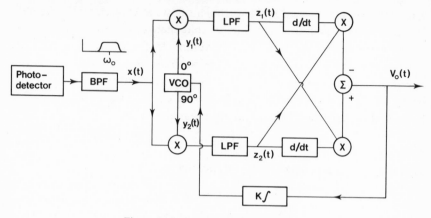

Figure 6.1.3. Autodyne frequency tracker.

Consider the bandpass-filtered Doppler signal as in equation (3.3.29):

$$x(t) = \kappa \sum_p K_p W(\beta \xi_p(t)) \cos D\xi_p(t)$$

where κ, K_p, β, D, and $W(\ )$ are all defined in Chapters 2 and 3, and $\xi_p(t)$ and $V_p(t) = d\xi_p(t)/dt$ are the instantaneous position and velocity of any (pth) scattering particle in the observation volume. Defining the output voltages of the VCO as

$$y_1(t) = A \cos \left[K \int V_0(t)\, dt \right]$$

$$y_2(t) = A \sin \left[K \int V_0(t)\, dt \right]$$

where K is the oscillator control constant, the output of the low-pass filters in the two branches is

$$Z_1(t) = \frac{A\kappa}{2} \sum_p K_p W(\beta \xi_p(t)) \cos \left[D\xi_p(t) - K \int V_0(t)\, dt \right]$$

$$Z_2(t) = \frac{A\kappa}{2} \sum_p K_p W(\beta \xi_p(t)) \sin \left[D\xi_p(t) - K \int V_0(t)\, dt \right]$$

(6.1.10)

and the input to the voltage-controlled oscillator is

$$V_0(t) = Z_1(t)\dot{Z}_2(t) - \dot{Z}_1(t)Z_2(t)$$

$$= [\omega_i(t) - KV_0(t)][Z_1^2(t) + Z_2^2(t)]$$

where $\omega_i(t)$ is the instantaneous frequency of the Doppler signal as given by equation (3.3.34). Thus, we have

$$V_0(t) = \frac{Z_1^2(t) + Z_2^2(t)}{1 + K[Z_1^2(t) + Z_2^2(t)]} \omega_i(t)$$

$$\simeq \omega_i(t)/K \qquad (6.1.11)$$

for large K; $\{V_0(t)\}$ therefore faithfully tracks the instantaneous frequency of the Doppler signal.

The acceptance bandwidth of the autodyne system is determined by the bandwidth of the low-pass filters in the two branches. As the output voltage $V_0(t)$ depends, to a certain extent, on the mean square signal level [proportional to $Z_1^2(t) + Z_2^2(t)$], it is possible to reduce the effect of signal drop-out by isolating the integrator in the feedback loop. This is achieved by continuously evaluating $Z_1^2(t) + Z_2^2(t)$ and comparing it with a preset level. If $Z_1^2(t) + Z_2^2(t)$ falls below the preset level, the integrator output is frozen, the integrator input is isolated, and the VCO is decoupled from any dc drift caused by the multipliers in the absence of a Doppler component on the input signal.

Since the autodyne circuit calculates the instantaneous frequency of the input signal and not the zero-crossing frequency, it does not lead to any bias errors in the measurement. The maximum tracking rate of the system is found to be proportional to the product of the gain K and the bandwidth of the low-pass filters, f_c. The noise power input is also restricted by the bandwidth of these filters; hence the performance of the autodyne system is far superior to the frequency discriminator of Figure 6.1.1.

Practical autodyne systems have been used to track Doppler signal frequencies up to 10 MHz with a long-term accuracy of around 0.2%.

6.2. *Processing Systems for Flows with Low Particle Concentrations*

To be effective the processing systems considered so far require a continuous Doppler signal. They rely on the presence of a large number of scattering particles in the flow to provide such a signal. In applications such as wind tunnel measurements or other gas flows, where artificial seeding is not possible and scattering particle concentration is exceedingly low, more sophisticated signal-processing techniques are employed. In this and the following sections we shall discuss two sytems which can be used for studying such flows, the photon correlators and the frequency-burst processing systems. Both these systems are capable of handling signals upto and beyond 20 MHz, the signals being in the form of a series of pulses for photon correlation and in the form of a series of bursts for the latter case.

One point worth stating at the outset is that with these systems the first-order statistics of the flow such as mean flow velocity and mean square turbulence level or the probability distribution of velocity (for the frequency burst processing system) can be easily measured. However, it is computationally difficult to obtain second-order statistics of the flow, such as turbulence microscales, or integral scales, or turbulence correlation.

Photon Correlators

Photon correlators and their use with LDV systems are a recent development. Their great advantage lies in facilitating flow measurements over a very large range of flow velocities, particularly under conditions where the intensity of scattered radiation is very low. Here we shall be concerned with the techniques for obtaining correlation functions in real time, while the theoretical aspects of estimating flow parameters from a record of photon count correlation have been covered in Chapters 4 and 5.

When the receiving optics in an LDV consists of a photomultiplier fitted with a discriminator unit, the output is a sequence of pulses representing a Poisson counting process. An estimate of the counting correlation for lag value sT is given by

$$\hat{R}(sT) \simeq \frac{1}{M} \sum_{k=1}^{M-|s|} N(kT, \overline{k+1}T)N(\overline{k+sT}, \overline{k+s+1}T)$$

$$s = 0, 1, 2, \ldots, L \tag{6.2.1}$$

for large M. Here $N(kT, \overline{k+1}T)$ is the numbers of pulses (or counts) observed in the time interval $(kT, \overline{k+1}T)$, T is the sampling time, MT is taken as the total observation time, and L is the total number of correlation lags.

Equation (6.2.1) may be recast into

$$\tilde{R}(sT, k+1) = \tilde{R}(sT, k) + N(kT, \overline{k+1}T)N(\overline{k-sT}, \overline{k-s+1}T)$$

$$s = 0, 1, 2, \ldots, L; \quad k = 0, 1, 2, \ldots \tag{6.2.2}$$

with the initial condition $\tilde{R}(sT, k) = 0$ for $k \leq s$ and all s, which yields

$$\tilde{R}(sT, M) = \sum_{k=1}^{M-|s|} N(kT, \overline{k+1}T)N(\overline{k+sT}, \overline{k+s+1}T) = M\hat{R}(sT)$$

According to equation (6.2.2) each new count $[N(kT, \overline{k+1}T)]$ over the current time interval $(kT, \overline{k+1}T)$ is multiplied by a delayed value $[N(\overline{k-sT}, \overline{k-s+1}T)]$ of the counting sequence, available in store, and the product is accumulated to the previous estimate $\tilde{R}(sT, k)$ of the counting correlation for lag value sT. In a hardware realization, equation (6.2.2) would represent the operation performed in each channel where a count correlation is accumulated for a specified lag value. However, such a hardware system would be exceedingly expensive and clearly impractical due to the high cost and complexity of incorporating a multiplier in each channel. An alternative would be to employ a single multiplier, so that the arithmetical operations of (6.2.2) are performed sequentially for each of the L lag values. Thus if T_m is the time taken to multiply two digital words, then an estimate of the complete autocorrelation function would be updated every LT_m sec. For real-time processing this sets an upper bound on the input sampling rate of the data, since the correlator would be incapable of coping with sampling rates greater than $1/LT_m$ sample/sec. Typically for a 50-channel correlator with a multiplier operating on 8-bit words at speeds of 250 nsec, the highest sampling rate which could be conveniently handled by the correlator is of the order of 80 000 sample/sec (i.e., signals with a bandwidth of 40 kHz), with the corresponding restriction on the minimum sampling time (T) of around 12.5 μsec. The frequency range of such a system would be far too low to be of any great use in LDV applications.

Clipped Correlators

In conventional correlators which operate on time series data, the computing effort is minimized by the use of clipping techniques. Here each new data point is multiplied by a delayed and hard-clipped value of past data points, and the products are accumulated. Systems based on these techniques are well known as relay correlators or polarity correlators (Watts, 1962; Jespers *et al.*, 1962). Thus for any data sequence $\{X_k\}$, a clipped correlation for lag value s is given by

$$\hat{R}_c(s) = \frac{1}{M-s} \sum_{k=0}^{M-s} X_k \operatorname{sgn}(X_{k+s}) \qquad s = 0, 1, 2, \ldots, L \qquad (6.2.3)$$

where

$$\text{sgn}\,(X_{k+s}) = 1 \qquad X_{k+s} > 0$$
$$= -1 \qquad X_{k+s} < 0$$

Hence

$$E[\hat{R}_c(s)] = E[X_k\,\text{sgn}\,(X_{k+s})]$$

It can be easily proved that for a zero mean Gaussian data sequence (Van Vleck and Middleton, 1966)

$$E[X_k\,\text{sgn}\,(X_{k+s})] = \int_0^\infty \int_{-\infty}^\infty X_k[p(X_k, X_{k+s}) + p(X_k, -X_{k+s})]\,dX_k\,dX_{k+s}$$

$$= \frac{1}{(2\pi)^{1/2}}R_x(s) \qquad \text{for all } s \tag{6.2.4}$$

Hence equation (6.2.3) leads to an unbiased estimate of the autocorrelation function. Similarly, an estimate of the cross-correlation function can be obtained if a Gaussian data sequence is cross-correlated with a hard-clipped version of another Gaussian sequence. The equation does not hold for non-Gaussian data. However, extensions may be found in Bogner (1965) and Knowles and Tsui (1967). Since most normally occurring data sequences are approximately Gaussian distributed, systems which exploit the relationship of equation (6.2.4) involve substantially reduced computing effort, since all multiplications are replaced by polarity changes and are therefore able to deal with very high data rates, in real time.

Similar to equation (6.2.4), another famous relationship called the *arcsine law* is sometimes used to further minimize computing labor. Here double clipping is used such that the correlation estimator is given by

$$\hat{R}_{cc}(s) = \frac{1}{M-s}\sum_{k=0}^{M-s}\text{sgn}\,(X_k)\,\text{sgn}\,(X_{k+s}) \qquad s = 0, 1, 2, \ldots, L \tag{6.2.5}$$

According to the arcsine law, for a Gaussian data sequence

$$E[\text{sgn}\,(X_k)\,\text{sgn}\,(X_{k+s})] = (2/\pi)\sin^{-1}\rho_x(s) \qquad \text{for all } s$$

where $\rho_x(s)$ is the normalized autocorrelation function of the sequence $\{X_k\}$. Thus $\rho_x(s)$ can be obtained from $\hat{R}_{cc}(s)$.

Several systems specifically designed to perform photon counting correlations now employ clipping procedures to minimize computing effort (Foord *et al.*, 1970; Jakeman *et al.*, 1970; Chen *et al.*, 1972). A clipped version of the counting sequence is obtained by comparing the counts per sampling interval with a preselected threshold or clipping level. If the threshold is exceeded, a binary 1 is stored, if not, a binary 0 is stored; and the correlation function is estimated as

$$\hat{R}_c(sT) = \frac{1}{M - |s|} \sum_{k=1}^{M-|s|} N(\overline{k + sT}, \overline{k + s + 1T}) N_c(kT, \overline{k + 1T})$$

$$s = 0, 1, 2, \ldots, L \qquad (6.2.6)$$

where

$$N_c(kT, \overline{k + 1T}) = 1 \quad \text{if } N(kT, \overline{k + 1T}) \geq q \quad \text{(preselected threshold)}$$

$$= 0 \quad \text{if } N(kT, \overline{k + 1T}) < q \qquad (6.2.7)$$

Recasting equation (6.2.6), we may achieve a direct hardware implementation of any channel of the correlator according to

$$\hat{R}_c(sT, k + 1) = \hat{R}_c(sT, k) + N(kT, \overline{k + 1T}) N_c(\overline{k - sT}, \overline{k - s + 1T})$$

$$s = 0, 1, 2, \ldots, L \qquad (6.2.8)$$

Figure 6.2.1 illustrates a multichannel counting correlator (Asch and Ford, 1973). The photomultiplier output is amplified and passed through a

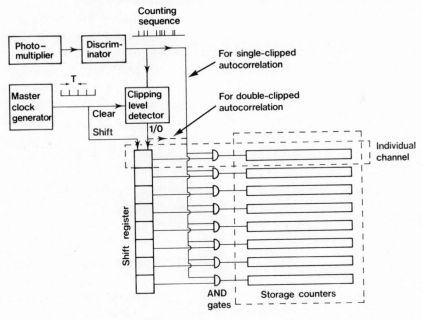

Figure 6.2.1. Photon counting correlator.

discriminator to shape the pulses. The pulses are then counted during each sampling time interval (T), in a threshold (or clipping level) detector, which acts as a limiter. At the end of each time interval the limiter feeds a 1 or a 0 to the shift register signifying a count greater or smaller than a predetermined threshold. Thus, the shift register maintains a record of the clipped counting sequence which is shifted along the register by signals from the sample time clock. The length of the register represents the number of channels in the correlator.

In parallel with the above operation, during each time interval, the input pulses are accumulated in a bank of counters via the AND gates, which are controlled by the stored values of the clipped sequence. Thus, each channel implements equation (6.2.8). The availability of parallel channels allows accumulation of several lag values of the clipped correlation function simultaneously. Since no multipliers are involved, the system operating times are only limited by the speeds of the logic circuitry. Photon correlators are now commercially available which allow a minimum sampling time of 50 nsecs, and can process, in real time, data rates up to 20 MHz and therefore can handle with ease Doppler signals lying within the megahertz range.

Double-clipped autocorrelations can easily be obtained by applying the clipped signal to both inputs of the AND gates which control the storage counters, as indicated in Figure 6.2.1. Single-clipped cross-correlation measurements can be performed by correlating a clipped counting sequence with another counting sequence applied directly to the input of the AND gates. For double-clipped cross-correlation an additional clipping level detector is required. An external delay unit is sometimes required to delay one sequence with respect to another in order to increase the range of lag values determined by the correlator. Double clipping of the counting sequence is particularly useful when the radiation incident on the photomultiplier consists of substantial contributions from side-wall flare or from background illumination in the vicinity of the flow.

In general the clipped photon correlator can operate for LDV setups with high scattering particle concentrations as well as for very low concentrations. In the former case there is a continuous stream of pulses or counts and the correlation estimates are updated at each sampling interval, with the counts during each interval making significant contributions to the correlation estimates in each channel. When the concentration is low, whenever a particle crosses the LDV observation volume, a significant number of counts are accumulated in all channels. These affect the shape of the correlation function. At all other occasions, spurious and random counts due to background radiation only add to the pedestal level of the correlation and accumulate in the channel corresponding to the zero lag estimate. These spurious counts do not, in any other way, change the shape of the correlation function. Thus the correlator, in time, estimates the correlation of the scattered intensity, after a large number of products have been accumulated to give statistical accuracy. As stated in Chapter 4, the count correlation estimate for the zero lag value and the pedestal level are usually discarded.

Measurement Accuracy

The relationships between clipped count correlations and the unclipped photon correlation have been extensively covered by Pike and his co-workers (Cummins and Pike, 1973). They have shown that for Gaussian radiation, the normalized single-clipped count correlation is

$$\rho_c(sT) = \frac{E[\hat{R}_c(sT)]}{E[N(kT, \overline{k+1T})]E[N_c(\overline{k+sT, k+s+1T})]}$$
$$= \frac{\overline{N}-q}{\overline{N}+1} + \frac{1+q}{1+\overline{N}}\rho(sT) \tag{6.2.9}$$

where q is the clipping level, $\overline{N} = E[N(kT, \overline{k+1T})]$ is the mean number of counts over the sampling interval, and $\rho(sT)$ is the normalized unclipped count correlation. Thus if the clipping level is chosen close to the mean count rate, the clipped autocorrelation would yield the desired count correlation, with the added advantage of requiring fewer computations. Note the similarity with the case of hard-clipped Gaussian sequences.

For the doubly clipped correlation function, with the clipping level set at zero counts, it has been proved (Jakeman and Pike, 1969) that the normalized correlation function $\rho(sT)$ is related to the clipped correlation $\rho_{cc}(sT)$ by

$$\rho_{cc}(sT) = \frac{(1+\overline{N})[2\overline{N} + (1-\overline{N})\rho(sT)]}{(1+\overline{N})^2 + \overline{N}^2(1-\rho(sT))} \tag{6.2.10}$$

which is a distorted function of the count correlation.

Further, as is usual with estimators of the form given in equation (6.2.1), the variance on the estimates for the unclipped, clipped, or doubly clipped count correlations is inversely proportional to the overall measuring time. Exact expressions for the variance of the count correlation estimates for the specific case of Gaussian–Lorentzian light have been obtained by Jakeman et al. (1971). These are too cumbersome to be included here.

It is important to note that the relationships (6.2.9)–(6.2.10) are only valid for Gaussian optical fields. For very low particle concentration this may not be necessarily true. For the case of non-Gaussian distributed fields, it is still possible to determine the intensity correlation by using clipping techniques. This may be achieved by introducing a variation on the clipping level, by either varying the clipping level randomly after each sampling interval according to a uniform distribution over a given range or alternatively by varying it linearly to follow a saw-tooth pattern. This may be proved by considering the conditional moment of the clipped correlation function of equation (6.2.6). Then we have

$$E[\hat{R}_c(sT)|q] = E[N(\overline{k + sT, k + s + 1}T) \cdot N_c(kT, \overline{k + 1}T)|q]$$

$$= \sum_{n_1 = 0}^{\infty} \sum_{n_2 = q}^{\infty} n_1 P(n_1, n_2; sT) \tag{6.2.11}$$

where

$$P(n_1; n_2; sT)$$

$$= \text{Prob}\,\{N(\overline{k + sT, k + s + 1}T) = n_1; N(kT, \overline{k + 1}T) = n_2\}$$

Considering a random clipping level q and defining its probability distribution as $P(q)$, we have

$$E[R_c(sT)] = \sum_{q=0}^{\infty} P(q) \sum_{n_1=0}^{\infty} \sum_{n_2=q}^{\infty} n_1 P(n_1, n_2; sT)$$

$$= \sum_{n_1=0}^{\infty} \sum_{n_2=0}^{\infty} n_1 P(n_1, n_2; sT) \sum_{q=0}^{n_2} P(q)$$

The second line is obtained by rearranging the summations. If the clipping level q is chosen to be uniformly distributed over a range much larger than the mean count rate, such that $P(q) = 1/Q$ for $q = 0, 1, 2, \ldots, Q$ and $P(q) = 0$ for q otherwise, with $Q \gg \bar{N}$, we have

$$E[R_c(sT)] \simeq \frac{1}{Q} \sum_{n_1=0}^{\infty} \sum_{n_2=0}^{\infty} n_1 n_2 P(n_1, n_2; sT)$$

$$\simeq (1/Q)R(sT) \tag{6.2.12}$$

which is the mean value of the unclipped count correlation. Hence the count correlation for non-Gaussian fields may be estimated by introducing a random variation on the clipping level of the correlator. The ramp variation presents an easy alternative for achieving a uniform variation on the clipping level. The former may be introduced by means of a pseudorandom binary sequence generator and the latter as the output of a counter with a cycle rate which should not coincide with any significant frequency of the Doppler signal.

6.3. Frequency-Burst Processing Systems

For low scattering particle concentration, the photodetected Doppler signal in the LDV takes the form of short sinusoidal bursts produced by individual particles moving across the observation volume (see Figure 3.1.1a). Frequency-burst processing systems are based on the principle that if the frequency of the bursts can be measured as they occur, then a record can be maintained of the instantaneous velocity of the medium. This is achieved by measuring with great precision the mean time interval between adjacent zero crossings of the signal burst (Brayton *et al.*, 1973).

Such a processing system is illustrated in Figure 6.3.1, where the following operations are performed: The photodetected signal is filtered and then the time duration of a specified number of cycles of the signal burst is determined with precision. This is compared with the duration of half the same number of cycles. If the former differs from twice the latter value by an amount greater than an acceptable percentage, the reading is rejected, otherwise the mean time period of the burst frequency is determined by appropriate scaling and then stored.

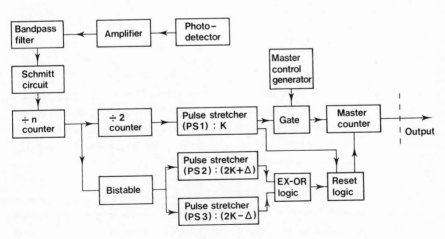

Figure 6.3.1 Frequency-burst processing system.

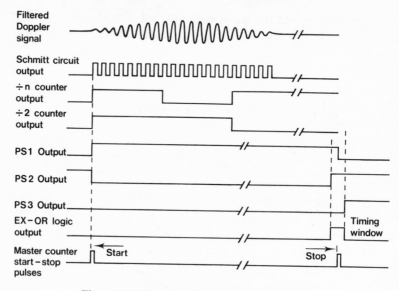

Figure 6.3.2. Waveforms in frequency-burst processor.

Usually the photodetected signal consists of the burst waveforms and other low-frequency components of the Doppler shifted radiation as well as additive wide-band noise. To remove the extraneous contributions the signal is amplified and bandpass-filtered.

The filtered signal is used to trigger a Schmitt circuit which records its zero crossings (see Figure 6.3.2). In a real fringe system the number of zero crossings per burst signal depends upon the number of fringes crossed by a scatterer as it moves across the observation volume. The threshold of the Schmitt trigger is suitably chosen to avoid triggering on the noise in the absence of the Doppler frequency component.

The Schmitt output is fed to a divide-by-n ($\div n$) counter which gives an output pulse of duration covering exactly n cycles of the Schmitt trigger output, and thus equals the time taken for a particle to produce n Doppler cycles. The $\div 2$ counter measures the time for $2n$ cycles of the Schmitt circuit, after which it is inhibited till the next set of measurements are made. It is usual to choose n as 8 or 10, corresponding to a system with 16 or 20 fringes. In Figure 6.3.2, n is taken as 8.

The output of the $\div 2$ counter is gated to a pulse stretcher which produces a pulse with exactly K times the $\div 2$ output pulse length. This is used to control the input gate to the main counter which accumulates pulses from a master clock generator (with clock rates up to 100 MHz). At the termination of the stretched pulse, the counter reading is a precise measure of the time duration of $2n$ cycles of the Schmitt circuit. By suitable scaling the mean period of the signal burst can be determined and recorded.

Pulse stretching can be achieved by means of precision analogue integrator circuits which ramp up to a voltage proportional to the input pulse length, and at the end of the pulse, discharge at a slower rate to give a long overall period directly proportional to the pulse length. Standard logic can then be used to shape the integrator output pulse.

If, during a signal burst, there is a change in signal frequency due to, say, a sudden phase change effected by noise fluctuations or signal amplitude variations, then it is necessary to detect and delete the corresponding frequency measurement. Brayton *et al.* (1973) have suggested the use of a pulse rate filter.

The output from the $\div n$ counter is applied to two bistables which are reset after the first n cycles of the Schmitt circuit. The bistable output is stretched by two pulse stretchers (PS2 and PS3) to slightly differing lengths. The stretched pulses when applied to the exclusive-or logic produce a timing window (pulse). For instance, for a pure sinusoidal input Doppler signal of period T, PS2 produces a pulse of duration $nT(2K + \Delta)$ and PS3 gives a pulse of width $nT(2K - \Delta)$. This leads to a timing window of width $2nT\Delta$ centered at time instant $2nKT$. The output of PS1 for the sinusoidal Doppler signal is a pulse of duration $2nKT$, which terminates within the timing window.

For any signal frequency variation within the duration of $2n$ cycles, when the trailing edge of the PS1 pulse does not lie within the timing window or within the acceptable range of variation depending upon choice of Δ, the reset logic is activated and the frequency reading in the counter is discarded as the signal is no longer considered as periodic. This technique ensures rejection of measurements corresponding to noise and other stray phase variations of the Doppler signal due to drift or dc shift.

The choice of Δ sets the data acquisition rate. Δ can vary between 0.5% and 10%. For a large value of Δ the data rate would be high but there would be a corresponding loss in accuracy of frequency measurement. A specific value of Δ is dictated by several conditions: input signal-to-noise ratio, particle concentration in the flow, and the speed of hardware associated with the frequency-burst processor.

An accepted reading is either passed on to a digital computer along with the time of occurrence of the signal burst for further processing or can be displayed after being averaged over several readings to give the mean value and the mean square deviation of the flow velocity. Alternatively, the reading can be converted through an analog-to-digital (A/D) converter for further analog processing.

The system can operate with equal facility on both continuous Doppler signals and signal bursts. The data sampling rate of the system depends upon the Doppler frequency and the mean rate of occurrence of signal bursts and is limited by the speed of the logic circuits. Thus the sampling rate may be given by $(T_1 + $ time for $2n$ Doppler cycles$)^{-1}$, where T_1 is the time to accumulate the reading in the counter and to reset all circuits. Brayton *et al.* (1973) have been able to measure burst signal frequencies up to 20 MHz, and one can envisage extensions up to 100 MHz.

Figure 6.3.3 gives a block diagram for an alternative frequency-burst system where the logic is considerably simplified to allow faster system response time. The Schmitt trigger and the $\div n$ and $\div 2$ counters perform in exactly the same way as in the previous processor. Here the main feature is an up–down counter which is used to determine the time difference between the first n cycles of the detected signal and the next n cycles.

The up–down counter is controlled by the $\div n$ counter output. It counts up during the first n cycles of the Schmitt circuit and accumulates counts from a master clocks generator, and it counts down during the next n cycles

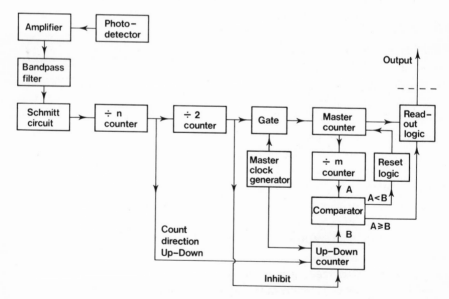

Figure 6.3.3. Frequency-burst processing system using up–down counter.

of the Schmitt circuit. The output from the ÷2 counter is used to inhibit the up–down counter at the end of $2n$ cycles. The final result in the up–down counter is exactly equal to the difference in binary, or one's complement binary, between counts accumulated during the first n cycles and the next n cycles of the Doppler signal. This number is then compared with a pre-selected fraction ($÷m$) of the counts accumulated in the main counter during the $2n$ cycles. The comparator and associated circuitry are only addressed at the end of the $2n$ cycles. If the difference exceeds the fraction, the master counter reading is rejected and all the circuits are reset. If not, the reading is scaled appropriately to give an average value of the time period of the signal burst and the result passed on for further analogue or digital processing as required.

Analogous to the Δ of the previous circuit, the $÷m$ counter establishes the tolerance or the deviation between the first n and the next n cycles of the Doppler signal. Typically for $m = \frac{1}{16}, \frac{1}{32}, \frac{1}{64}$, etc., the tolerance would be approximately 6%, 3%, 1.5%, etc. Obviously the smaller the value of m, the greater would be the accuracy of measurement, and the larger would be the data rejection rate.

With high-speed digital logic such a processor is capable of measuring burst frequencies up to 30 MHz. Some commercial systems based on similar frequency-burst techniques quote operating ranges up to 100 MHz.

In general, by using the processer output it is possible to compute the correlation function of the Doppler signal frequency and hence that of the flow, from a very *large* record of (a) the burst frequencies and (b) the occurrence times of the bursts. Autocorrelations calculated from a short record would be distorted by biasing errors due to the random arrival times of the bursts (i.e., of the particles at the observation volume), and the occurrence time distribution would have to be considered before a reliable estimator for the correlation function could be established.

6.4. *Laser Doppler Signal Simulators*

Traditionally, frequency-modulated sine wave generators have been used for testing frequency-detection systems since most applications, such as those in communications, involved the detection of information from a frequency- or phase-modulated sinusoidal carrier. The LDV Doppler signal differs significantly from such a signal. As shown in Chapter 3, the filtered Doppler signal can be represented as a narrow-band carrier, randomly frequency-modulated when turbulence conditions are studied. To evaluate the performance of various LDV signal processing systems it is therefore necessary to generate a signal that can closely simulate, statistically, the Doppler signal, and, in particular, produce frequency variations which reflect *known* fluid velocity changes.

It is not too difficult to simulate a narrow-band FM noise carrier; for instance, such a signal would be produced by passing white noise through a voltage-tuned filter with a center frequency controlled by an external modulating signal. However, it is essential that the simulated signal maintain an important characteristic of the Doppler signal, namely, that at all time instants, whatever the instantaneous Doppler frequency, the ratio of the carrier bandwidth to center frequency remain constant. This constant is fixed by the terms of the optical parameters of the setup [see equations (3.2.17)–(3.2.18)]. For instance, when the mean Doppler frequency is high, i.e., the observed fluid velocity is high, the ambiguity noise bandwidth which is inversely proportional to the passage time of particles across the observation volume, is also large, and when the mean Doppler frequency is low, the ambiguity noise bandwidth is small. This condition holds even when the flow velocity past the LDV observation volume varies rapidly due to turbulence effects.

Figure 6.4.1 illustrates a system for simulating a bandpass-filtered LDV signal with a mean shift frequency which can be externally modulated. The

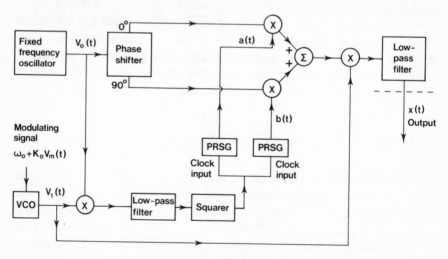

Figure 6.4.1. Doppler signal simulator.

circuit exploits the property of pseudorandom sequence generators (PRSG) of producing what is effectively band-limited white noise with a cutoff frequency (say $\frac{1}{2}\Delta\omega_p$) directly proportional to the input clock rate (say, ω_p, $\omega_p \doteq K_1\Delta\omega_p$, with K_1 a constant). Thus if the output sequence of a PRSG, after smoothing, is mixed with its input clock signal, then we have a narrow-band signal with a bandwidth directly proportional to its center frequency. By varying the clock rate we can produce an FM narrow-band carrier similar to the Doppler signal under turbulence. This method was first suggested by Wilmshurst (1972).

In the circuit two oscillators are used, one is set to a nominal frequency (say ω_i), and the other is a voltage-controlled oscillator to which any modulation can be applied to simulate instantaneous frequency variations. The arrangement shown allows the instantaneous frequency to be swept down to zero.

Consider the constant-frequency oscillator output to be $V_0(t) = \cos\omega_i t$ and that of the VCO as $V_1(t) = \cos[(\omega_0 + \omega_i)t + K_0\int V_m(t)\,dt]$, where K_0 is the VCO voltage-to-frequency conversion constant and $V_m(t)$ is the input modulating signal corresponding to any desired frequency variation. If $a(t)$ and $b(t)$ are the two output signals from the PSRG's, then the simulator output signal is

$$x(t) = a(t)\cos\left[\omega_0 t + K_0\int V_m(t)\,dt\right] + b(t)\sin\left[\omega_0 t + K\int V_m(t)\,dt\right] \quad (6.4.1)$$

It may be seen that the input clock rate to the PRSG has an instantaneous frequency of $\omega_0 + K_0V_m(t)$, the desired Doppler frequency. Hence, the instantaneous bandwidth of $a(t)$ and $b(t)$ is proportional to this frequency. The proportionality constant depends upon the length of the shift registers involved. By an appropriate choice of hardware this constant can be made as close as possible to the LDV signal bandwidth-to-center frequency ratio dictated by equations (3.2.14) and (3.2.15), and thus any Doppler signal characteristics can be simulated. A suitable arrangement of the shift registers ensures that the signals $a(t)$ and $b(t)$ are uncorrelated. The squarer adjusts the input level to the PRSG's.

Note the similarity of equation (6.4.1) with (3.1.17), for zero input modulation, and note that the two branches in the circuit which generate the two orthogonal components of the Doppler signal can be easily identified.

No attempt is made in the simulation to shape the spectrum of the signal $x(t)$ to be identical to that of the LDV Doppler signal since it is more important to have a facility for generating signal frequencies and bandwidths bearing known and prespecified relationships. Further, in most signal-processing systems, it is the signal frequency and its variation, rather than the exact spectral shape that dictate their performance. A system such as in Figure 6.4.1 would facilitate their testing. For further details see Wilmshurst (1972).

6.5. *Ambiguity Noise Reduction*

It has been shown that with an LDV system in conditions of high seeding concentration the instantaneous frequency, as measured by a frequency tracker, shows small fluctuations termed ambiguity noise. A large part of the text has been concerned with the analysis of ambiguity noise; however, in conclusion, it seems appropriate to point out that systems have been devised for reducing this effect. These make use of two separate frequency trackers operating in parallel. Oldengarm (1972), for example, describes an optical system in which two beams originating from the same laser are symmetrically focused into the flow (as in the real fringe method) and impinge directly onto two photodetectors on the detection side, one beam on each detector. Each detector then observes the direct beam together with scattered light from the other beam, and therefore the two detectors produce signals with the same Doppler frequency. However, since the scattering particles are generally of random size and shape, the two signals will have partially correlated phase and amplitude. If the frequencies of the two photodetector signals are tracked (i.e., with two frequency trackers), the result is two outputs which contain the same information about the velocity fluctuations but which have only partially correlated ambiguity noise components. If the velocity statistics are now calculated by cross-correlating the two tracker outputs rather than autocorrelating the output from a single tracker, the ambiguity noise effect is reduced. In fact it would be completely eliminated if the two ambiguity noise components were uncorrelated and also if the velocity signal was independent of the ambiguity noise fluctuations. This can easily be seen as follows.

Suppose the instantaneous frequencies from the two detectors are

$$\omega_1(t) = \omega_u(t) + \omega_{n1}(t)$$

$$\omega_2(t) = \omega_u(t) + \omega_{n2}(t)$$

where subscript *u* refers to the component caused by the velocity fluctuations and subscript n refers to the ambiguity noise component. Then the cross correlation is

$$E[\omega_1(t)\omega_2(t + \tau)] = E[\omega_u(t)\omega_u(t + \tau)] + E[\omega_u(t)\omega_{n2}(t + \tau)]$$
$$+ E[\omega_{n1}(t)\omega_u(t + \tau) + E[\omega_{n1}(t)\omega_{n2}(t + \tau)]$$

The first term on the right-hand side of the above equation is the true velocity correlation, and the second and third terms can safely be assumed negligible. The last term, which represents the major source of error, will hopefully be much smaller than the cross-product term produced when either $\omega_1(t)$ or $\omega_2(t)$ is autocorrelated. Thus the cross correlation of the outputs from the two detectors gives a better representation of the velocity correlation than the autocorrelation of the signal from a single detector. Note, however, that the velocity correlation is a time-averaged quantity and the cross-correlation technique does not eliminate the uncertainty associated with the measurement of an instantaneous velocity fluctuation.

References

Abbiss, J. B., *et al.* (1972), Laser anemometry in an unseeded wind tunnel by means of photon correlation spectroscopy of backscattered light, *J. Phys. D* **5**, L100–L102.

Adrian, R. J., and Goldstein, R. J. (1971), Analysis of a laser Doppler anemometer, *J. Phys. E* **4**, 505–511.

Anderson, L. K., and McMurtry, B. J. (1966), High speed photodetectors, *Proc. IEEE* **54**, 1335–1349.

Angus, J. C., *et al.* (1969), Motion measurement by laser Doppler techniques, *Ind. Eng. Chem.* **61**, 8–20.

Asch, R., and Ford, Jr., N. C. (1973), Design of an ideal digital correlation computer, *Rev. Sci. Instrum.* **44**, 506–508.

Ashley, L., and Cobb, C. (1958), Single particle scattering functions for latex spheres in water, *J. Opt. Soc. Am.* **48**, 261–268.

Batchelor, G. K. (1970), *An Introduction to Fluid Dynamics*, Cambridge University Press, London.

Beck, M. S., Lee, K. T., and Stanley-Wood, N. G. (1973), A new technique for evaluating the size of particles flowing in a turbulent fluid, *Powder Tech.* **8**, 85–90.

Bedi, P. S. (1971), A simplified optical arrangement for the laser Doppler velocimeter, *J. Phys. E* **4**, 27–28.

Bedi, P. S., and Thew, M. T. (1972), Localized velocity and turbulence measurement in turbulent swirling flows using laser Doppler anemometry, in *Electro-optic Systems in Flow Measurement, University of Southampton, 25th–26th September, 1972*, Southampton.

Bénard, C. (1972), Incoherent and chaotic bunching effects, *J. Phys. (Paris)* **33**, 1027–1036.

Bendat, J. S., and Piersol, A. G. (1971), *Random Data Analysis and Measurement Procedures*, Wiley–Interscience, New York.

Bendjaballah, C., and Perrot, F. (1971), Photoelectron statistics of laser light modulated by Gaussian noise, *Opt. Commun.* **3**, 21–22.

Birch, A. D., *et al.* (1973), The application of photon correlation spectroscopy to the measurement of turbulent flows, *J. Phys. D* **6**, L71–L73.

Blackman, R. B., and Tukey, J. W. (1958), *The Measurement of Power Spectra*, Dover, New York.

Blake, K. A. (1972a), Simple two-dimensional laser velocimeter optics, *J. Phys. E* **5**, 623–624.

Blake, K. A. (1972*b*), New developments of the NEL laser velocimeter and the treatment of data, in *Electro-optic Systems in Flow Measurement, University of Southampton, 25th–26th September, 1972*, Southampton.

Bloom, A. L. (1965), Noise in lasers and laser detectors, *Spectra-Phys. Laser Tech. Bull.* **4**.

Bloom, A. L. (1966), Gas lasers, *Proc. IEEE* **54**, 1262–1276.

Bogner, R. E. (1965), New relay correlation method, *Electron. Lett.* **1**, 53.

Born, M., and Wolf, E. (1959), *Principles of Optics*, Pergamon Press, Oxford.

Bossel, H. H., Hiller, W. J., and Meier, G. E. A. (1972*a*), Noise cancelling signal difference method for optical velocity measurements, *J. Phys. E* **5**, 893–896.

Bossel, H. H., Hiller, W. J., and Meier, G. E. A. (1972*b*), Self-aligning comparison beam method for one-, two-, and three-dimensional optical velocity measurements, *J. Phys. E* **5**, 897–900.

Bourke, P. J., Brown, C. G., and Drain, L. E. (1971), Measurement of Reynolds shear stress in water by laser anemometry, *DISA Inf.* **12**, 21–24.

Bradshaw, P. (1971), *An Introduction to Turbulence*, Pergamon, Oxford.

Brayton, D. B., and Goethert, W. H. (1971), A new dual-scatter laser Doppler-shift velocity measuring technique, *ISA Trans.* **10**, 40–50.

Brayton, D. B., Kalb, H. T., and Crosswy, F. L. (1973), Two-component dual-scatter laser Doppler velocimeter with frequency burst signal readout, *Appl. Opt.* **12**, 1145–1156.

Brodkey, R. S. (1967), *The Phenomena of Fluid Motion*, Addison-Wesley, Reading, Mass.

Buchhave, P. (1973), Light collecting system and detector in a laser Doppler anemometer, *DISA Inf.* **15**, 15–20.

Chen, S. H., Tartaglia, P., and Polonsky-Ostrowsky, N. (1972), A new method for the clipped intensity correlation measurement, *J. Phys. A* **5**, 1619–1623.

Chenoweth, A. J., Gaddy, O. L., and Holshouser, D. F. (1966), Carbon disulfide travelling-wave Kerr cells, *Proc. IEEE* **54**, 1414–1429.

Christie, J., Burns, J. G., and Ross, M. A. S. (1972), Development of a spark discharge method of flow measurement, in *Electro-optic Systems in Flow Measurement, University of Southampton, 25th–26th September, 1972*, Southampton.

Clarke, K. K., and Hess, D. T. (1971), *Communication Circuits: Analysis and Design*, Addison-Wesley, Menlo Park, Calif.

Cooper, J., and Greig, J. R. (1963), Rapid scanning of spectral line profiles using an oscillating Fabry–Pérot interferometer, *J. Sci. Instrum.* **40**, 433–437.

Costas, J. P. (1950), Periodic sampling of stationary time series, M.I.T. Res. Lab. Electron. Tech. Rep. 156.

Cramer, H. (1963), *Mathematical Methods of Statistics*, Princeton University Press, Princeton, N.J.

Cummins, H., *et al.* (1963), Frequency shifts in light diffracted by ultrasonic waves in liquid media, *Appl. Phys. Lett.* **2**, 62–64.

Cummins, H. Z., and Pike, E. R. (1973), eds., *Photon Correlation and Light Beating Spectroscopy*, Plenum, New York.

Davenport, W. B., Johnson, R. A., and Middleton, D. (1952), Statistical errors in measurements of random time functions, *J. Appl. Phys.* **23**, 377–388.

Degiorgio, V., and Lastovka, J. B. (1971), Intensity-correlation spectroscopy, *Phys. Rev. A* **4**, 2033–2050.

Deighton, M. O., and Sayle, P. A. (1971), An electronic tracker for the continuous measurement of Doppler frequency from a laser anemometer, *DISA Inf.* **12**, 5–10.

Doob, J. L. (1953), *Stochastic Processes*, Wiley, New York.

Drain, L. E. (1972), Coherent and noncoherent methods in Doppler optical beat velocity measurement, *J. Phys. D* **5**, 481–495.

Drain, L. E., and Moss, B. C. (1972), The frequency shifting of laser light by electro-optic techniques, in *Electro-optic Systems in Flow Measurement, University of Southampton, 25th–26th September, 1972*, Southampton.

Durrani, T. S., and Nightingale, J. M. (1972), Data windows for digital spectral analysis, *Proc. IEE (GB)* **119**, 343–352.

Durrani, T. S., and Greated, C. A. (1973a), Frequency domain analysis of laser Doppler signals for estimation of turbulence parameters, *Proc. IEE (GB)* **120**, 913–918.

Durrani, T. S., and Greated, C. A. (1973b), Statistical analysis and computer simulation of laser Doppler velocimeter systems, *Trans. IEEE* **IM-22**, 23–34.

Durrani, T. S., and Greated, C. (1973c), Application of photon correlation analysis to wind tunnel measurements, *International Congress on Instrumentation in Aerospace Simulation Facilities, Cal. Tech., 1973*, Pasadena, Calif., 210–218.

Durrani, T. S., and Greated, C. A. (1974a), Theory of LDV tracking systems, *Trans. IEEE,* **AES-10**, 418–428.

Durrani, T. S., and Greated, C. (1974b), Statistical analysis of velocity measuring systems employing the photon correlation technique, *Trans. IEEE* **AES-10**, 17–24.

Durrani, T. S., and Greated, C. (1975), Spectral analysis and cross-correlation techniques for photon-counting measurements on fluid flows, *Appl. Opt.* **14**, 778–786.

Durrani, T. S., Greated, C. A., and Wilmshurst, T. H. (1973), An analysis of simulators and tracking systems for laser Doppler velocimeters, *Opto-electron.* **5**, 71–89.

Durst, F., and Whitelaw, J. H. (1973), Light source and geometric requirements for the optimization of optical anemometry signals, *Opto-Electron.* **5**, 137–151.

Eliasson, B., and Dandliker, R. (1974), A theoretical analysis of laser Doppler flowmeters, *Optica Acta* **21**, 119–149.

Engelund, F. A. (1968), *Hydrodynamik*, Danish Technical University Press, Copenhagen.

Fage, A., and Townend, H. C. H. (1932), An examination of turbulent flow with an ultra microscope, *Proc. R. Soc. A* **132**, 656–677.

Farmer, W. M., and Brayton, D. B. (1971), Analysis of atmospheric laser Doppler velocimeters, *Appl. Opt.* **10**, 2319–2325.

Fisher, M. J., and Krause, F. R. (1967), The crossed-beam correlation technique, *J. Fluid Mech.* **28**, 705–717.

Fleury, P. A., and Boon, J. P. (1973), Laser light scattering in fluid systems, in *Advances in Chemical Physics*, ed. by I. Prigogine and S. A. Rice, Vol. **XXIV**, Wiley–Interscience, New York, 1–93.

Foord, R., et al. (1970), Determination of diffusion constant of Haemoganin at low concentration, by intensity fluctuation spectroscopy of laser light, *Nature* **227**, 242–245.

Foord, R., et al. (1974), A solid-state electro-optic phase modulator for laser Doppler anemometry, *J. Phys. D* **7**, L36–L39.

Foreman, J. W. (1967), Optical path length difference effects in photomixing with multimode gas laser radiation, *Appl. Opt.* **6**, 821–826.

Gaster, M. (1964), A new technique for the measurement of low fluid velocities, *J. Fluid Mech.* **20**, 183–192.

George, W. K., and Lumley, J. L. (1973), The laser Doppler velocimeter and its applications to the measurement of turbulence, *J. Fluid Mech.* **60**, 321–362.

Goodman, J. W. (1968), *Introduction to Fourier Optics*. McGraw-Hill, New York.

Gordon, E. I. (1966), A review of acoustooptical deflection and modulation devices, *Proc. IEEE* **54**, 1391–1401.

Greated, C. A. (1970), Measurement of Reynolds' stresses using an improved laser flowmeter, *J. Phys. E* **3**, 753–756.

Greated, C. A. (1971*a*), Noise reduction in a laser velocimeter, *J. Phys. E* **4**, 261–262.

Greated, C. A. (1971*b*), Velocity measurement in air with a scattering interferometer, *International Congress on Instrumentation in Aerospace Simulation Facilities, Rec. IEEE* 151–156.

Greated, C. A. (1971*c*), Resolution and back scattering optical geometry of laser Doppler systems, *J. Phys. E* **4**, 585–588.

Greated, C. A. (1975), Application of photon correlation spectroscopy to the measurement of highly turbulent fluid flows. *The Engineering Uses of Coherent Optics, University of Strathclyde 8–11 April*, ed. by E. R. Robertson, Cambridge University Press, London.

Hallermeier, R. J. (1973), Design considerations for a 3-D laser Doppler velocimeter for studying gravity waves in shallow water. *Appl. Opt.* **12**, 294–300.

Hay, J. S., and Pasquill, F. (1957), Diffusion from a fixed source at a height of a few hundred feet in the atmosphere, *J. Fluid Mech.* **2**, 299–310.

Helstrom, C. W. (1968), Estimation of modulation frequency of a light beam, *NASA Rep.* **SP-217**, *M.I.T.–NASA Workshop on Optical Space Communications, Williams College, Aug. 4–17, 1968*, Williamstown, Mass.

Hiller, W. J., and Meier, G. E. A. (1972), The scattered light beam method, *Electro-optic Systems in Flow Measurement, University of Southampton, 25th–26th September, 1972*, Southampton.

Hinze, J. O. (1959), *Turbulence*, McGraw-Hill, New York.

Hinze, J. O. (1972), Turbulent fluid and particle interaction, *Prog. Heat Mass Trans.* **6**, 433–452.

Holland, L. (1956), *Vacuum Deposition and Thin Films*, Chapman and Hall, London.

Huffaker, R. M. (1970), Laser Doppler detection systems for gas velocity measurements, *Appl. Opt.* **9**, 1026–1039.

Hughes, A. J., O'Shaughnessy, J., and Pike, E. R. (1972), Long range anemometry using a CO_2 laser, *Electro-optic Systems in Flow Measurement, University of Southampton, 25th–26th September, 1972*, Southampton.

Iten, P. D., and Dandliker, R. (1972), A sampling FM wideband demodulator, *Proc. IEEE* **60**, 1470–1475.

Jackson, D. A., and Paul, D. M. (1970), Measurement of hypersonic velocities and turbulence by direct spectral analysis of Doppler shifted laser light, *Phys. Lett.* **32A**, 77–78.

Jackson, D. A., and Paul, D. M. (1971), Measurement of supersonic velocity and turbulence by laser anemometry, *J. Phys. E* **4**, 173–177.

Jakeman, E., and Pike, E. R. (1969), Spectrum of clipped photon-counting fluctuations of Gaussian light, *J. Phys. A* **2**, 411–412.

Jakeman, E., Pike, E. R., and Swain, S. (1970), Statistical accuracy in the digital autocorrelation of photon counting statistics, *J. Phys. A* **3**, L55–L59.

Jakeman, E., Pike, E. R., and Swain, S. (1971), Statistical accuracy in the digital autocorrelation of photon counting fluctuations, *J. Phys. A* **4**, 517–534.

James, J. F., and Sternberg, R. S. (1969), *The Design of Optical Spectrometers*, Chapman and Hall, London.

Jespers, P., Chu, P. T., and Fettweis, A. (1962), A new method to compute correlation functions, *Trans. IRE* **IT-8**, S106.

Jonsson, L. (1974), Laser velocity meter for water flow, Dept. of Hydraulics, Lund Institute of Technology, Lund, Sweden, Bulletin Ser. A, No. 32.

Jordan, J. R. (1973), A correlation function and time delay measuring system designed for large scale circuit integration, *Measurement and Process Identification by Correlation and*

Spectral Analysis. 1. Measurement and Control, University of Bradford, 2–4 January, Bradford, U.K.

Kaminow, I. P., and Turner, E. H. (1966), Electro-optic light modulators, *Proc. IEEE* **54**, 1374–1390.

Karchmer, A. M. (1972), Particle trackability considerations for laser Doppler velocimetry, NASA Tech. Memo No. TMX-2628.

Kendall, M. G., and Stuart, A. (1961), *The Advanced Theory of Statistics,* Griffin, London, Vol. 2.

Kerker, M. (1969), *The Scattering of Light and Other Electromagnetic Radiation,* Academic, New York.

Kittel, C. (1958), *Elementary Statistical Physics,* Wiley, New York.

Knowles, J. B., and Tsui, H. T. (1967), Correlating devices and their estimation errors, *J. Appl. Phys.* **38**, 607–612.

Kofoed-Hansen, O., and Wandel, C. F. (1967), On the relation between Eulerian and Lagrangian averages in the statistical theory of turbulence, Danish Atomic Energy Commission, Roskilde, Denmark, RISO Rep. No. 50.

Kogelnik, H. (1950), Imaging of optical modes–resonators with internal lenses, *Bell Syst. Tech. J.* **43**, 455–493.

Kreid, D. K. (1974), Laser Doppler velocimeter measurements in non-uniform flow: error estimates, *Appl. Opt.* **13**, 1872–1881.

Lacoss, R. T. (1971), Data adaptive spectral analysis methods, *Geophysics,* **36**, 661–675.

Lading, L. (1972), A Fourier optical model for the laser Doppler velocimeter, *Opto-Electron.* **4**, 385–398.

Lading, L. (1973), Analysis of a laser correlation anemometer, *Turbulence in Liquids, University of Missouri, 10–12 September, 1973,* Rolla, Missouri.

Lanz, O., Johnson, C. C., and Morikawa, S. (1971), Directional laser Doppler velocimeter, *Appl. Opt.* **10**, 884–888.

Leaver, K. D., and Chapman, B. N. (1971), *Thin Films,* Wykeham, London.

Lee, A., Greated, C. A., and Durrani, T. S. (1974), Velocities under periodic and random waves, *14th International Coastal Engineering Conference, Danish Hydraulic Institute,* Copenhagen.

Lennert, A. E., *et al.* (1970), Laser applications for flow field diagnostics, *Laser J.* 19–27.

Leslie, D. C. (1973), *Developments in the Theory of Turbulence,* Clarendon, Oxford.

McComb, W. D. (1973), The turbulent dynamics of an elastic fibre suspension: a mechanism for drag reduction, *Nat. Phys. Sci.* **241**, 117–118.

Maissel, L. I., and Glang, R. (1970), *Handbook of Thin Film Technology,* McGraw-Hill, New York.

Mandel, L., and Wolf, E. (1965), Coherence properties of optical fields, *Rev. of Mod. Phys.* **37**, 231–287.

Manning, R. (1973), Symmetric transforms for the laser velocimeter, *J. Phys. D* **6**, 1173–1187.

Mayo, W. T. (1970), Spatial filtering properties of the reference beam in an optical heterodyne receiver, *Appl. Opt.* **9**, 1159–1162.

Mazumder, M. K. (1970), Laser Doppler velocity measurement without directional ambiguity by using frequency shifted incident beams, *Appl. Phys. Lett.* **16**, 462–464.

Melchoir, H., Fisher, H. B., and Arams, F. A. (1970), Photodetectors for optical communication systems. *Proc. IEEE* **58**, 1466–1486.

Melling, A., and Whitelaw, J. H. (1973), Seeding of gas flows for laser anemometry, *DISA Inf.* **15**, 5–14.

Meneelly, C. T., She, C. Y., and Edwards, D. F. (1972), Measurement of flow and turbulence distribution of a free jet by laser photon spectroscopy, *Opt. Commun.* **6**, 380–382.

Middleton, D. (1960), *An Introduction to Statistical Communication Theory*, McGraw-Hill, New York.

Mishina, H., and Asakura, T. (1974), A laser Doppler microscope, *Opt. Commun.* **11**, 99–102.

Monin, A. S., and Yaglom, A. M. (1971), *Statistical Fluid Mechanics*, ed. by J. L. Lumley, M.I.T. Press, Cambridge, Mass.

Oldengarm, J. (1972), Reduction of the ambiguity noise level in laser Doppler velocimetry using a cross-correlation technique. *Electro-optic Systems in Flow Measurement, University of Southampton, 25th–26th September, 1972*, Southampton.

Olson, D. E., Iliff, L. D., and Sudlow, M. F. (1972), Some aspects of the physics of flow in the central airways, *Bull. Physio-path Resp.* **8**, 391–408.

Papoulis, A. (1965), *Probability, Random Variables, and Stochastic Processes*, McGraw-Hill, New York.

Papoulis, A. (1968), *Systems and Transforms with Applications in Optics*, McGraw-Hill, New York.

Parzen, E. (1960), *Modern Probability Theory and Its Applications*, Wiley, New York.

Parzen, E. (1962), *Stochastic Processes*, Holden-Day, San Francisco.

Paul, D. M., and Jackson, D. A. (1971), Rapid velocity sensor using a static confocal Fabry–Pérot and a single frequency argon laser, *J. Phys. E* **4**, 170–172.

Philip, J. R. (1967), Relation between Eulerian and Lagrangian statistics, *Phys. Fluids Suppl.* 569–571.

Picinbono, B. (1971), Statistical properties of random modulated laser beams, *Phys. Rev. A* **4**, 2398–2407.

Rice, S. O. (1944, 1945), Mathematical analysis of random noise, *Bell Syst. Tech. J.* **23**, 282–332; **24**, 46–156.

Rice, S. O. (1948), Statistical properties of a sine wave plus random noise, *Bell Syst. Tech. J.* **27**, 109–157.

Rice, S. O. (1963), Noise in FM receivers, in *Time Series Analysis*, ed. by M. Rosenblatt, Wiley, New York.

Rizzo, J. E. (1972), Velocity measuring interferometers. *Electro-optic Systems in Flow Measurement, University of Southampton, 25th–26th September, 1972*, Southampton.

Robben, F. (1971), Noise in the measurement of light with photomultipliers, *Appl. Opt.* **10**, 776–796.

Rouse, H., ed. (1959), *Advanced Mechanics of Fluids*, Wiley, New York.

Rousseau, M. (1971), Statistical properties of optical fields scattered by random media with application to rotating ground glass, *J. Opt. Soc. Am.* **61**, 1307–1316.

Rudd, M. J. (1969), A new theoretical model for the laser Doppler meter, *J. Phys. E* **2**, 55–58.

Saffman, P. G. (1963), An approximate calculation of the Lagrangian autocorrelation coefficient for stationary homogeneous turbulence, *Appl. Sci. Res. A* **11**, 245–255.

Saffman, P. G. (1965), The lift on a small sphere in a slow shear flow, *J. Fluid Mech.* **22**, 385–400.

Saleh, B. A. (1973), Statistical accuracy in estimating parameters of the spatial coherence function by photon counting techniques, *J. Phys. A* **6**, 980–986.

Stumpers, F. L. H. M. (1948), Theory of frequency modulation noise, *Proc. IRE* **36**, 1081–1092.

Tartaglia, P., and Chen, S. H. (1973), The spatial coherence factor in light scattering from a system of independent particles, *Opt. Commun.* **7**, 379–383.

Tatarski, V. I. (1967), *Wave Propagation in a Turbulent Medium*, Dover, New York.

Taub, H., and Schilling, D. B. (1971), *Principles of Communications Systems*, McGraw-Hill, New York.

Tennekes, H., and Lumley, J. L. (1972), *A First Course in Turbulence*, M.I.T. Press, Cambridge, Mass.

Thompson, D. H. (1968), A tracer-particle fluid velocity meter incorporating a laser. *J. Phys. E* 1, 929–932.

Townsend, A. A. (1956), *The Structure of Turbulent Shear Flow*, Cambridge University Press, London.

Troup, G. J. (1972), *Photon Counting and Photon Statistics, Progress in Quantum Optics*, Pergamon, Oxford, Vol. 2, Pt. 1.

Van de Hulst, H. C. (1957), *Light Scattering by Small Particles*, Wiley, New York.

Van der Pol, B. (1946), The fundamental principles of frequency modulation, *IEEE J.* Pt. III, **93**, 153–158.

Van Vleck, J. H., and Middleton, D. (1966), The spectrum of clipped noise, *Proc. IEEE* **54**, 2–19.

Vasilenko, Y. G., *et al.* (1972*a*), Laser velocity meters—a comparative study. *Opt. Laser Tech.* 270–272.

Vasilenko, Y. G., *et al.* (1972*b*), The development of optical Doppler techniques for measuring flow velocities, *Electro-optic Systems in Flow Measurement, University of Southampton, 25th–26th September, 1972*, Southampton.

Wang, C. P. (1972), A unified analysis of laser Doppler velocimeters, *J. Phys. E* **5**, 763–766.

Wang, C. P. (1974), Doppler velocimeter using diffraction grating and white light, *Appl. Opt.* **13**, 1193–1195.

Wang, C. P., and Snyder, D. (1974), Laser Doppler velocimetry: experimental study, *Appl. Opt.* **13**, 98–103.

Watrasiewicz, B. M. (1970), Improved signal-to-noise ratio in the laser velocimeter, *J. Phys. E* **3**, 823.

Watts, D. G. (1962), A general theory of amplitude quantization with applications to correlation determination, *Proc. IEE (GB)* **109C**, 209–218.

Wilmshurst, T. H. (1972), A signal simulator for testing laser Doppler fluid flow velocimeter systems, *J. Phys. E* **5**, 1205–1208.

Wilmshurst, T. H., and Rizzo, J. E. (1974), An autodyne frequency tracker for laser Doppler anemometry, *J. Phys. E* **7**, 924–930.

Wilmshurst, T. H., Greated, C. A., and Manning, R. (1971), A laser fluid-flow velocimeter with wide dynamic range, *J. Phys. E* **4**, 81–85.

Wong, E. (1971), *Stochastic Processes in Information and Dynamical Systems*, McGraw-Hill, New York.

Yeh, Y., and Cummins, H. (1964), Localized fluid flow measurements with an He–Ne laser spectrometer, *Appl. Phys. Lett.* **4**, 176–178.

Zohar, S. (1969), Toeplitz matrix inversion, *J. Ass. Comput. Mach.* **16**, 592–601.

Author Index

Subject Index